The Clot Thickens

*The enduring mystery
of heart disease*

Dr Malcolm Kendrick

Published by Columbus Publishing Ltd 2021
www.columbuspublishing.co.uk

ISBN: 978-1-907797-76-7
Rev: 20211025

Design and typesetting by Raffaele Bolelli Gallevi

Brand and product names are trademarks or registered trademarks of their
respective owners.

The content of this book is intended to inform, entertain and provoke your thinking.
This is not intended as medical advice. It may, however, make you question current
medical and nutritional advice.
That is your choice. It's your life and health in your hands.
Neither the author nor the publisher can be held responsible or liable for any loss or
claim arising from the use, or misuse, of the content of this book.

COLUMBUS PUBLISHING

Reviews

"Malcolm Kendrick's masterly survey of the enduring mystery of heart disease reads like a detective story. With great verve he marshals the evidence for the two main contending theories, exonerates the presumed suspect and makes a formidable case for thrombogenesis (blood clotting) as the perpetrator. Witty, provocative and entertaining, 'The Clot Thickens' packs a powerful scientific punch. Highly recommended."

Dr James Le Fanu, Doctor, Journalist, Author of
The Rise and Fall of Modern Medicine

"For everyone who believes that there is more to heart disease than avoiding fat or taking a statin this book will confirm your thinking. 'The Clot Thickens' strips away the idea that high cholesterol is the key underlying cause of heart disease. Replacing it with evidence exposing the true culprits.

"Entertaining, understandable, and fascinating, this unique and cutting-edge work (I call it a 'living text book') shows that for decades the causes of heart disease have simply been swept under the table. Whether you have heart disease, know someone with it, if you fear it, or you are just interested in it, this meticulously researched book will shake up every aspect of your thinking. It will also help you to understand exactly what you can do to reduce your risk."

Lucy Johnston, Health and Social Affairs Editor, Sunday Express

"Science evolves by being challenged. Not by being followed. Malcolm Kendrick, proves once again, he is not a follower. 'The Enduring Mystery of heart disease – The Clot Thickens' clearly questions the current cholesterol causes cardiovascular disease paradigm held by most doctors. Anyone stating that 'we', as a medical profession, have heart disease worked out, has stopped the scientific method in its tracks. They have stopped questioning and thinking. That's a worry for patients everywhere."

Dr Gary Fettke, M.B.,B.S.(UNSW), F.R.A.C.S., F.A.Orth.A

"What I really liked about this book (in addition to the title!) is Dr Kendrick's logical, evidenced approach to the true causes of heart disease, paired with pragmatic information as to what each of us can do to actually live longer. The good news is so much of our fate is in our own hands, as I know so well from my own clinical work helping people with T2 Diabetes to 'cut the carbs'. Here is an experienced clinician who just wants you to live longer. READ THE BOOK!!"

Dr David Unwin, M.D UK

"Whether you agree or disagree with the Author's conclusions, what shines through is his decades of dedicated, independent investigation into the possible causes of heart disease. His style of writing is humorous and at times irreverent but engaging throughout. And it is always good to debate our pool of knowledge so we can try to make sense of it ourselves."

Dr Rob Lawson., Chairman British Society of Lifestyle Medicine

'To anyone aware of the contradictions and misconceptions involved in the official medical view of cholesterol, Dr Malcolm Kendrick is a hero. A fearless, independent voice challenging the official, and vastly profitable, theory that heart disease is the result of too much of it.

"To support his case, Kendrick has been diving for decades into the arcane regions of cholesterol biology, returning with findings which demonstrate that the official theory is profoundly flawed. He reports them in detailed but clear, non-specialist prose, spiced with humour. For his pains he has been effectively medically excommunicated.

"Undaunted he has been developing an alternative theory, set out in his new book 'The Clot Thickens'. It describes the essential changes in your system that make heart disease more likely, complete with an arsenal of references. This is serious research."

Jerome Burne, Award winning medical journalist

"Malcolm Kendrick is a rare beast. A natural skeptic, contrarian and a GP obsessed for his entire adult life with the causes of heart disease. This book is his Hegelian antithesis to the collective dogma of modern Cardiology. He presents a witty 'Poirot-like' walk through the potential culprits responsible for the development of coronary artery disease. Has he spotted major clues that all the major researchers in the world have failed to? We may never know!

However, his researched opinions should be given credit and future academic consideration."

Dr Scott W Murray, MBChB, BSc, MRCP, MD, Consultant Cardiologist Venturi Cardiology; Past President of the British Association of Cardiovascular Prevention and Rehabilitation (BACPR)

"Malcolm Kendrick's new book brings to mind the quote from Thomas Huxley when he first learned of Darwin's theory of evolution: 'how extremely stupid (of me) not to have thought of that'. What Kendrick presents is nothing less than a unifying theory of heart disease, that explains why everything from sickle cell disease to diabetes to a stressful lifestyle increases cardiovascular risk (and he does it with a large dollop of humour). After decades stuck in the blind alley that is the LDL hypothesis, this book is a revelation. It should be read by anyone with even a slight interest in understanding heart disease and what they can do to protect themselves from it."

Dr Sebastian Rushworth, M.D. Sweden

"In 'The Clot Thickens', Malcolm Kendrick mounts a high caliber fusillade against the diet-heart-cholesterol hypothesis and, as the title suggests, presents the alternative: the role of the thrombogenic process. The medical establishment maintains extensive political Kevlar and it is not clear where things will go but the reader is provided a broad view of the medicine that bears on the interaction between coagulation and heart disease. There's something to learn for everybody even those of us who have worked in related fields and who have followed previous warriors in this battle. When I first read Uffe Ravnskov's pioneering 'Cholesterol Myth's', I thought 'it can't be this bad. I have to go back and read the original literature.' I did and it was that bad. I never understood how the cholesterol idea could be sustained. In 'The Clot Thickens', Kendrick, a colleague and fellow admirer of Ravnskov, points out the limitations of the likely alternative at that time (bacterial or viral infection). He provides extensive evidence on the more compelling role of damage to the circulation and the role of thrombosis (clotting) and inhibition of fibrinolysis (clot breakdown). A far-ranging discussion with good straight-forward definitions of medical terms and includes some tantalizing stories to send you to the thorough set of references."

Professor Richard Feinman, Professor of biochemistry and medical research. State University of New York

"For 30 years, Dr Malcolm Kendrick has been obsessed with what really causes heart disease (spoiler alert – because it's not cholesterol). He has built hypotheses and then knocked them down in a genuinely scientific search for the truth. A chance breakthrough led to him looking for the process by which heart disease forms and suddenly all the single causes made sense. This book describes how Dr Kendrick established the explanation that withstands scrutiny and what it is. Having read so much of his work over so many years, I think he's got there. I really think he has."

Dr Zoë Harcombe, Author, presenter & researcher.

Acknowledgements

I have been studying cardiovascular disease for many years now, and during that time I have been fortunate enough to meet a number of inspirational and supportive individuals. There is Dr. Uffe Ravnskov, who brought together doctors and researchers under the banner of The International Network of Cholesterol Sceptics (THINCS). Within this network are those who do not believe that cardiovascular disease is caused by a raised blood cholesterol. We few, we happy few, we band of brothers.

Uffe is a man of great integrity, and wisdom. For decades now he has fought an often-lonely battle against the cholesterol hypothesis. As did the, now sadly departed, Professor Paul Rosch. Chairman of the board of the American Institute of Stress and Professor of medicine and psychiatry at New York Medical college. He changed my thinking about cardiovascular disease, turned me round, and pointed me in the correct direction. For which I am eternally grateful.

There is, of course, my family. They have put up with my madcap thoughts for far too many years. They have also attacked and criticised my ideas and made them stronger. But most of all they have been my rock, keeping me grounded in the real world, stopping me from flying too close to the sun.

There was Elspeth Smith, a lecturer and researcher at Aberdeen University, who taught me to think about cardiovascular disease in a completely different way. In my opinion, her research should have changed the world. But it did not. She never gained the recognition that she deserved. I hope this book goes some way to redressing the balance in her favour.

Then, there was my father. He once ripped a page out of a maths textbook in front of me, announcing *'Well, that is complete rubbish.'* Which, amongst other things, gave me the confidence to challenge the established order. Without that, I would never have dared to take up arms against a sea of cardiovascular troubles.

Contents

Introduction

"It does not matter who you are, or how smart you are, or what title you have, or how many of you there are, and certainly not how many papers your side has published, if your prediction is wrong then your hypothesis is wrong. Period."

Richard Feynman

Why would you want to read a book about heart disease? Because you've been diagnosed with it, and are desperate to know what's happening? Because you've reached an age when you're worried about it, and want to avoid it? Because someone you know, and love, is suffering from it? Some, we few, we happy few, simply because we are fascinated.

Why did I become so fascinated? Well, I am a doctor, and doctors are supposed to pay some kind of attention to various illnesses. Added to this, heart disease kills more people than any other disease in the whole wide world. So, this further sharpened the focus.

From a personal perspective, I am Scottish. When I was at medical school, Scotland had the highest rate of deaths from heart attacks in the world. We saw a constant flood of patients arriving in hospital, some survived, some did not. Although, by this time, it had almost become background noise. Middle-aged men had heart attacks, it's what happens. The circle of life.

So, yes, for quite some time, we Scots were *the* world champions at dropping dead from heart attacks… *'och MI the noo, Jimmy.'* We were just ahead of Northern Ireland.

Mind you, it had taken us a while to get there. After the second world war the Americans led the world, and they clung on for quite some time. Then, during the swinging 60s, Finland overtook the US. Then it was us, bonnie Scotland.

Okay, you can argue the figures, and if there is one thing that I have learned about studying heart disease it is that the figures sure can be argued. However, Scotland was definitely in the premier league. Maybe truly world champions.

But why? What on earth were we doing that no-one else was managing, at least not quite as well? England wasn't too far away but, nah, in truth, they were never really that close. France, part of the Auld Alliance with Scotland – against England of course – they had one fifth our rate. Hardly even out of the starting blocks, whilst we were staggering over the finish line, clutching our chests and gasping for breath.

What could the French be doing wrong, to be so far behind? After all they smoked like chimneys, they drank like fish, they ate pâté de foie gras, and steak bleu – very much an acquired taste. They slathered everything in butter, and cream. They had never even come across the concept of a vegetarian meal.

Ever tried ordering a vegetarian meal in France 40 years ago? The chef just took the meat off the dish with a disdainful flourish, and you ate whatever pitiful, skanking fare was left. At least that is what I was told by others who had experienced the French approach, or l'approche français. I am not vegetarian. Indeed, I was far more likely to eat the meat and throw away the vegetables. *'Chef, remove these pitiful legumes from my dish.'*

I have been to France many times. Love it. I am not quite sure why I don't live there now. Probably because they won't let me in, especially post-Brexit. One thing I did observe during my travels is that they most certainly did not have a low saturated fat diet. Unless they all went home and secretly munched on carrot sticks, broccoli, and kale, whilst no-one was looking. I suspect not.

Instead, French recipe books were full of half litres of cream to make this, and half a kilo of butter to make the roux sauces. Yum, yum. So, when I was told that the main cause of heart disease was eating too much fat, animal fat, saturated fat, I must admit I was a soupçon sceptical.

Despite the existence of the French Paradox – yes, that is what it was called – you will know that it was decreed, very early on, that the main cause of heart disease was eating too much saturated fat. This raised your cholesterol level, and the excess cholesterol was then deposited in your arteries, narrowing them down until one, or more, would eventually block. Causing a heart attack, or stroke, or suchlike.

This comes under the general heading of the *'diet-heart hypothesis'*. Or the cholesterol hypothesis. Or the diet-heart/cholesterol hypothesis. It flips this way and that, depending on which way the wind blows. A veritable will o' the wisp.

This hypothesis was first proposed as far back as the late nineteenth century. However, it was not until the 1950s that it really gained traction, firstly in the US. Mainly due to the laser focus, and drive, of one man, Ancel Keys. He became known as 'Mr Cholesterol' – and featured on the front cover of TIME magazine.[1]

Promoted mercilessly by Keys, and his rapidly growing band of supporters, the diet-heart hypothesis spread around the world and achieved the status of 'inarguable fact.' On a par with – moon orbits Earth.

There is just one teensy weensy little problem. It is wrong. In fact, both parts of it are wrong. Heart disease has nothing to do with eating saturated fat, nor does it have anything to do with cholesterol in the bloodstream.

It is due to something else entirely. Yes, please just hold onto both thoughts in the *'pending further examination'* tray, and do not simply dismiss them because they sound wrong. Perhaps more importantly, they probably feel wrong. Mad even.

I admit that it took me quite a while to change my thinking. I cannot expect anyone to simply go – *'Crikey. Now that you mention it, I realise that you are obviously right. Everything that everyone else has said about diet and cholesterol for the last fifty years is wrong.'*

Instead, what I am going to do is take you on a little trip to explain why the diet-heart/cholesterol hypothesis is wrong. Then I will guide you on a different journey, to a far more interesting place. Namely, what actually does cause heart disease, and perhaps even more importantly how to stop it happening – to you.

This leans heavily on alternative thinking about heart disease that was actually proposed several years before the cholesterol hypothesis was even a twinkle in anyone's eye. In fact, it was first thought of in 1852 by one Karl von Rokitansky. He called it the *'encrustation hypothesis.'* This was seven years before the Origin of Species was published. Yes, there truly is nothing new under the sun.

Before proceeding any further, I need pause briefly and clear up some of the terminology that I will be using in this book. Because it can all become horribly confusing. The first thing to mention is that there is no such thing as 'heart disease'. Or, at least, this is such a broad term that it is of no practical use whatsoever, as it covers hundreds of different conditions. Most of which have nothing to do with what we commonly call *'heart disease.'*

Instead, what I am taking about here is a specific condition that affects the larger arteries in your body. The disease itself is a thickening and narrowing, which is most often called atherosclerosis. The narrowings themselves are usually called atherosclerotic plaques. There can be one or two plaques throughout all your arteries, or there can be hundreds of them, that can merge together.

The most likely place for atherosclerotic plaques to be found is within the arteries that supply blood to the heart. The coronary arteries. They are called coronary arteries because they are said to encircle the heart like a crown. '*A coronation of blood vessels*' to quote some textbook or other. I think you need a damned good imagination to see that.

Because plaques are most often found in the coronary arteries, and the most common way to die from atherosclerosis is a heart attack, one of the terms used to describe atherosclerosis is coronary artery disease (CAD). Sometimes coronary heart disease (CHD).

However, atherosclerosis can affect arteries anywhere in the body. Arteries in the neck, leading to strokes... a cerebral infarction. Arteries supplying the kidneys, leading to kidney damage... renal/kidney infarction etc. etc.

Because plaques can be found in arteries in most parts of the body, an alternative title is cardiovascular disease (CVD). Unfortunately, this is not entirely accurate either. Atherosclerosis is not a 'vascular' disease; it is purely an 'arterial' disease. I say this because it never affects the veins, and veins make up at least half your blood vessels – or half of your *vasculature*. Neither does it affect the smaller arteries, called arterioles.

There is also an entirely separate section of your vascular system, which is only very rarely affected by atherosclerosis. What I am talking about here is the system of blood vessels within the lungs, known as the 'pulmonary circulation'. The right side of your heart pumps blood round the lungs. It then arrives at the left side, which then pumps it round the rest of your body. Whereupon it arrives back at the right side again.

The blood supply to the main part of your body is called the 'systemic circulation.' Therefore, if you want to be fully accurate, the disease I am discussing should be called systemic-large-artery-disease (SLAD). Because that is what it is. I've never called it that, and no-one has ever used this term in the history of medicine. In addition, it does sound a bit daft. Although, you never know, it could catch on.

Having said all of this, rather than being fully accurate, I tend to use the rather sloppy term, cardiovascular disease (CVD). Occasionally calling it heart disease, or coronary heart disease (CHD), or atherosclerosis – sometimes atherosclerotic plaques. Happily, though inaccurately, flipping around between them. Well, if everyone else can do it...

In fact, it is a recurring theme of this book that medical terminology is horribly inaccurate and terribly confusing. Try looking up the word 'lesion' some time.

Why is the diet-heart cholesterol hypothesis wrong?

Back to the matter in hand. The diet-heart/cholesterol hypothesis. Part one of the hypothesis is that saturated fat in the diet raises the cholesterol level. Part two is that a raised cholesterol level causes SLAD. Sorry, cardiovascular disease.

Of course, if a raised cholesterol level doesn't cause heart disease, then the first part of the hypothesis becomes somewhat irrelevant. There's little point even discussing it. Who cares if saturated fats raise cholesterol, if cholesterol doesn't cause cardiovascular disease? A good question.

However, I suspect you may feel I was guilty of hitting the fast-forward button if I simply ignored the entire saturated fat issue. There are still endless warnings about it, how damaging it is, and how we should avoid it like the plague. Therefore, I suppose that I must begin by looking at saturated fat, and how it has no impact on cholesterol levels.

Unfortunately, we run smack bang into another terminology problem that I also need to sort out before going any further. Which is that no-one actually has any such thing as a cholesterol level. This is because cholesterol cannot float free in the blood, as it is not water soluble, and therefore cannot be blood soluble.

Because of this somewhat inconvenient chemical fact, cholesterol has to be transported around in teeny weeny little spheres called lipoproteins (lipid + protein = lipoprotein). Which are about the size of a virus.

There are several different types of lipoprotein. The biggest is called a chylomicron, the smallest is called a high-density lipoprotein (HDL). The one that is currently blamed for cardiovascular disease is known as low-density lipoprotein (LDL). It is often referred to as 'bad' cholesterol. Although, of course, it is not cholesterol at all. It is a minute lipid + protein sphere, which carries cholesterol within it, amongst many other things.

Just to give you some idea of the scale of things I am talking about here. If a low-density lipoprotein were the size of a human being, a standard sized human cell would be about the size of an Olympic sports stadium.

And just for another rough size comparison. If a high-density lipoprotein were the size of a pea, a low-density lipoprotein would be the size of a golf ball, and a chylomicron would be the size of a basketball (Figure 1). I have included a few other lipoproteins here, that I will discuss later, including the very low density lipoprotein (VLDL), and the intermediate density lipoprotein (IDL).

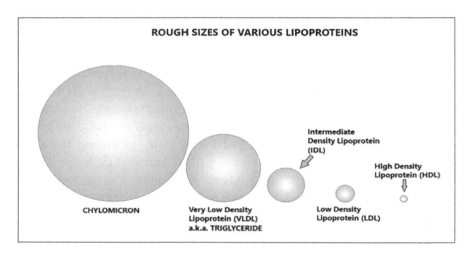

Figure 1

Why saturated fat cannot raise cholesterol/LDL levels

First a brief bit of history. After the second world war, terror stalked the US as an explosion in the rate of heart attacks scoured the land. It seemed to have appeared from nowhere, and it was wiping out hundreds of thousands of middle-aged men. Women were mainly spared, or at least the proportion seemed to be in the order of around 10 to 1. Men to women. (Whether this is true or not, I am not certain, but we shall let it go).

At the time this caused a major panic. Heart disease was killing well over a million people a year. Which makes COVID19 look exceedingly tame in comparison.

No-one knew where it had come from, or why. Researchers were tripping over themselves to find answers. Step forward Ancel Keys, with his ready prepared diet-heart hypothesis. This was a man who had jumped straight to the top of Mount Assumption. He returned with a tablet of stone with the words 'saturated', and 'fat', carved upon it.

Bathed in the bright glow of scientific certainty, he simply *knew* what caused heart disease. It was saturated fat in the diet. And lo, he became a man on a mission; a mission to convince the world that he was right.

In the absence of any obvious alternatives, his idea was taken up with great vigour. Something needed to be done, and this was certainly something. Saturated fat consumption could be reduced, and all would be well. 'Huzzah!' Shouted all the animals around the world. The land-based ones anyway.

Studies were set up, committees organised. Although, in the way of such things, there was no immediate change the eating habits of the average American man, or woman. Which provides a perfect example of the fact that the time lag from the research world to the real world, can usually be measured in decades.

Which means that it took some time before we arrive at the single most important event in the demonisation of saturated fat. This was the Senator McGovern's Dietary Committee of 1977. A congressional hearing where various experts met up to lay down dietary guideline rules, for the prevention of heart disease.

In truth, although it was nearly 30 years since the hypothesis was trumpeted by Keys, the participants were still far from unanimous about the connection between saturated fat and cardiovascular disease.

"When the US government introduced "Dietary Goals for the United States", they did not have unanimous support. The guidelines, which urged the public to cut saturated fat from their diet, were challenged by a number of scientists in a Congressional hearing. The findings were not based on sufficient evidence, they argued.

"They were ignored. Dr Robert Olson recounts an exchange he had with Senator George McGovern, in which he said: 'I plead in my report and will plead again orally here for more research on the problem before we make announcements to the American public.' McGovern replied: 'Senators don't have the luxury that the research scientist does of waiting until every last shred of evidence is in.'"[2]

Senator McGovern might as well have said. *'Listen son, we know that saturated fat raises cholesterol and causes heart disease, we don't need any damned evidence.'*

And the simple fact is that they didn't really have any damned evidence, at least no damned evidence that would stand up in a court of law, or science. However, they still managed to find saturated fat guilty, as charged... as expected. Some people would call this proper, strong, leadership. Make a decision and go with it.

I would call it monumental stupidity. Science and politics are not comfortable bed fellows. In fact, they mix very badly. Politicians demand immediate, simplistic answers. Scientists, at least true scientists, want to get at the truth. There is very rarely much overlap.

Indeed, strip aside the bluster and the confirmation bias, and the reality is that dietary guidelines were taken up enthusiastically around the world, despite a complete lack of any real evidence. A fact highlighted by an article, published in the *BMJ*, entitled:

"Evidence from randomised controlled trials did not support the introduction of dietary fat guidelines in 1977 and 1983: a systematic review and meta-analysis."

The researchers looked at all the evidence available to those who created the dietary guidelines at the time. They found that there was exactly, and precisely... none.

*"CONCLUSION: Dietary recommendations were introduced for 220 million US and 56 million UK citizens by 1983, **in the absence of supporting evidence from RCTs**"* [3]

An RCT is short for, a randomised controlled trial. They are considered the gold-standard form of medical research. The type of research that can either confirm, or refute, your hypothesis. In 1977, such trials did not exist.

Okay, you might think, there was no good evidence before this committee met. But surely there must be some in the four decades since then? Again, the answer is no. Nothing, zip, nada. [4] It remains a fact that there was not, and is not, any randomised controlled trial evidence to support the dietary guidelines, or the demonisation of saturated fat. None.

I am aware that people may find it impossible to believe that hugely influential guidelines can be put together by 'experts,' then promoted around the world, based on nothing more than a tentative scientific hypothesis. It sounds preposterous. Well, I suppose it is preposterous, but it also happens to be true.

Unfortunately, it is rather difficult to present this lack of evidence. *'Ladies and Gentlemen, here is the complete lack of evidence to support the diet-heart hypothesis. I now proudly present you with – nothing at all... Tada!"* Small sigh of disappointment from the audience.

Rather than spend too much time looking at the complete and utter lack of evidence, I going to switch to theory, where I will attempt to explain why it was never possible for saturated fat to raise blood cholesterol levels in the first place. By cholesterol levels I mean, of course, LDL-cholesterol levels.

The diet-heart hypothesis, like any hypothesis, has to rest on a basic understanding of the science underlying it. In this case it came into being purely through the process of reverse engineering. By which it was believed that a raised cholesterol caused heart disease, and something must be raising it. Because it couldn't just go up all by itself... could it?

What could that something be? It was decreed that it must be found in the diet. In fact, when he began his research, Ancel Keys was convinced that it was cholesterol in the diet that raised cholesterol levels. Which sounds sensible. Substance X in the diet, raises the level of substance X in the blood. Well, it sounds sensible if you ignore the critical fact that you do not actually have any substance X floating about in the blood.

Yes indeed, this was Keys original 'cholesterol' hypothesis. Cholesterol in the diet, raises blood cholesterol levels. He then carried out a number of cholesterol feeding experiments on humans, and found that dietary cholesterol did absolutely nothing. Here is his direct quote from a scientific symposium in 1954:

"The evidence – both from experiments and from field surveys – indicates that cholesterol content, per se, of all natural diets has no significant effect on either the cholesterol level or the development of atherosclerosis in man." [4]

You might think this should have blown the cholesterol hypothesis straight out of the water. But it did not. Keys simply decreed that, sorry, it is not cholesterol in the diet that raises the cholesterol level. It is saturated fat. *'Oops, silly me.'* Mind you, I suppose it is the sort of mistake that any idiot could make?

I mean, when he first came out with the diet-heart/cholesterol hypothesis in 1948, he did not even know that there was such a thing as a low-density lipoprotein. There were just 'lipoproteins.' All lumped together and called cholesterol. The first time anyone knew that were many different types of lipoprotein was in around 1950.

Fat and cholesterol synthesis itself, and how they are both transported around the body, only became untangled during the 1960s. Which means that Keys had no real idea about fat metabolism, or how or where lipoproteins were made, or what controlled their levels. All that he had was *the* answer. Saturated fat raises cholesterol level and causes heart disease. All facts must now be made to fit. In Figure 2 we can see what a saturated fat looks like, in comparison to unsaturated and the, so-called, super-heart healthy polyunsaturated fats.

The Structure of fatty acids - which are often (inaccurately) called 'fats'

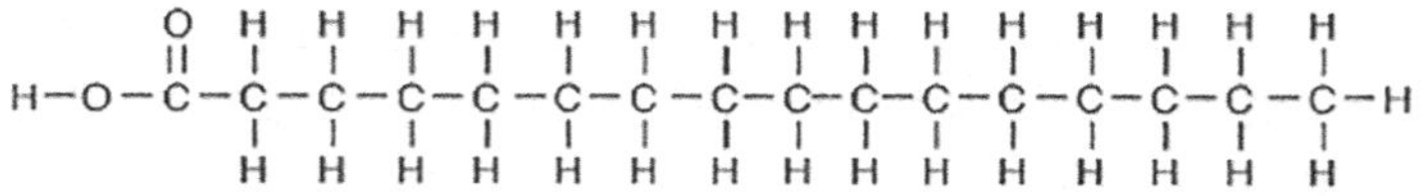

Saturated fatty acid - all carbon atoms have two hydrogen atoms attached

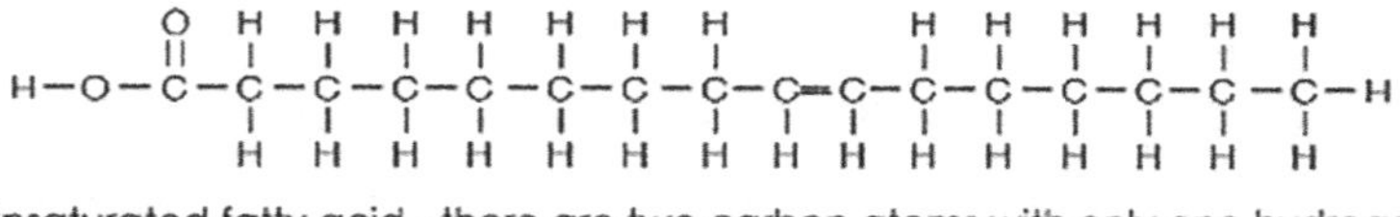

Unsaturated fatty acid - there are two carbon atoms with only one hydrogen atom attached (The carbon atoms are not fully 'saturated' with hydrogen atoms)

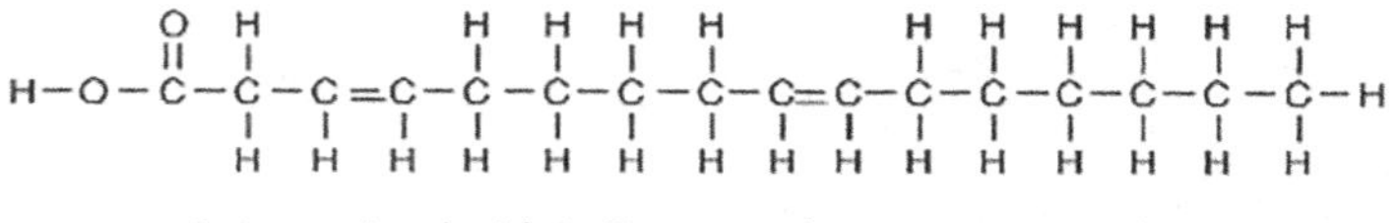

Polyunsaturated fat - There are two, or more, carbon atoms with only one hydrogen atom attached

---

Figure 2

Today, we know virtually everything there is to know about fat metabolism, and it is now beyond doubt that saturated fat consumption cannot raise LDL levels. It is not simply unlikely, it is impossible. There is no mechanism within the body for it to do so. Yes, a rather bold, hubristic statement. But I have seen nothing to contradict it, and it is supported by the science.

The reasons why saturated fat cannot raise LDL levels

We begin with the knowledge that the body is exceptionally good at keeping the level of all substances that float about in the bloodstream under tight control. If the level of anything rises too high, mechanisms are triggered to bring the level back down, and vice-versa. The technical term for this is a *'negative feedback loop'*. The overall system of keeping everything under control is known as homeostasis.

For saturated fat to drive LDL levels up, and keep them at a damaging level, it must first be overcoming homeostasis. Or, to put it another way, 'excess' saturated fat consumption overwhelms the metabolic and physiological control systems designed to keep us alive, and healthy. Is this possible, or likely?

My attempt to answer this question starts by first asking, what happens when we eat saturated fat? The first step is that it binds to bile salts in the bowel. Bile salts are a form of mildly adapted cholesterol which are made in the liver and released from the gall bladder when you eat fat.

Without bile salts, fat cannot be absorbed, and it simply passes straight through and out the other end. I can assure you that the end result is not pleasant in any way, shape, or form. The medical term is steatorrhea (fatty poo), otherwise described as 'pale, bulky and offensive'. And it sure is offensive.

Once bound with bile salts, saturated fat is absorbed into the gut wall, where it is then packed into the very large lipoprotein known as a chylomicron. Once this has been filled up with fats, the chylomicron travels up a special tube called the thoracic duct. At the end of which it is released directly into the blood stream.

Directly into the bloodstream.

It does not, and this is a mission critical point, pass through the liver. Straight into the bloodstream it goes, to begin its journey around the body.

15

As chylomicrons bumble their way around the body, they are stripped of their fat content by cells they brush up against, primarily fat cells. Which means that they gradually shrink down, and down. Eventually they become about the size of an LDL molecule. At which point they are known as *'chylomicron remnants'*. These remnants are absorbed back into liver and are then broken down into their constituent parts.

Which means that only a very small percentage of the fat that you eat can end up in the liver. The vast, vast, majority travels straight from the bowel to fat cells (adipose tissue). Whereupon fats are stored in the form of triglycerides*.

A TRIGLYCERIDE - ofen inaccurately called a 'fat' [Very Low Density Lipoproteins (VLDLs) can also be called triglycerides - just to make things impossible to understand]

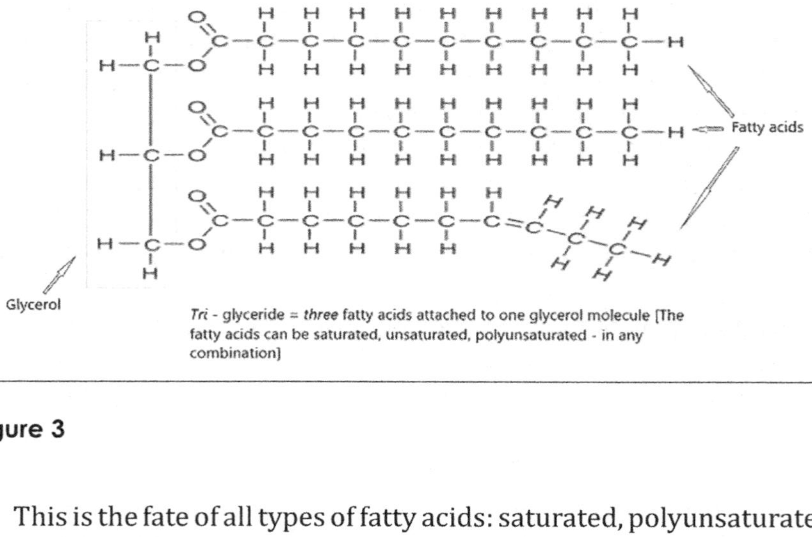

Glycerol

Fatty acids

Tri - glyceride = three fatty acids attached to one glycerol molecule [The fatty acids can be saturated, unsaturated, polyunsaturated - in any combination]

Figure 3

This is the fate of all types of fatty acids: saturated, polyunsaturated, or monounsaturated. There is nothing unique about saturated fat in the way that it is absorbed, transported around the body, and then stored.

---

* Figure 3 shows that a triglyceride is made up of three fats (fatty acids) attached to a single glycerol molecule – a glycerol molecule is one half of a glucose molecule. This structure allows fatty acids to be packed very tightly together, taking up much less space. This structure also prevents the fatty acids from being acids. The body doesn't like 'acidy' things floating about and does what it can to neutralise them.

At this stage in the journey, I would like you to sharpen a pencil and write down the following key fact. Nothing in the absorption, transport, and storage of dietary fat, saturated or otherwise, has anything to do with LDL a.k.a. 'bad cholesterol' in any way shape or form. Got that? You mean you have lived all your life and you didn't know this? Don't worry, you can have virtually the entire medical profession to keep you company.

Which leads on to the next question. Where *are* LDLs made, and what do they do if they don't transport dietary fat around the body? The answer to the first part of question is that LDLs are not really made anywhere, not directly. They only come into existence when very low-density lipoproteins (VLDLs) shrink down in size.

Sorry, but I have to add this lipoprotein to this tale. Very low-density lipoproteins (VLDLs) are manufactured in the liver. They contain both fats and cholesterol which are, mainly, synthesized there. (To add to the confusion, VLDLs are usually called 'triglycerides'... don't ask why. They just are).

The role of a VLDL is to transport fatty acids out of the liver and deliver them to fat cells. As with chylomicrons, VLDLs travel around the body getting stripped of fatty acids, gradually reducing in size.

Just to confirm that when people use the term 'fats', they really mean 'fatty acids'. Unfortunately, when people use the term fat, they also mean triglycerides. When they say fat cells, they also mean adipose tissue. Many people also call cholesterol a fat. I am sorry... medical terminology. Thud... head hits desk. *'This is a banana, which is actually an apple, sorry an orange. Well, they are all fruits aren't they. Don't be so picky.'*

Moving on, once VLDLs have shrunk down to their smallest size, via being an intermediate density lipoprotein, they have transformed themselves into LDL molecule. Thus, an LDL molecule is simply what is left of VLDL molecule, once it has shed a sufficient amount of fat.

Very low-density lipoprotein → shrinks → Intermediate density lipoproteins → shrinks → Low-density lipoprotein.

The vast majority of LDL molecules that come into being through this process are simply pulled out of the circulation by LDL receptors in the liver. Although a certain amount of LDL – containing cholesterol – does remain free, floating about in the blood.

Cells that require additional, life-giving cholesterol, manufacture an LDL receptor, which they then wave about in the bloodstream. The receptor will bind to a passing LDL molecule. At which point the entire *'LDL/LDL receptor complex'* is drawn into the cell and broken down.

Another way of looking at this system is that the job of VLDL is to take fatty acids from the liver and distribute it around the body for storage. Then, once a VLDL has shrunk down into an LDL, the second role takes over, which is to provide cholesterol to cells that need it.

In whatever way you view these lipoproteins, the key takeaway fact is that VLDLs are the only source of LDLs. Thus, for the LDL level to rise, the VLDL level must go up first. Which leads to the next question. What makes VLDL levels go up? Well, as I hope is now clear, it is not, and never could have been saturated fat consumption.

Instead, what causes VLDL levels to rise is eating carbohydrates. Yes, carbohydrates. Bread, pasta, potatoes, fruit, rice, cornflakes, sugar and suchlike. Just to remind you that all these different forms of carbohydrate are made up of simple sugars stuck together, end to end.

Therefore, in whatever form you choose to eat your carbohydrates, they are all broken down within the gut into their constituent simple sugar building blocks – largely glucose and fructose. These molecules, and any other form of sugar, are transported directly into the liver. The liver will then decide upon their fate.

(When it comes to fructose, there is huge and very heated debate about what happens to it. It appears that some/most is converted to fat, some is converted to glucose, and some is simply broken down into things called ketone bodies and burned up. For the sake of this discussion, fructose is either used to create new fatty acids, or is converted to glucose. Which means that we are really restricting this discussion to glucose, as everything ends up here – one way or another).

Moving on. If you eat a lot of carbohydrate, in whatever form: bread, potatoes, crunchy nut corn flakes, sugar itself, you end up with a liver full of glucose molecules. The liver now has three choices about what to do with it. Store it as glycogen (a molecule that consists of hundreds of glucose molecules stuck end to end – a glucose polymer), release it gradually into the circulation, or convert it into fat.

The liver can pack away about 500 calories of glycogen, or thereabouts. Once this 500 calorie limit has been reached, the liver is full. If you keep on eating carbohydrates, what happens next? What happens next is the only thing that can possibly happen. Which is that the liver is forced to convert the excess glucose into fat, or else it would end up as a massive cube of glucose.

In humans, the process of converting sugar into fat within the liver, is called lipogenesis (*lipo* = fat. *Genesis* = creation). The more complete scientific term is *de novo* lipogenesis (creating fats from 'novo' new).

Just to prove that I am not simply making all of this up, here follows a quote. It is a bit jargon heavy, but I think it is worth including. If the first bit about acetyl-CoA is a bit bamboozling, just focus on the final sentence:

*"**De novo lipogenesis** is the biological process by which the precursors of acetyl-CoA are synthesized into fatty acids [fats]. In human subjects consuming diets higher in fat (> 30 % energy), **lipogenesis is down regulated** and extremely low; typically < 10 % of the fatty acids secreted by the liver. **This percentage will increase when dietary fat is reduced and replaced by carbohydrate.**"*[4]

This is simply confirmation of the bleeding obvious. Namely that any excess glucose must be converted to fat by *de novo* lipogenesis (DNL) – because there is nothing else that can happen to it. One further thing I need to mention here is that all new fats synthesized in the liver are *saturated* fats, and only saturated fats (mostly palmitic acid C16:0). The liver does not make unsaturated fats – possibly too unhealthy?

The most important fact here is that, if you eat a lot of fat, the liver reduces its fat synthesis This, in turn, means that the VLDL level will fall.

On the other hand, if you eat carbohydrates the VLDL level rises.

"Low-fat, high-carbohydrate (LF/HC) diets commonly elevate plasma triglyceride (TG) concentrations."[5]

Key points

- Eating more fat/saturated fat reduces VLDL production.

- Eating more carbohydrate increases VLDL production.

Which is, of course, the exact opposite of what we are led to believe. I occasionally amuse myself by asking what would happen if someone came up with the diet-heart hypothesis today. It would simply be laughed out of court. *'Do you understand anything about fat metabolism? Clearly not.'*

You may be now wondering the following. If carbohydrates raise VLDL levels, which they do, why does this not greatly increase LDL levels? More VLDL must mean more LDL. This would be true, except for the fact that the liver monitors LDL levels, and if they rise, it simply removes excess LDL from circulation. This is the process of homeostasis in action. Doing what it does.

Saturated fat vs. unsaturated fat

There is another issue here which I feel obliged to cover. Which is that a number of studies have shown that the LDL level can fall when saturated fats are replaced by polyunsaturated fats. This has been seen often enough for me to believe that it may even be true. Given what I have written above, how can this fact possibly be explained?

After all, as discussed above, the body deals with all fats we eat in the same way. They are absorbed in the gut, packed into chylomicrons, then stuffed into fat cells – the end. Nothing different there.

There is though, an explanation for this finding, and it is the following. In the vast majority of studies where saturated fats have been replaced by polyunsaturated fats, the polyunsaturated fats used came from plant oils. Plant oils contain a high proportion of stanols, which are the plant equivalent of cholesterol.

One of the chemicals in Figure 4 below is a stanol, the other is cholesterol. You can try to guess which one is which. (Clue, the one on the right is cholesterol).

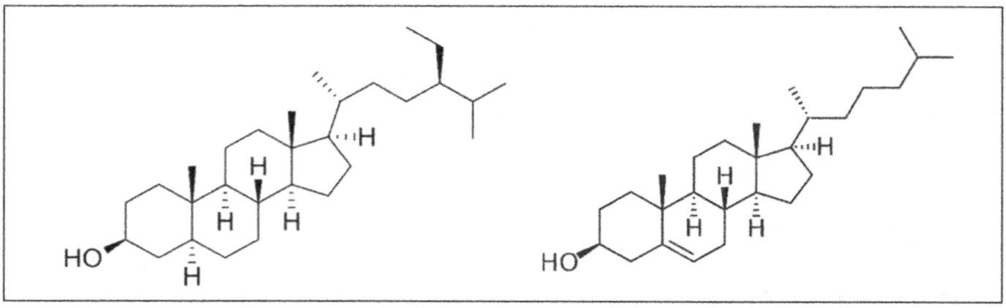

Figure 4

It has long been known that stanols can lower LDL levels. A fact that is heavily advertised by Benecol, and the manufactures of other such 'low fat' spreads. The reason why this happens is because stanols compete with cholesterol for absorption, resulting in reduced LDL levels. Early drugs that lowered LDL, before statins, used the same basic principle of blocking cholesterol absorption from the guts.

With less cholesterol available from the diet, the liver pulls more LDL molecules out of the bloodstream in order to create VLDLs – which need both fatty acids and cholesterol to be constructed.

Therefore, the fall in LDL with polyunsaturated fats has nothing to do with reducing saturated fat consumption – although this is the explanation that is universally promoted. Instead, it was the added plant stanols that produced this effect.

In essence, the studies which claim to show that you can lower LDL by reducing saturated fat consumption, falls foul of the old two variables problem.

By which I mean, if you change two variables in an experiment, at the same time, you cannot say which of them was responsible for the effect. In this case, was LDL lowered by the reduction in saturated fats, or the increase in plant stanols? I am going for the stanols. Stanols are often called sterols, the terms are interchangeable – this is probably to add even more confusion. ['*You say stanols, I say sterols, let's call the whole thing off*'].

The power of an idea

Despite what I have written above, the idea that saturated fat raises LDL levels remains pretty much unchallenged. In truth, it has never been more powerful than it is today. This just confirms how powerful a simple idea can be. Saturated fat raises the LDL level – end of.

Once implanted, it is almost impossible to shift. Indeed, whatever I have written here, however strong the science, many people will still be battling away to find flaws to prove that I am wrong. '*But what about odd numbered polyunsaturated fats, or...*

A recent conference in Switzerland, organised by the *British Medical Journal* (*BMJ*), and a Swiss Insurance company Swiss Re discussed the dietary guidelines and the role of saturated fat. I was invited, but could not attend, as I was working.

Zoë Harcombe, who shares my concerns about the diet-heart hypothesis, did attend and she shared the takeaway messages:

"At the recent Swiss Re/The BMJ Food for Thought conference, the closing speakers tried to find some agreement on dietary fat guidelines...

"Fiona [Fiona Godlee, editor of the BMJ] *started with: 'The point about saturated fat is: the evidence is now looking pretty good, but the guidance hasn't shifted... there doesn't seem to have been an enormous 'mea culpa' from the scientific community that we got it so wrong. That does surprise me.'*

"Salim [Salim Yusuf, cardiologist and epidemiologist] *replied: 'We got brainwashed by a very questionable study, called The Seven Countries Study, many years ago and it was ingrained in our DNA and generations of us were brought up with that... Somebody said that you need to wait for guidelines committees to die before you can change the guidelines committees'!*

"Fiona then said: 'Maybe one outcome of this meeting would be for this meeting to say 'that's gone now', the science has changed. Am I right Salim? Am I right Dariush? It seems to be that should be an outcome of some sort from this meeting.'

"Alas, the UK guidelines committee shows no signs of such change, let alone the 'mea culpa' that Fiona suggests might be in order." [5]

Yes, everyone got it wrong. The editor of the British Medical Journal was virtually pleading with people to change the guidelines. *'That's gone now.'* A reference to saturated fat consumption. Yet nothing changes.

But what of the mass of evidence in support of the diet-heart hypothesis I hear you cry? Surely there must be supportive data, which simply overwhelms these puny negative studies? *'Kendrick, you are just picking and choosing'*. In fact, I am not. There was, and is, no evidence. To quote Salim Yusuf *'We got brainwashed...'* And we remain brainwashed. Just in case you are wondering if Salim Yusuf is a trusted source. Here from the journal *Cardiovascular Research*:

"Dr Salim Yusuf is Distinguished Professor of Medicine and Clinical Epidemiology & Biostatistics at McMaster University in Canada. He is also Executive Director of the Population Health Research Institute at McMaster University, Chief Scientist at Hamilton Health Sciences, Past-President of the World Heart Federation, and Senior Advising Editor of Cardiovascular Research."

Anyway, you may now be thinking, so what if saturated fat doesn't raise LDL levels? We still know that raised 'cholesterol' levels cause heart disease. That, at least, is beyond doubt. Isn't it?

Why a raised cholesterol does not cause heart disease

To be frank, it didn't take me long to cast aside the idea that saturated fat had anything to do with cardiovascular disease. The evidence was clearly complete scientific gibberish. However, it took me a lot longer to discard part two of the cholesterol hypothesis.

I mean, when you first come across it, this part of the hypothesis sounds like the purest common sense. Atherosclerotic plaques are full of cholesterol – at least we are repeatedly told this is true (although it is not really the case). The only place this cholesterol could possibly have come from is the bloodstream, isn't it? So, a higher level will obviously lead to cardiovascular disease.

Study after study also seemed to confirm the link between high cholesterol levels and cardiovascular disease. Children with a genetic condition known as familial hypercholesterolaemia (FH), who have super-high levels of LDL, could die before the age of five from cardiovascular disease.

Statins, drugs that lower cholesterol, also reduce cardiovascular disease. International experts are also pretty much of one voice. Cholesterol – or LDL, or whatever you decide to call it – causes cardiovascular disease. And so on and so forth, until the evidence stretches over the horizon. Then right round the world to smack you on the back of the head again.

'Who but a bumbling fool, who understands nothing of science, could possibly suggest that this hypothesis is wrong? Who but the most ridiculous idiot? Who, but some strange and misguided buffoon... I call upon you, reveal yourself, and be ready for approbation to rain down upon your extraordinarily dense skull.'

'Ahem...' (Small squeaky voice) *'That would be me.'*

Yes, when I first became convinced that cholesterol had nothing to do with cardiovascular disease, I became uncomfortably aware that I was very much in a small and select club. A club so select indeed, that it appeared to contain but one member. Me.

There were actually others, but I did not know they existed. Decades ago, Dr George Mann set up the Veritas society to challenge the cholesterol hypothesis. He has since been pretty much written out of history, even though he played a central role in setting up the original, massively influential Framingham study. The source from which all heart disease guidelines have flowed.

He, like others, who disagreed became ghosts in the machine. In much the same way, powerful evidence contradicting the cholesterol hypothesis was simply not published.

For example, a major dietary trial was done, between 1968 and 1973. It was called the Minnesota Coronary Experiment (MCE). It was large scale, with over 9,000 participants, it was even a randomised controlled trial (RCT). Yes, the gold standard.

As found in earlier studies, replacing saturated fats with polyunsaturated fats reduced the cholesterol level. However, and this is key, it had precisely no impact on cardiovascular disease.

More disturbingly, the greater the fall in the cholesterol level, the more people died. Yes, you did just read that. For each 1% **fall** in cholesterol there was a 1% **increase** in the risk of death.

"There was a 22% higher risk of death for each 30 mg/dL (0.78 mmol/L) reduction in serum cholesterol."

As the authors of this study commented.

"Available evidence from randomized controlled trials shows that replacement of saturated fat in the diet with linoleic acid [a polyunsaturated fat] *effectively lowers serum cholesterol **but does not support the hypothesis that this translates to a lower risk of death from coronary heart disease or all causes.**"* [6]

Again, the careful language of the clinical study. I would have called it. *'If you lower the cholesterol level with polyunsaturated fats, people are more likely to die.'* But that is not the sort of title that ends up published in the *New England Journal of Medicine*. Can't imagine why.

There is a further fascinating, and deeply disturbing thing about this study. It was completed in 1973. However, if you do decide to look up the reference I provided, you will find that it was not actually published until 2016. A delay of more than 40 years. How so? Does this represent the most lengthy and rigorous proof reading and peer review process in the history of scientific research?

No.

The story of how the data were eventually discovered, was written up in an article in *Scientific American* called: *"Records found in dusty basement undermine decades of dietary advice."* The article itself is worth a read. I include the first three paragraphs.

"If biology has an Indiana Jones, it is Christopher Ramsden: he specializes in excavating lost studies, particularly those with the potential to challenge mainstream, government-sanctioned health advice.

"His latest excavation – made possible by the pack-rat habits of a deceased scientist, the help of the scientist's sons, and computer technicians who turned punch cards and magnetic tape into formats readable by today's computers – undercuts a pillar of nutrition science.

"Ramsden, of the National Institutes of Health, unearthed raw data from a 40-year-old study, which challenges the dogma that eating vegetable fats instead of animal fats is good for the heart. The study, the largest gold-standard experiment testing that idea, found the opposite, Ramsden and his colleagues reported on Tuesday in the BMJ" [7]

What we have here, gentle reader, is a study completed in the early 1970s, which showed that there was indeed a connection between polyunsaturated fat consumption and the cholesterol level. However, it completely refuted the diet-heart/cholesterol hypothesis. In super short summary, what was discovered was that:

Increased polyunsaturated fat intake → **reduced** cholesterol levels→ **increased** risk of death.

Something noted in other studies. This time with regard to heart disease: *"Plant sterols lower cholesterol but increase risk for coronary heart disease."* [8]

Karl Popper has a term to describe a finding such as the Minnesota Coronary Experiment. He called them black swans. If your hypothesis is that all swans are white, finding more and more white swans modestly increases the possibility that your hypothesis is correct. However, finding one black swan immediately and absolutely refutes your hypothesis. End of.

However, it is difficult to refute a hypothesis if the black swan has been hidden in the back of a garage for 40 years. Which is exactly what happened with the MCE study. I think it is important to mention that the lead investigator of the MCE study was the one and only Ancel Keys. I wonder why the study was not published…

Other unpublished data, from the same time period, found exactly the same thing. The Sydney Diet Heart Study was considerably smaller, but still a randomised controlled study. Again, the researchers replaced saturated fats with polyunsaturated fats. Again, the cholesterol levels fell.

Again, these data were not published at the time, but the results were, as follows.

For those in the study who replaced saturated fats, with polyunsaturated fats:

All-cause mortality   =   1.62 (62% increase)

Cardiovascular mortality =   1.70 (70% increase)

Heart disease mortality   =   1.74 (74% increase)[9]

The conclusions of the, eventually published, study were succinct. I have spelled out acronyms in full.

"Substituting linoleic acid [a polyunsaturated fat] *in place of saturated fatty acids* [saturated fats] *increased all-cause, cardiovascular and coronary heart disease mortality. Advice to increase linoleic acid or unspecified polyunsaturated fats merits reconsideration."*

'*Merits reconsideration...*' These results directly contradict everything we are told about saturated fats, and polyunsaturated fats. Yet, all we get is *'merits reconsideration'*. Is hiding data that you don't want people to see, the same as simply lying about it? Discuss. I know what I think.

As you can see, the reality is that there *was* powerful randomised controlled trial evidence in the 1970s about saturated fat and cholesterol levels. Evidence that could have been used at the congressional hearings, but clearly was not.

How many more trials found the same thing? Hard to say. When people bury the results of their research, one imagines that it very often stays buried.

Of course, when I first started to become obsessed with cardiovascular disease, I knew nothing of these hidden figures. However, I had been looking closely at the basic science. Things were simply not adding up.

One thing that stood out for me is that cholesterol plays a critical role in human health. If this were not so, the liver would not be bothered to churn out about five grams a day. All day, every day. Yes, the liver manufactures a poison to kill us all.

Cholesterol stabilises all cell membranes throughout the body allowing them to carry out thousands of important metabolic processes. It is critical for the support and health of neurones. It is used to make new synapses in the brain. It acts as the backbone for essential hormones, and vitamin D, etc. etc.

Could this substance really be the chemical of doom? Of course, you can argue that it is not cholesterol that we should be worried about, it is the low-density lipoprotein – LDL.

Again, though, why would this benign little molecule cause such havoc. I really could not see any clear mechanism of action. Or at least no mechanism of action that made a great deal of sense.

In fact, I became more concerned that if the cholesterol level was too low then we could run into problems. For example, I had come across a genetic condition called Smith-Lemli-Opitz-Syndrome (SLOS) which results in very low cholesterol synthesis, low LDL levels, and suchlike.

It is not common, by any manner of means, but it can result in such nasty things as microcephaly (a very small brain), mental retardation, heart defects, fused toes, extra fingers underdeveloped genitals in males, early death – and suchlike. Very unpleasant indeed. Yes, you certainly need your cholesterol.

I was not the only one to have concerns about the impact of a low cholesterol level. I turned my attention to a study published in 1992, just after statins first launched. It was a report from a major conference called '*Low blood cholesterol; mortality associations.*' Which took place a couple of years earlier, in 1990.

This conference was convened because it had been noted that low cholesterol levels had been associated with a higher death rate – not in all studies, but in many studies.

As statins charged over the horizon, there was a concern that lowering cholesterol might increase the death rate (overall mortality rate), even if there was a benefit in cardiovascular disease. There is not much point in lowering the risk of death from one disease if you simply increase deaths from other diseases at the same time. In medicine we call this – a complete bloody waste of time.

It was a big old study, and a big old report. It came under the umbrella of the National Heart Lung and Blood Institute, which is the most influential cardiovascular organisation in the US. It develops guidelines, decides on which treatments to be used, and suchlike.

There isn't really an equivalent in the UK. Think of it as a combination of the royal colleges of medicine and suchlike, and the National Institute of Care & Health Excellence (NICE), with a bit of department of health thrown in – sort of. Anyway, that is the background. What did they find?

Below are two graphs (Figure 5 and Figure 6). The first figure is for men, the second is for women. They show the data on overall morality (risk of death), at different levels of cholesterol. There were four groups. Those with 'low' cholesterol, those with 'optimal' levels, those with 'high' levels, and those with 'very high' levels. These were defined as follows.

Low   < 4mmol/l (<160 mg/dl[*])

Optimal   4–5 mmol/l (160–199 mg/dl)

High   5–6.2 mmol/l (200–240 mg/dl)

Very high > 6.2 mmol/l (>240 mg/dl)

I should add that both graphs were set to a risk of one, at the 'optimal' cholesterol level. One means 'average' risk of death. Anything below one means a lower-than-average risk, anything above one means a higher risk. On this graph 1.15 means a 15% greater chance of dying – of anything.

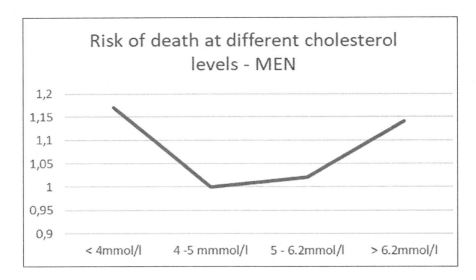

Figure 5

---

* In the US, they use different units to the UK, and the rest of the world. Because…. Well, they do.

As you can see, the lowest risk of death occurred when the cholesterol level was between four to five, 'optimal'. So far, so good. It rises very slightly as the cholesterol level goes up to six(ish) and then rises again above 6.2. However, as you can see, the greatest risk of death occurs at the lowest levels of cholesterol. When the cholesterol levels are below 4, the death rate is 17% higher.

Next, is the graph for women.

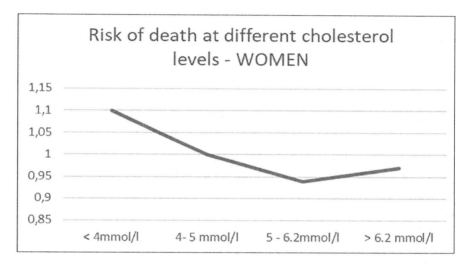

Figure 6

A somewhat different pattern. However, exactly as with men, the highest risk of death was found at the lowest cholesterol levels. With women a 'high' cholesterol level, that is between five to six, was associated with the lowest risk of death. Taking this one step further, there was also a lower risk of death when the cholesterol was above 6.2, in comparison to when the level was between 4 and 5 a.k.a. 'optimal'.[10]

In truth, these changes in risk are not that great. One point one, one point two. On these graphs it might look fairly dramatic, but in reality, you are talking about very small absolute alterations in risk. Two or three months in life expectancy, in total.

I will mention just one more study here, from Norway. It was called the Nord-Trøndelag Health Study, shortened to HUNT2, for reasons that are not clear. Data were gathered from just over 50,000 people over a period of 10 years. Which represents over half a million years of observation. In short, it was a massive study.

What they found was that, in men, a high cholesterol level made no real difference to life expectancy. However, when they looked at women, the higher the cholesterol level, the longer they lived – and they also suffered far less cardiovascular disease (CVD).

The difference was highly significant – there was a 40% risk reduction in mortality for women with the highest cholesterol levels. The conclusion of their paper was carefully politically worded.

*"Our study provides an updated epidemiological indication of possible errors in the CVD risk algorithms of many clinical guidelines. If our findings are generalizable, clinical and public health recommendations regarding the 'dangers' of cholesterol should be revised. This is especially true for women, for whom moderately elevated cholesterol (by current standards) may prove to be **not only harmless but even beneficial.**"* [11]

By moderately elevated, they meant up to 7 mmol/l, which is now considered dangerously high. If you had this level in the UK, or US, you would immediately be diagnosed as having familial hypercholesterolaemia (FH) and started on an emergency statin.

Anyway, I looked at studies like this, and others. Then I asked myself, what seemed to me a very reasonable question. Why the *#$# %$ &#$# are we trying desperately to lower the cholesterol level with drugs? A question that no-one has ever satisfactorily answered. At least not to my mind.

What I found more frustrating was that no-one seemed remotely interested in answering this question. There was often an awkward silence, as if someone had broken wind loudly in front of the Queen. If I pressed on, people just started to become rather angry. Ranging from somewhat irate, heading towards incandescent, then full on Chernobyl.

The consequences of questioning the diet heart hypothesis

There are, I have discovered, two areas of medicine that absolutely cannot be questioned. Number one... I will allow you to guess at, not that difficult in truth. It's a word beginning with vaccines. Number two, and not that far behind, is the cholesterol hypothesis. It is an unbelievably touchy subject.

I first became aware of the strength of feeling around this area when I learned of Dr Uffe Ravnskov. A doctor who has never believed that cholesterol (or LDL) causes cardiovascular disease. He set up a loose network of doctors and scientists called The International Network of Cholesterol Sceptics (THINCS).

Uffe is a man of great moral courage, and a good man, who I have found to be straight as an arrow. He wrote a book called *The Cholesterol Myths* in 1991. What then took place was covered by Tom Naughton, a very funny guy, bright as a button, and also a cholesterol sceptic.

"When the Cholesterol Myths was published in 1991, the experts treated it like any other threat to conventional wisdom: they ignored it or mocked it, without ever bothering to actually dispute the arguments presented in it. Editors of medical journals simply asked the established health authorities if Ravnskov was correct; when the authorities said no, the editors wrote him off as a lone kook. In Finland the experts actually burned the book on live TV. I suppose Ravnskov should be grateful that putting heretics on a rack is frowned upon in modern societies." [12]

Yes, they burned Uffe's book. I mean, what more perfect metaphor could be found than the burning of a book. Of course, in this case it was not a metaphor – it actually took place. I mean… what the.

Others in our little tribe included Professor Kilmer McCully. He had been studying homocysteine (a breakdown product of various proteins). He discovered that children with abnormally high homocysteine levels were far more likely to develop atherosclerosis and die of CVD, often at a very young age. He was a researcher at Harvard at the time.

For a while, in the early 70s he published away merrily, and was pursuing his ideas without any problems. Then the roof fell in. Here is part of an article discussing the attacks that McCully suffered. Not only was he booted out of Harvard, but the attacks by Harvard University continued once he had gone. Here are a few paragraphs from a *New York Times* article on what happened to him.

*"Thomas N. James, a cardiologist and president of the University of Texas Medical Branch who was also the president of the American Heart Association in 1979 and '80, is even harsher [regarding the treatment of McCully]. 'It was worse than that you couldn't get ideas funded that went in other directions than cholesterol,' he says. 'You were intentionally discouraged from pursuing alternative questions. **I've never dealt with a subject in my life that elicited such an immediate hostile response.**'*

"It took two years for McCully to find a new research job. His children were reaching college age; he and his wife refinanced their house and borrowed from her parents. McCully says that his job search developed a pattern: he would hear of an opening, go for interviews and then the process would grind to a stop. Finally, he heard rumors of what he calls 'poison phone calls' from Harvard. 'It smelled to high heaven,' he says.

"McCully says that when he was interviewed on Canadian television after he left Harvard, he received a call from the public-affairs director of Mass. General. 'He told me to shut up,' McCully recalls. 'He said he didn't want the names of Harvard and Mass. General associated with my theories.'" [13]

That, my friends, is what happens to you when you dare to question the almighty cholesterol hypothesis. As you can imagine, this makes things somewhat tricky for those who want to pursue alternative ideas. You get attacked, funding is withdrawn, you are disowned by your own university and hounded by them for years afterwards. You become a pariah a 'denier'. Not a particularly comfortable place to be.

Perhaps the first person to be ruthlessly attacked for questioning the cholesterol hypothesis, at least the dietary part, was John Yudkin. A UK professor, and nutritional researcher. He believed that sugar, not fat, was a cause, even *the* cause of heart disease. He wrote a book called *Pure, White and Deadly*. He was then turned on by, none other than, the sainted Ancel Keys.

Here from an article in the *Guardian* newspaper

"Ancel Keys was intensely aware that Yudkin's sugar hypothesis posed an alternative to his own. If Yudkin published a paper, Keys would excoriate it, and him. He called Yudkin's theory 'a mountain of nonsense' and accused him of issuing 'propaganda' for the meat and dairy industries. 'Yudkin and his commercial backers are not deterred by the facts,' he said. 'They continue to sing the same discredited tune.' Yudkin never responded in kind. He was a mild-mannered man, unskilled in the art of political combat.

"That made him vulnerable to attack, and not just from Keys. The British Sugar Bureau dismissed Yudkin's claims about sugar as 'emotional assertions'; the World Sugar Research Organisation called his book 'science fiction'. In his prose, Yudkin is fastidiously precise and undemonstrative, as he was in person. Only occasionally does he hint at how it must have felt to have his life's work besmirched, as when he asks the reader, 'Can you wonder that one sometimes becomes quite despondent about whether it is worthwhile trying to do scientific research in matters of health?'" [14]

Yes, of course, as it turns out there was an entire industry in the background supporting Keys. They even set up a quasi-scientific organisation called the Sugar Research Foundation. Amazingly, their research always manged to find that sugar was wonderful and health giving.

Indeed, people should get out there and eat more more sugar. Feed it to your kids, stuff it down. Who needs teeth, just look at those gleaming dentures, gaze upon the joy of the ever-expanding waistlines of the population. Gasp in amazement as diabetes takes over the nation. Healthy, healthy, healthy.

For many years, the sugar foundation spent large sums of money promoting the idea that fat was the cause of heart disease. Their tireless work behind the scenes was reviewed in a paper in the *Journal of the American Medical Association (JAMA)*:

"We examined Sugar Research Foundation (SRF) internal documents, historical reports, and statements relevant to early debates about the dietary causes of coronary heart disease, and assembled findings chronologically into a narrative case study. The Sugar Research Foundation sponsored its first coronary heart disease research project in 1965, a literature review published in the New England Journal of Medicine, which singled out fat and cholesterol as the dietary causes of coronary heart disease and downplayed evidence that sucrose consumption was also a risk factor. The sugar research foundation set the review's objective, contributed articles for inclusion, and received drafts. The sugar research funding and role was not disclosed. Together with other recent analyses of sugar industry documents, our findings suggest the industry sponsored a research program in the 1960s and 1970s that successfully cast doubt about the hazards of sucrose while promoting fat as the dietary culprit in coronary heart disease." [15]

Harvard researchers were also co-opted to the cause of promoting sugar, whilst demonising fat. John Hickson, an industry executive, discussed a plan to shift public opinion "*through our research and information and legislative programs.*" Hickson proposed countering the alarming findings on sugar with industry-funded research. "*Then we can publish the data and refute our detractors.*"

"In 1965, he enlisted the Harvard researchers to write a review that would debunk the anti-sugar studies. He paid them a total of $6,500, the equivalent of $49,000 today. Mr. Hickson selected the papers for them to review and made it clear he wanted the result to favor sugar. Harvard's Dr Hegsted reassured the sugar executives. 'We are well aware of your particular interest,' he wrote, 'and will cover this as well as we can.'

33

"As they worked on their review, the Harvard researchers shared and discussed early drafts with Mr. Hickson, who responded that he was pleased with what they were writing. The Harvard scientists had dismissed the data on sugar as weak and given far more credence to the data implicating saturated fat. 'Let me assure you this is quite what we had in mind, and we look forward to its appearance in print,' Mr. Hickson wrote."

Dr Glantz indicated that *"after the review was published, the debate about sugar and heart disease died down, while low-fat diets gained the endorsement of many health authorities. By today's standards, they behaved very badly."* [16]

Well, well, surprise, surprise. Money lurking in the background once more. It must be said that the sums of money involved were rather puny. Nowadays, if you want a Harvard researcher to write a scientific paper it will cost you a bloody sight more than that. Most of them don't get out of bed for less than $10,000 a day.

But it is not just money that has distorted the entire area. Religion has also played a major role. The Seventh Day Adventist Church has been a long term, and highly significant, player in nutritional research.

"The emphasis on health ministry within the Seventh-day Adventist (SDA) movement led to the development of sanitariums in mid-nineteenth century America. These facilities, the most notable being in Battle Creek, Michigan, initiated the development of vegetarian foods, such as breakfast cereals and analogue meats.

"The Seventh Day Adventist Church still operates a handful of food production facilities around the world. The first Battle Creek Sanitarium dietitian was co-founder of the American Dietetics Association which ultimately advocated a vegetarian diet. The Seventh Day Adventist Church established hundreds of hospitals, colleges, and secondary schools and tens of thousands of churches around the world, all promoting a vegetarian diet.

"As part of the 'health message,' diet continues to be an important aspect of the church's evangelistic efforts. In addition to promoting a vegetarian diet and abstinence from alcohol, the Seventh Day Adventist church has also invested resources in demonstrating the health benefits of these practices through research. Much of that research has been conducted at Loma Linda University in Southern California, where there have been three prospective cohort studies conducted over 50 years." [17]

The Seventh Day Adventists also gave us that tasteless crunchy object known as the cornflake. As described in an article in the Smithsonian Magazine *"The Secret Ingredient in Kellogg's Corn Flakes Is Seventh-Day Adventism,"*

"...few know the story of the two men from Battle Creek, Michigan, who created those famously crispy, golden flakes of corn back in 1895, revolutionizing the way America ate breakfast: John Harvey Kellogg and his younger brother Will Keith Kellogg.

"Fewer still know that among the ingredients in the Kellogg's' secret recipe were the teachings of the Seventh-day Adventist church, a homegrown American faith that linked spiritual and physical health, and which played a major role in the Kellogg family's life.

"For half a century, Battle Creek was the Vatican of the Seventh-day Adventist church. Its founders, the self-proclaimed prophetess Ellen White and her husband, James, made their home in the Michigan town starting in 1854, moving the church's headquarters in 1904 to Takoma Park, outside of Washington, D.C. Eventually, Seventh-day Adventism grew into a major Christian denomination with churches, ministries and members all around the world. One key component of the Whites' sect was healthy living and a nutritious, vegetable and grain based-diet." [18]

Money and religion, now that's what I call a powerful combination. Then, when statins arrived on the scene, with their unique ability to significantly lower cholesterol levels, the full might of the pharmaceutical industry put its shoulder to the wheel. This is no mere billion-dollar industry, this is a trillion-dollar industry. There is also the trillion-dollar low-fat food industry.

So, no, there is not a great, evil, shadowy global worldwide cabal, promoting the cholesterol hypothesis. But there are massive players here, all very much on one side of the argument. Many of them well-meaning, others far less so.

Battling against all this is the science. At least I believe it is the science. On the side of science there are the dreadful inconvenient things called – the facts.

The definitive review

In our attempt to fight nonscience with science we happy few, we band of brothers at THINCS got together to assemble all the data we could find on LDL levels and the risk of death.

Our plan was to present *the* definitive study. Was LDL truly damaging? Was it harmless? Or could it even, possibly, whisper the idea in darkened corridors, be beneficial.

We restricted our analysis to the 'elderly', defined as those over 60, because this is the age group where well over 90% of all deaths from CVD occur. Which makes it the place where most of the data lie. Studying LDL levels, and rates of death, in 20-40-year-olds is almost completely pointless, because almost no-one dies of heart disease in this age group.

Anyway, our study was then published in the *BMJ Open*, and here is what we found:

*"High LDL-C is **inversely** associated with mortality in most people over 60 years. This finding is inconsistent with the cholesterol hypothesis (i.e., that cholesterol, particularly LDL-C, is inherently atherogenic). Since **elderly people with high LDL-C live as long or longer** than those with low LDL-C, our analysis provides reason to question the validity of the cholesterol hypothesis."*

We used very careful wording, stripped of any emotion, as demanded by the high priests of medical research and journal publication. I would like to have called the paper '*Hello world. Surprise! If you have a high cholesterol level, you will live longer than everyone else.*'

Instead, it was actually called "*Lack of an association or an inverse association between low-density-lipoprotein cholesterol and mortality in the elderly: a systematic review.*" Yawn.[19]

Did it have any effect? Has it had any effect? Well, it was the most widely read paper in the *BMJ Open* for six months – in a row. Which means that a lot of doctors know precisely what it said. What was the impact? Well, statin prescribing has continued to boom worldwide. It has never been higher than it is now.

So, in 2018, we tried again. This time analysing LDL and cholesterol levels and, looking more specifically at cardiovascular disease this time:

"The idea that high cholesterol levels in the blood are the main cause of CVD is impossible because people with low levels become just as atherosclerotic as people with high levels and their risk of suffering from CVD is the same or higher. The cholesterol hypothesis has been kept alive for decades by reviewers who have used misleading statistics, excluded the results from unsuccessful trials and ignored numerous contradictory observations."[20]

As we also mentioned:

"Despite the fact that LDL-C is routinely referred to as the 'bad cholesterol', we have shown that high LDL-C levels appear to be unrelated to the risk of CVD, both in FH (familial hypercholesterolaemia) individuals and in the general population and that the benefit from the use of cholesterol-lowering drugs is questionable. Therefore, a systematic search for other CVD risk factors is an important topic for future research."

This was the second most downloaded paper by the medical publisher Taylor Francis in that year. Taylor Francis is the second biggest medical publishing house in the world. The effect, once again… nothing.

I could go on, and on and on, quoting paper after paper, study after study, demonstrating that LDL is unrelated to CVD, or overall mortality. I tried this in two previous books. *The Great Cholesterol Con* and *A Statin Nation*. Others within THINCS have written many books, and papers.

Unfortunately, none of this has had any discernible impact. Which, I must say, has been a tad on the disappointing side.

Over the years, I have found that blowing up the cholesterol hypothesis with facts is easy. However, as with the later terminator movies, after you have blown it into smithereens, the hypothesis simply re-forms and starts chasing after you again. Even worse, as with a 1950s B Movie, attacking the monster simply makes it stronger. It feeds off your energy.

Eventually I came to realise, long before we at THINCS wrote these papers, that the transient satisfaction of giving the cholesterol hypothesis a damn good kicking was merely a distraction. It was never going to get us anywhere.

"The most difficult subjects can be explained to the most slow-witted man if he has not formed any idea of them already; but the simplest thing cannot be made clear to the most intelligent man if he is firmly persuaded that he knows already, without a shadow of doubt, what is laid before him."

Leo Tolstoy

It became increasingly clear, at least to me, that facts were never going to get the job done. At least, not until there was somewhere else for the thinking to go. What we needed, was an alternative hypothesis. An attractive hypothesis.

'You think it is cholesterol that causes cardiovascular disease. But here is another hypothesis which, I believe, fits the facts rather better. I humbly lay it before you and ask for your kind consideration of this matter.'

Then, at least there would be another planetary body in the Solar System. A different gravity well to attract that thinking rather than everything, always, coalescing back around planet cholesterol.

If not cholesterol, what can be the cause?

So, what does cause atherosclerosis. I have been pondering this question for well over 30 years now. I have to say that cardiovascular disease is a most tricky little blighter to get a handle on. Whenever I thought I had found a cause, *the* cause, I came across a nasty little fact that contradicted everything. Back to square one.

I looked at other people's ideas. Uffe Ravnskov, and a few others in THINCS, favour an infectious disease hypothesis. I must admit that there are some good theoretical reasons for this.

For example, you can find the remnants of bacteria in atherosclerotic plaques. Plaque structure can also look much like areas of damage caused elsewhere in the body by infectious agents e.g., tuberculosis.

In addition, the rise and fall of cardiovascular disease within countries can look like the sweep of an infectious disease epidemic. At least it can, in a certain light. With a following wind.

However, to my mind, the infectious disease hypothesis is an idea whose wings separate from the fuselage long before take-off. Mainly because the pattern of CVD across a hundred years, or so, looks absolutely nothing like any infectious disease epidemic in history. Not even remotely. Yes, CVD did start to rise sharply about a hundred years ago and has been falling since... in many Western countries.

But that's about as good as it gets. Japan has never had a high rate of CHD, ever. However, the Japanese, when they moved to the US, developed much the same rate of CHD as the surrounding population. So, is this infectious agent, or agents, unable to travel from one country to another? You have to move to another country to get infected. Bong!

Another problem with the infectious disease hypothesis is that you can find populations living cheek by jowl, that have vastly different rates of cardiovascular disease. The most extreme example is probably Australian aboriginals. Young aboriginal women have a rate of cardiovascular disease that is up to 13 times higher than that of the surrounding female population. By surrounding I mean, living in the same towns and cities.[21]

In the US it is the other way around. Certain immigrant populations, especially Muslims, have five times the rate of CVD of the surrounding population. I don't think it is remotely plausible to suggest that we have an infectious agent capable of picking out specific ethnic groups, whilst leaving others alone?

It would also have to be an agent that infects men far more than women – at least in some places. At one point, in New Zealand, in the 1970s, men had fifteen times the rate of CVD of women – who were living in the same houses. Whereas, in Brazil men and women had almost identical rates of CVD. In reality the moment you start picking at it, the infectious disease hypothesis unravels completely.

Frustratingly, and I have found it extremely frustrating, you can suggest almost any possible cause for CVD, gather together what looks like a terrific case. Then, inevitably, the contradictions arrive, like a shoal of piranha, ready to tear your ideas to shreds. This entire area is an enormous jigsaw puzzle. To misquote Churchill. '*CVD is a riddle wrapped in a mystery inside an enigma.*'

Moving away from individual causes, I started to look in more detail at the other risk factors. Here, for example, is the latest risk calculator for use in the UK called Qrisk3.[22] It is more complex than previous risk calculators, and it asks you for information on 20 different factors. They are, in no particular order of importance:

- Age
- Sex
- Smoking
- Diabetes
- Total cholesterol/HDL ratio
- Raised blood pressure.
- Variation in two blood pressure readings
- BMI
- Chronic kidney disease

- Rheumatoid arthritis

- Systemic Lupus Erythematosus (SLE)

- History of migraines

- Severe mental illness

- On atypical antipsychotic medication

- Using steroid tablets

- Atrial fibrillation

- Diagnosis of erectile dysfunction

- Angina, or heart attack in first degree relative under the age of 60

- Ethnicity

- Postcode

It is true that all of these factors are directly, or indirectly, associated with cardiovascular disease. Some exceedingly tenuously, for example, postcode.

The problem here is to try to explain how these very different things all cause the same disease. How does a history of migraines link to, say, chronic kidney disease? What about rheumatoid arthritis, and postcode? Raised blood pressure and severe mental illness. Smoking, and erectile dysfunction. Someone, anyone?

The current solution to this is to state that cardiovascular disease is *multifactorial*. No need to think beyond that. Just find the important risk factors, then deal with each one separately. This, of course, works up to a point. Stop smoking, keep the blood pressure down, control diabetes and the risks will definitely fall.

However, in the end, you cannot just bring a whole bunch of factors together, declare that the disease is multifactorial, and attempt to convince yourself that you have created a scientific hypothesis.

"Science is built up of facts, as a house is built of stones; but an accumulation of facts is no more a science than a heap of stones is a house."

Henri Poincaré

40

No, in order to understand cardiovascular disease, you have to be able to explain exactly how, for example, rheumatoid arthritis and smoking can both lead to exactly the same thickenings and narrowing of the large arteries.

And you have to do this for more than the 20 factors on Qrisk3. As far back as 1981, a compilation of 246 items were gathered together and published in a paper, entitled: *"A survey of 246 suggested coronary risk factors."* [23]

How many would there be today. Thousands, I would imagine. Some can probably be ignored, but we would still be left with a massive number. I could drop in around 50 off the top of my head: Kawasaki's disease, sickle cell disease, the use of Avastin (an anti-cancer drug), raised homocysteine, antiphospholipid syndrome, high levels of lead (the heavy metal), air pollution, recreational use of cocaine... etc.

So many... so damned many.

At one point, to amuse and distract myself, I decided to find out how many possible interactions there could be between the 246 risk factors suggested in 1981. The number is 246 x 245 x 244... x 2 x 1. Which is otherwise known as 246 factorial.

That number is:

84780974778285342816238561455548417281371633003839326661430688854748332432645855971589581923646740532744232968263007178950382481022666893846537522142147850161951901643121125830684398460001868068469912200342991286010101141191392319487892821710751341634617090843411664746702478340313383473092162970369088223992057355126790671309657612172941416384285875155292305115666276413405937332063747327791827249414222286766453720875008000000000000000000000000000000000000000000000000000000000000

There is not even a way to describe a number that enormous. To quote Donald Trump, it is probably the biggliest number ever. More than ten-duotrigintillion. Far greater than a googolplex. Mightier, even, than Skewe's number. Yes, I looked these all up on Google. I also found a website to calculate 246 factorial. Truly, this is an age of wonders.

Even if you restrict yourself to Qrisk3, with its relatively puny 20 factors, the figure is:

2,432,902,008,176,640,000 possible interactions.

Two-point four quintillion. Almost as much money as Elon Musk makes – this week anyway. Yes, the 20 factorial number is a lot smaller. However, it is realistically beyond the power of computation. Certainly, beyond controlling all the variables in a clinical trial.

Whichever way you look at it, multifactorial simply means... incomprehensible. It also means irrefutable. With two point four quintillion possible interactions, any and all contradictions, to anything, can be argued away. '*Aha, but did you consider* (insert factor, or factors of your choice here)'.

Turning the problem around, was it ever going to be possible to bring all the factors into a coherent hypothesis? I presumed it had to be possible, as something *had* to connect them. This thought was the only thing that kept me going at times as I disappeared down various blind alleyways.

I must say that there were long periods where I gave up, and decided it was completely impossible. An unsolvable Rubik's cube. Or at least unsolvable by me. Time to move on and achieve world peace, or faster than light space travel, or an anti-gravity machine – all of which had to be easier than working out what causes atherosclerosis.

Then, one fine day, I was gently pointed onto a completely different way of thinking by Professor Paul Rosch at a cardiovascular conference. A very great man with a very great brain. He suggested that I needed to stop searching for a cause, or causes, or *the* cause.

Instead, I should consider cardiovascular disease to be a process. Or, to put it another way, I needed to fully understand the mechanism of arterial damage, before jumping to any premature conclusions as to what causes it, then desperately attempt to back-fill a theory around that. Wrong way round. See under, diet-heart hypothesis.

This represented my lightbulb moment. No longer was I a bluebottle bashing brainlessly against a windowpane. Hoping that my 500th attempt to fly straight through an impenetrable glass barrier would be successful... when the previous 499 had been miserable failures.

I came to understand that the pane of glass I had been fruitlessly battering against was the '*single cause*' model of disease. In truth, I didn't realise that this was my error. Like almost everyone else, I had been programmed into believing that, in the end, all diseases have a single, necessary, cause. I just needed to find out what it was. Batter, batter.

In my defence, this way of looking at diseases appeared to be the only righteous path, the only true way. Why would anyone think in a different fashion? After all, the single/necessary cause model had been incredibly effective in medical breakthroughs for centuries.

It underpinned the successful search for infectious agents such as TB – caused by the tuberculous bacillus. Malaria – caused by the malaria parasite... carried by mosquitos. Syphilis, gonorrhoea, smallpox, polio, diphtheria, rabies, leprosy... The great scourges of mankind, the diseases that killed millions and millions over the years. They present in many different and complex ways, with hundreds of different signs and symptoms, but they all had one necessary cause.

Using the single cause approach, other terrible diseases such as rickets, and scurvy, and pellagra and beriberi were also found to have a single necessary cause. In these cases, it was the lack of a single vitamin. A different vitamin in each case.

The amazing success of this approach has created this unquestioned single cause paradigm. A way of looking at diseases that has become almost like the air you breath, something you don't even notice is there. In fact, I am certain that most researchers do not even consider that they are looking at cardiovascular disease in one way. Thinking about how you are thinking about things, is always difficult.

In the end, the thing that I call the *single factor paradigm*, even if no-one else does, has led us to a place of almost perfect irony. Unable to find *the* single necessary cause. By which I mean the factor, or agent, without which the disease cannot occur – it was decreed that cardiovascular disease is caused by multiple single factors.

So, instead of having a coherent model, we have just ended up with an ever-lengthening list of risk factors for cardiovascular disease. The mainstream view is encapsulated in this quote from the *American Journal of Hypertension*:

> *"Coronary heart disease is clearly a multifactorial disease with risk factors that tend to cluster and interact in an individual to determine the level of coronary risk."* [24]

Sounds clever, but it is just describing a large pile of stones.

At this point the late lamented Paul Rosch stepped in. He pointed out to me over dinner that you must discard the single cause model. Instead, view CVD as a *process,* because that is the only way it can make any sense.

Let me use an analogy here, which should become clear later on in this book. The analogy is rust on the bodywork of a car. The bodywork on most cars will not rust until the paintwork is damaged in some way. Unless, like me, you bought an Alfasud in your reckless youth. This rusted so fast that, on a still winter's morning, you could hear the rust ripping through the metalwork – a sharp crackling sound.

In general, though, unless you bought an Alfasud – other fast rusting Italian models were available at the time – you needed to damage the paintwork for rust to form. How can this happen?

There are a multitude of possible causes. A stone flying up from the road, another car hitting yours, reversing into an unseen low wall, a tin of baked beans falling out of the shopping bag onto the door. A key missing the lock then scratching the paintwork, a sharp bush by the roadside, a windsurf board falling off the roof rack, the roof rack itself falling off. The list is very long – virtually endless.

On the face of it, a stone and a tin of baked beans have almost nothing in common. Not in structure, nor function, nor anything else. The only connection they have is they are both capable, in certain circumstances, of damaging the paintwork on a car.

When you look at them in this light, and only in this light, then you have it – the connection. It is not what they are, it is what they can do. It is not structure or function but 'process' that links them, and that process is damage to the paintwork,

Using process thinking, it finally became possible to connect all of the risk factors: smoking, migraines, chronic kidney disease, diabetes… and everything else. Whilst, on the surface some of them appear a million miles apart they can all be linked, very neatly together once you look at them in the correct way.

Which means that the correct answer to the question, what causes CVD? Is that there is no answer to this question. The question is, and always should have been, what is the process of cardiovascular disease? Once you can answer this, you can work out how different factors can all cause atherosclerosis in the same way. Once you understand this, you can then work out how to stop it – pretty much dead in its tracks. I hope.

PART 1

The process of cardiovascular disease

CHAPTER 1

The competing hypothesis – blood clots (the thrombogenic hypothesis)

It may come as a surprise to know that there have been two main ideas about cardiovascular disease battling it out for well over 150 years. In truth, it has been a bit of a one-sided contest. The cholesterol hypothesis has become so dominant that it now stands alone, unquestioned and unchallenged – indeed virtually unquestionable. Such is the way of the world. To the victor go the spoils, and they also get to rewrite history to suit themselves.

However, if you do decide to pull the curtain back, and peer round the corner, there has always been an alternative hypothesis lurking just out of sight. It has never caught the public imagination. In truth, it has had virtually no impact on the views of the mainstream medical profession. Although, over the years, it has been championed quite vigorously, in various guises.

The main problem is that it is incompatible with the cholesterol hypothesis. I have seen attempts made to weld them together, but they are rather half-hearted, and splinter under a little pressure.

Which means that you either believe one, or the other. I happen to believe in the other. I hope to convince you that the other is correct, which will make two of us. Maybe three if you include my mum – although I suspect she is just saying it to make me feel better.

The alternative hypothesis – blood clots (the thrombogenic hypothesis)

(This is the Readers' Digest format. More detail will follow).

The alternative hypothesis is that blood clots, and blood clotting, are the key players in cardiovascular disease. From start, to finish.

By which I mean that atherosclerotic plaques, the thickenings and narrowings in arteries, are the remnants of blood clots, formed on the arteries themselves. Or to put it another way, blood clots that have been created on, then incorporated into, artery walls.

The process starts when the lining of the artery wall is damaged in some way. This stimulates the formation of a blood clot (thrombus) which covers over the area, rather like a scab does when you damage your skin. A new layer of arterial lining then grows over the top of the thrombus, which effectively draws it into the artery wall. In most cases, the remnant thrombus is then fully broken down and removed.

However, if there is an increased rate of damage, or bigger or tougher blood clots are formed, or the repair systems are not working so well, then repeated blood clotting at the same spot, will lead to plaques getting bigger. Eventually, they will severely narrow the artery and constrict blood flow.

Over many years of growth, plaques can end up in a whole range of different forms. They can be tough and fibrous, known as _fibro_atheroma. They can develop an almost liquid core, like a boil, with a thin covering. These are often called 'vulnerable' plaques. Such plaques are the dangerous ones, as they are more liable to rupture, exposing the plaque contents to the bloodstream. This is an extremely powerful trigger for further blood clotting.

A bit of good news about plaques is that, after decades, they normally pass through the vulnerable stage and begin to calcify. Literally, become full of calcium. This can make them, and the surrounding artery stiff, almost like a concrete pipe. In this calcified form plaques are significantly less dangerous than earlier versions, in that they are far less likely to rupture, triggering a heart attack, or stroke.

How much of the above is controversial?

Almost everything I have written above would be accepted without much of a murmur by the mainstream medical community. For instance, the idea that plaque 'rupture' creates a thrombus that can block an artery. This is pretty much unquestioned as the cause of most heart attacks.

It is also widely accepted that thrombus formation, on top of an already existing plaque, can make plaques suddenly jump in size. Here, for example, is a passage from a paper in the journal *Atherosclerosis*. This is about as mainstream a publication as you can get in CVD research. The paper was called: *"The role of plaque rupture and thrombosis in coronary artery disease."*

> *"In addition, **plaque rupture and subsequent healing is recognized to be a major cause of further rapid plaque progression.**"*[25]

However, the very idea, *the very idea*, that thrombi could possibly have a role in starting the plaque in the first place is dismissed, virtually out of hand. It is LDL which does this, and LDL alone. LDL infiltrates the arterial wall to start the process, then a gradual build-up of LDL keeps the plaque growing. It is only at the later stages when blood clotting may take over – or have some role to play.

It seems a strange disease that can start as one process, and then transform itself into another one, halfway through? Personally, I prefer the single process model. It makes life easier. Also, if you really start thinking about the '*plaques represent the build of one molecule of LDL at a time*' concept, you find your thinking ends up at some very strange places indeed.

Just to take you down a little thought experiment for a short meandering journey. In a coronary artery, an average sized plaque is about three millimetres in diameter. Perhaps somewhat smaller than you thought. An LDL molecule is around 20 nanometres in diameter. A nanometre is one millionth of a millimetre.

Therefore, and trust me on this, to fill a three-millimetre plaque full of LDL molecules, you would need somewhere in the region of three-point five quadrillion (3,500,000,000,000,000) of the little blighters. That, as you may have noted, is a very large number indeed. It also makes you realise just how small an LDL molecule is. I find everything gets difficult to visualise on a micro level.

To try to overcome this difficulty, I often like to bring things into a scale we can more readily visualise. As mentioned earlier, using a human scale, if an LDL molecule were the size of a human being, then a typical cell lining an artery (endothelial cell) would be the equivalent of an Olympic sized sports stadium. A three-millimetre plaque would have the surface area of a city the size of Chicago, or the Isle of Wight. If you cut the plaque down the middle.

I don't know if that makes things less mind-boggling, or more?

Moving this thought experiment along. An average plaque takes about 40 years to develop. This is very nearly 15,000 days. Therefore, if you want to build a three-millimetre plaque, you need 250 million LDL molecules to be added to the plaque each and every day.

(In this thought experiment I am assuming none of the LDL molecules get removed, they just stay there. I am also assuming that there is nothing else in a plaque other than LDL molecules).

This equates to around 2,500 molecules joining the plaque each second. Just sit and think about that for a while. I did, and the carefully considered scientific conclusion that I came to was – it's bonkers.

It's not bonkers because that rate is ridiculously fast. In fact, a rate of 2,500 per second, is not remotely high. On a molecular scale the human body does things at speeds that are almost inconceivably fast.

For example, there are enzymes within all cells that can catalyse reactions at more than one million times a second. DNA snipping enzyme can open, then close, a strand of DNA 36,000 times a second. I am never quite sure who managed to count that fast.

Which means that transporting 2,500 molecules across endothelial cells and into the plaque beneath is not fast. In fact, on that scale it is inconceivably, glacially, get a bloody move on, slow.

In addition, this is not 2,500 LDLs filing patiently through a single sports stadium entrance, one by one. It is the equivalent of 2,500 human beings walking across a surface area of nearly 400 square kilometres. Or the equivalent of one person entering an Olympic stadium every four seconds.

The final conclusion is that, in order to build a three-millimetre plaque, over 40 years, one LDL molecule would have to pass through one endothelial cell every three or four seconds. Which is a completely and utterly ridiculous concept.

In addition, and far more problematic, is the idea that LDL molecules can enter one side of an endothelial cell, travel straight though, and pop out the other side. You could as easily force a tennis ball though one side of a blue whale, run round (or swim round) and wait for it to emerge on the side opposite. Not that I have ever tried to do this, but I assume it would be tricky.

The simple fact is that cells don't allow anything to enter without a reason (we shall leave viruses out of this discussion as they hijack cell mechanisms to do this). Cells are extraordinarily careful about what they allow in, and what they don't. There are receptors and gates and channels, each one designed to allow entry of one thing, and one thing only. Down to the size of individual atoms, such as sodium, or potassium.

Then, once a substance has been granted entry, each cell has to decide whether or not they are going to transport that substance from one side to the other. Finally, there are complex mechanisms required to eject it out the other side.

So, you need a receptor, or a 'gate' to allow the substance in. Then you need a transportation system to get the substance across. Then an ejection mechanism, to pop it out the other side. Technically, this is an 'endocytosis' (getting the thing in), 'transcytosis' (moving it through) and 'exocytosis' (popping it out other side).

You think this can all happen by accident? Or that LDL forces its way into a cell, battles heroically across, then chops a hole in the other side of the cell membrane to escape? (Note to editor, insert music to *The Great Escape* here).

Yes, of course, there are LDL receptors. They are made within a cell when it feels the need for some additional cholesterol. Once made, these receptors effectively become the entrance that allows LDL entry. Which simply demonstrates how difficult it is to get an LDL molecule into a cell, unless the cell wishes to grant it entrance. Sorry, it is not difficult, it is impossible. Once inside the cell, the LDL is broken down into its constituent parts. Often the receptor is also broken down, but not always.

The whole process can be seen in Figure 7. LDL arrives, links to an LDL receptor and is drawn inside the cell (endocytosis). Enzymes arrive to break down the LDL (and often the receptor as well). Cholesterol and fatty acids are released into the cell. In some cases, the intact receptor shuttles back to the cell surface.

However, even if you do manage to get an LDL molecule into the cell and put a lock on the systems designed to break it down into its component parts, you then have to get LDL back out of a cell again – on the other side? Good luck with that. You would need an 'inside-out' LDL receptor, pointing backwards into the cell itself. Such structures do not, as far I have been able to ascertain, exist. Nor has anyone even suggested that they do.

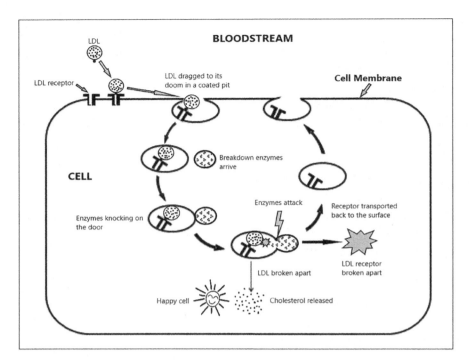

Figure 7

So, if LDL molecules cannot simply pass straight through endothelial cells – and they can't – what else can explain LDL getting into an artery wall? At present, although this is usually left fuzzy, the explanation is that LDL molecules can slip *between* endothelial cells, then into the artery wall beneath.

At this point, I shall change my analogy from a blue whale to terraced houses.

Endothelial cells are not detached homes on a posh housing estate, with plenty of space between to walk through from front to back. No, instead, endothelial cells are terraced houses. Somewhat more downmarket I am afraid.

These terraced houses are firmly cemented together on both sides, and there is no gap of any sort between them. If you want to reach the back garden of a terraced house, you are required to knock on the front door, walk through, and go out the back door again. You cannot squeeze between them, using a non-existent corridor.

In the same way, if you want to get from one side of an endothelial cell to the other, you must pass through the cell. You cannot pass between cells. They are sealed together with things called tight junctions. A whole series of strong, interlinked, protein bridges. This, I should add, is not up for debate, it is simply scientific fact.

*"Tight junctions prevent the passage of molecules and ions through the space between plasma **membranes of adjacent cells**, so materials must actually enter the cells (by diffusion or active transport) in order to pass through the tissue."* [26]

If this were not the case. If there were no barriers to prevent substance simply moving across from the blood to the spaces between cells, and vice-versa, life simply could *not* exist. To quote from a paper in the journal *'Tissue Barriers'* yes indeed, there is such a journal:

*"Physiological barriers provide the framework for a boundary between circulating blood and interstitial fluid, **a pre-requisite for mammalian life**."* [27]

'A pre-requisite for mammalian life'. Last time I looked; human were mammals, and most of us are alive. Which means that, for the LDL/cholesterol hypothesis to be true, it requires that fundamental processes, that are required to sustain life… simply do not exist.

Just to give you one example of what happens if you loosen the tight junctions between cells, we can look at the Ebola virus. With Ebola infection the tight junctions are opened up. So, the barrier function is lost. Blood can escape into the tissues, and organs, and things go rapidly downhill from there.

This leakage is the reason why Ebola is also known as a form of haemorrhagic fever. Blood appears in the cornea, so your eyes become bloodshot. You cough up the blood that that has escaped into your lungs. Your tongue falls off. Your urine is filled with blood from your kidneys, your bowel motions turn black, and then…. Bang, dead, from haemorrhaging.

Ebola provides a good example of the importance of tight junctions. Open them up… and die.

"Ebola patients experience a breakdown in endothelial barrier integrity that leads to massive fluid losses and vascular collapse." [28]

That would be where the *'pre-requisite for mammalian life'* comes in.

Yes, indeed, if you don't think about it in any great depth, the idea that LDL molecules pass from the blood and then into the arterial wall behind, seems pretty straightforward. Logical, common sense even. However, once you start examining the actual processes required for this to happen, you begin to realise that the idea is completely and utterly ridiculous.

It simply cannot happen. If LDL could pass straight into the arterial wall, then so could almost everything else in the bloodstream. Very shortly after that, you would be dead.

What is inside a plaque?

Okay, maybe that was all too theoretical. Is it backed up by the facts? Despite what I have written I probably still need to convince you that plaques are not made up of LDL. Instead, they are the remnants of blood clots.

You may think this must have been sorted out years ago… decades even. Despite what I have written above this, surely, cannot even be a question. Plaques are full of cholesterol. This is simply a known fact, isn't it? In truth, it is not.

It's certainly true that there is cholesterol in a plaque, some plaques – possibly even most plaques. However, there are an awful lot of other things trapped in there as well, which are not cholesterol, and have absolutely no connection to LDL, or cholesterol, in any way, shape or form.

There are red blood cells, fibrin, platelets, white blood cells, smooth muscle cells, calcium, collagen etc. etc. etc. How did they get in there?

Almost the only thing beyond any question is that a plaque is not just a big lump of cholesterol stuck inside the artery wall. Plaques, if you start picking away at them, are rather complicated and messy old things. Here is what one group of researchers found, when they examined plaques in a group of old people.

These were 'end-stage' plaques, and they consisted of:

- fibrous tissue (87 ± 8%)

- calcific deposits (7 ± 6%)

- pultaceous debris (5 ± 4%)

- foam cells (1 ± 1%)[29]

Yes, I had to go and look up *'pultaceous debris'* myself. I had never come across this term before, anywhere, ever. Maybe I missed that lecture. The medical definition of pultaceous is *'having a soft consistency: pulpy.'* Which doesn't really help much in knowing what it consists of.

I quite like the word though, I have dropped pultaceous into one or two conversations in an effort to sound more intelligent. Not worked thus far, but I haven't entirely given up hope up yet. *'Ah yes, this cake is highly pultaceous, if I may be so bold.'*

I also realise that unless you are medically trained, you're never going to have heard of any of the other things on that list either. Fibrous tissue? Yes, that is tissue that is fibrous, whatever exactly that means – many different things as I have discovered. The point I wanted to make here though was very simple, and it is as follows. Can you see the word cholesterol?

The obvious answer is that, no, you cannot. To be honest, when I came across this paper, I wasn't particularly trying to find support for the observation that *'there is often no cholesterol in a plaque'*. I was just doing one of my many wide-angled searches which started with the words *'main contents of atherosclerotic plaques.'* You can try searching around in this area for yourself if you like.

I suspect that, like me, the thing you will soon discover is that it is remarkably difficult to get to the bottom of what's inside an atherosclerotic plaque. The technical term for this is plaque morphology. Obviously, I have dug rather deeper than most, and spoken to pathologists and interventional cardiologists and read 10,000 papers, and walked 500 miles to be the one that...

Having done all this, I still don't think that I can truly answer the question. What are plaques made of? Not with any certainty. Some years ago, the *American Heart Association* (*AHA*) made the most exhaustive attempt to try to answer this. If you want to try battling your way through a real page turner, try reading this little beauty:

"A Definition of Advanced Types of Atherosclerotic Lesions and a Histological Classification of Atherosclerosis: A Report From the Committee on Vascular Lesions of the Council on Arteriosclerosis, American Heart Association." [30]

That, I should add, was only part three. Trouble sleeping, well you can read the entire three-part series if you want. Loss of consciousness will be rapid. But if you do manage this heroic feat, you will find that there is remarkably little mention of LDL, or cholesterol. Equally, once you have wearily turned the last page, you will be left absolutely none the wiser as to what plaques are made of. Let's just say that... it's complicated.

Anyway, here is a list of various things the American Heart Association said could be found lurking within a plaque. At least this is a list of the headers they used to describe them (jargon alert):

- Smooth muscle cells

- Macrophages

- Lymphocytes

- Lipid, lipoprotein, and fibrinogen in the extracellular matrix

- Proteoglycans

- Collagen

- Elastin

- Calcium

Lipids and lipoproteins get one mention, I suppose. As for cholesterol – silence was the stern reply. Yet, if you look at sites such as WebMD, their writers feel able to make a statement such as the following:

*"**Cholesterol plaques** form by a process called atherosclerosis. Another name for atherosclerosis is 'hardening of the arteries.' **LDL or 'bad cholesterol' is the raw material of cholesterol plaques.** Progressive and painless, atherosclerosis grows **cholesterol plaques** silently and slowly. The eventual result is blocked arteries, which places blood flow at risk."* [31]

'Cholesterol plaques! My giddy aunt, and what a malarkey Mr Copperfield, and no doubt.' Statements like this are specifically designed to leave you in absolutely no doubt that atherosclerotic plaques consist of a big lump of LDL/cholesterol. Which is, of course, the most complete and utter balls. I could have used a ruder word.

Does this mean that plaques are what remains of incorporated thrombi instead? Obviously, I believe so, or I wouldn't have written this book. However, before moving on to look at that issue in more detail, I want to cover three major observations about plaques. Observations that have been used as unquestioned support for the cholesterol hypothesis. They are:

- Fatty streaks

- Cholesterol crystals

- Finding LDL within plaques

For decades this 'terrible triad' has been used to underpin the case against cholesterol. What I intend to show you is that these observations provide no such evidence. Instead, when turned round, they end up fully supporting the thrombogenic hypothesis instead.

Fatty streaks

Fatty streaks are widely considered to be the earliest version of atherosclerotic plaques. You start with a fatty streak, it grows, and grows, and eventually you have a large, complex plaque on your hands. Here is one passage, amongst the many thousands that I could have chosen:

*"Atherosclerosis begins in childhood as **deposits of cholesterol and its esters**, referred to as **fatty streaks**."* [32]

The argument used here is simple, and also seemingly inarguable. LDL is full of cholesterol and its esters. Fatty streaks are deposits of cholesterol and its esters. Fatty streaks are the first abnormality you see on the artery wall, and they grow into larger more complex plaques.

'Therefore, I put it to you that LDL is guilty of this, the most heinous crime of causing fatty streak, then plaques, and thus CVD...'

There is a murmur around the court as the defence lawyer rises to question the cardiology expert. For yes, it is he, Atticus Finch...

Atticus: *'Can I simply ask if anyone has actually seen a fatty streak turn into an atherosclerotic plaque.'*

Expert: *'There is no need sir, it is simply a known fact.'*

Atticus: *'So I shall take that as a no.'*

Expert: *(Affronted) 'Do you have any evidence that fatty streaks do not become plaques?'*

Atticus: *(Reaches into his briefcase). 'As a matter of fact, my dear sir. I do. If I may refer the court to a detailed study of fatty streaks and atherosclerotic plaques by Velican and Velican'. (Atticus clears his throat).*

The Velicans studied the arteries of many hundreds of children and adults who had died from accidents, and if I may quote from their research article, the snappily entitled Progression of coronary atherosclerosis from adolescents to mature adults (Theatrical pause).

Among the four types of early atherosclerotic lesions investigated, only the fatty streaks did not show this direct conversion to a lesion of possible clinical significance.' [33]

Yes, the Velicans were extremely clear. Having looked at hundreds and hundreds of arteries, and thousands of plaques, they found absolutely no evidence that fatty streaks demonstrate any form of conversion into plaques. Indeed, it is something that never happens. You very rarely see the word 'never' in a scientific paper.

The work of the Velicans and other researchers was brought together in the book: 'Factors in Formation and Regression of the Atherosclerotic Plaque,' (which included the work of the Velicans). Another page turner:

"Juvenile-type fatty streaks are the earliest lesions that can be recognized by macroscopic inspection of aortas of children... Holman reported that **they were already present in all children aged more than 3**, *increased rapidly in area between ages 8-15, and reached a maximum at age 20.*

"For many years it was widely believed that they [fatty streaks] *were the precursors of fibrous plaques.... However, there is now evidence from many different sources* [including the work of the Velicans] *that suggests that* **fatty streaks and fibrous plaques develop by separate and independent pathways**.

"They, [the Velicans], *record many significant morphological observations.* **They did not observe conversion of fatty streak into atherosclerotic plaques** *and concluded that the two types of lesions developed as* **unrelated pathological processes**. *'Advanced' fatty streaks exhibiting cell disintegration and accumulation of extracellular lipid were first encountered in the 26-30 age group and increased fairly rapidly over the next decade, but again they did not observe 'further transitional stages between advanced fatty streaks and atherosclerotic plaques.'*

"In the third decade lipid became abundant in the plaques [not the fatty streaks] in the form of foam cells which were particularly associated with areas of insudation. and small pools of extracellular lipid: there was also **'progressive involvement of microthrombi in the early steps of plaque formation.'"***

Another extremely important point in that passage is the fact that fatty streaks are present in *all* children by the age of three. This is at a time when their LDL levels are far, far, lower than found in any adult, and, at this age, they have no other 'classical' risk factors for heart disease either.

Indeed, fatty streaks can even be found in the foetus, where the LDL level is less than a third of the adult level. Which kind of knocks a high LDL as a cause of CVD on the head. LDL can initiate plaque development when the level is one third than that found in any adult population on the planet. Hmmmm, don't think so.

However, the main takeaway from this research is that fatty streaks, whatever they may contain, and however they form, simply *do not* become atherosclerotic plaques. Which means that one of the major pillars supporting the LDL hypothesis crumples into a heap of dust.

On the other hand, their findings were entirely supportive of the thrombogenic hypothesis. I say this because their other main observation was that clinically significant plaques have layer upon layer of small blood clots within them. They called this finding *'incorporated microthrombi.'* As described in the following passage.

*"In addition, particular cycles of evolution towards advanced lesions [clinically significant plaques] appeared.... Their obstructive character was related to both **successive incorporation of microthrombi**** and the onset of large lipid deposits."*

I make that one nil to the thrombogenic hypothesis, even using a video referee.

Cholesterol crystals

Here I have an admission to make. Cholesterol crystals are indeed found in many atherosclerotic plaques. Yes, cholesterol in a plaque,

---

* insudation is the term used for the accumulation of a substance derived from the blood. I have also found that this word goes down badly in conversations. Almost as badly as pultaceous.

** a microthrombus is simply a small blood clot – or maybe the remnants of a, once larger, clot.

who'd have thought we should ever live to see such a thing. In fact, the description of cholesterol crystals takes us right back to the genesis of the cholesterol hypothesis, and Rudolf Virchow himself.

He was one of the first researchers to study diseased arteries in any detail, and he did so as far back as the mid-nineteenth century, along with Karl von Rokitansky, remember him? They knew each other well. Although, from reading between the lines, they were not best buddies. The pupil, Virchow, became the master. Basic plot structure for 'A Star is Born.' Never ends well, although I am not entirely sure which one was Lady Gaga.

Virchow's attention was drawn to white sharp pointy things that can be seen within many plaques. He identified these as cholesterol crystals, and he proposed that they were a vital plaque component. Although he never believed that cholesterol caused plaques. He noted that the appearance of cholesterol was a much later stage phenomenon.[34]

Despite what I have written earlier about the lack of cholesterol in many plaques, this observation has been repeatedly confirmed. Those cholesterol crystals really are there, and they are present in many plaques, but how did they get there? The answer appears obvious. LDL molecules are full of cholesterol, crystals are made of cholesterol. Ergo, the cholesterol came from LDL. Simple.

This sounds like the purest common sense. But be careful, as Einstein is said to have said: 'Common sense is the collection of prejudices acquired by age eighteen.' He knew that you need to be extremely careful about jumping to conclusions. Especially those based on the first thing that pops into your mind.

Science is often highly counter-intuitive. The most damaging scientific move is to jump to the immediate and apparently obvious answer. It may feel right, because it fits in nicely with everything else you think you know, but it may also be utterly wrong. Fast thinking vs. slow thinking. Emotion vs. thought. Confirmation bias.

So, what could be wrong with the idea that the building blocks of cholesterol crystals arrive inside LDL. To answer this, we need to go back to a bit of basic chemistry. Yes, I know, that's a phrase to strike fear into the heart of most readers, but please bear with me. This will be relatively painless – I hope.

It is true that an LDL molecule carries both cholesterol and fats inside it. To be more accurate, as mentioned before, they are not fats, but fatty acids. Fat, or fats, are generic terms used to describe all types of 'fatty molecule'. Chemically, there is no such thing as a 'fat'. Clear? Probably not.

Anyway, it is fatty acids which are the basic molecule that makes up all forms of, what we have decided to call, fat. God, I hate scientific terminology. Can we please call things by one, accurate, name, and not have a hundred different names for the same thing... please?

"'When I use a word,' Humpty Dumpty said in rather a scornful tone, 'it means just what I choose it to mean – neither more nor less.' 'The question is,' said Alice, 'whether you can make words mean so many different things.' 'The question is,' said Humpty Dumpty, 'which is to be master – that's all'".

Back to cholesterol. The critical issue here is that virtually none of the cholesterol in an LDL is 'free'. The vast majority is chemically bound to a fatty acid. This creates a chemical compound known as a *'cholesterol ester'*. Cholesterol + fatty acid = *cholesterol ester.*

The basic chemical equation for any ester is:

$$acid + alcohol = ester.$$

You do not need to know much more than this, although you might be wondering, where on Earth does the alcohol come from, to make the 'cholesterol ester?' The answer is that cholesterol can also be chemically 'defined' as having a part of it acting as an alcohol; it just means that it contains a specific chemical group called an 'OH' or hydroxyl group.

"Cholesterol is a sterol [a combination steroid and **alcohol**] *and a lipid found in the cell membranes of all body tissues and transported in the blood plasma of all animals."* [35]

Yes indeed, scientific terminology is just so horribly imprecise. Cholesterol can be called a steroid, an alcohol, or a lipid. It can also be a stanol and a sterol – depending on which of its characteristics you use to define it. Whichever classification you decide to pop cholesterol into, you cannot change the fact that you have cholesterol *esters* carried within LDL, *not* free cholesterol molecules.

The reason why this is of critical importance is that you cannot make cholesterol crystals from cholesterol esters. To make a cholesterol crystal you need pure cholesterol.

Aha, the plot thickens – about time you might be thinking. So, where can you get pure cholesterol from, if not LDL? The answer is perhaps surprising. It certainly surprised me once I tracked it down. Pure cholesterol can be found in red blood cells (RBCs), otherwise known as erythrocytes.

"About 40% of the weight of the erythrocyte [red blood cell] *is composed of **lipid***. The red cell membrane is comprised of a cholesterol rich phospholipid bilayer. **Cholesterol** is intercalated between the phospholipid molecules."* [36]

Yes, coming in from the left field is the observation that red blood cells (RBCs) are composed of 40% fat. Not only that, but they also contain a very high concentration of free cholesterol. The highest concentration of any tissue in the body – apart from, maybe, synapses in the brain. Which means that red blood cells, not LDL, are the source of the free cholesterol in plaques.

"The cholesterol in foam cells [damaged macrophages found in plaque] *is mostly esterified. However, **the proportion of free cholesterol in atherosclerotic plaques is markedly high. Therefore, it is logical to suggest that cholesterol present in plaques might be derived from other sources...** It has been observed that erythrocyte membranes were present in the necrotic core of advanced atherosclerotic plaques. **Further studies have shown that erythrocyte membranes contribute to a significant increase of cholesterol accumulation in atherosclerotic plaques, since these membranes contain large amounts of cholesterol."** [37]*

This rather changes the angle of attack does it not? Cholesterol crystals, and much of the other cholesterol found in plaques, arrived there as the free cholesterol found in red blood cells, not LDL. Yes, Einstein was right. Do not jump to conclusions. It is a quick and easy journey, but a long cold trudge back to base.

Next question, how do red blood cells find themselves in artery walls?

The answer is immediately obvious. Red blood cells make up a large part of the volume of all blood clots. They are both drawn into clots as they form, and they play an active role in binding clots together, also

---

* Just in case you were wondering, lipid is just another name for a fat. But course, there is no such thing as a fat... sigh. *Intercalated* means fits within, or lies within.

preventing them from being broken apart. It is the main reason why blood clots look red.

"Red Blood Cells (RBCs) may perform a dual role, both helping to stem bleeding but at the same time contributing to thrombosis in a variety of ways, including when the tightly packed array of RBCs in a contracted clot blocks blood flow and resists dissolution." [38]

Why do scientists all have to head for the thesaurus when they write papers. *'Resists dissolution...'* Have you ever heard anyone use those words in a spoken sentence? Perhaps when Winston Churchill was talking about antidisestablishmentarianism. Otherwise, no. *Resists dissolution* means resists breakdown, or stops it being split apart.

God, the dreadful passive voice of medical writing. All emotion, all excitement and interest sucked away, leaving a bloodless corpse. Who decided that scientific writing must be so flat and dry? For example, the dreaded phrase *'The experiment was carried out.'* Who carried it out? Where did they carry it? Did they need to use a lorry? Was it heavy?

Who did the experiment anyway? Was it you? If so, why not just say *'we did this experiment'*. Nope, it must be *'the experiment was carried out.'* Even though that does not make anything more accurate in any way – simply more boring. Another commonly used phrase is the following. *'These results suggest that.'* Result can't suggest anything, they are simply numbers on a piece of paper. It is only you, Mr Researcher, who can suggest things.

Do people honestly believe writing is made more accurate and scientific in this way? No personal pronouns, ever. I, you, her, we, she, him, they. Such emotive words must not pollute our ascetic work of impersonal purity. No-one ever does anything in science. We didn't do an experiment, perish the thought, *'it was done'*. How, by itself? By the Borg? By the unknowable spirit of God?

And breathe....

Anyway, there you go, getting back on track. For decades, people have looked at cholesterol crystals in plaques and assumed that they must have come from 'cholesterol' in the blood a.k.a. LDL. This has been a major pillar in support of the LDL/cholesterol hypothesis.

However, if you look more closely, that piece of evidence too, becomes dust. The cholesterol required to make cholesterol crystals must have come from red blood cells. The red blood cells, in turn, arrived as a key component of blood clots.

Does this observation obliterate the LDL hypothesis? Certainly not on its own.

After all, the mainstream view reluctantly accepts the fact that plaques can indeed rupture, blood clots then cover over the exposed area, then get dragged in. Thus, clots can become part of plaques. So, finding red blood cells in plaques does not, entirely, contradict the LDL hypothesis. Although it does confirm that cholesterol crystals arrive later on in the plaque development – as noted by Virchow.

In order to fully contradict the hypothesis, we need to move on to a more mission critical question. Do we actually have any LDL in plaques? Gasp, what do you mean? Is the man completely mad? Of course, there is LDL in plaques. Of course? Over to you Poirot.

Low density lipoprotein in plaques

Just to remind you. Here is the mainstream message about LDL, cholesterol and plaques once more.

> "**Cholesterol plaques** form by a process called atherosclerosis. Another name for atherosclerosis is 'hardening of the arteries.' **LDL or 'bad cholesterol' is the raw material of cholesterol plaques.** Progressive and painless, atherosclerosis grows **cholesterol plaques** silently and slowly. The eventual result is blocked arteries, which places blood flow at risk."[39]

Ho hum. If you keep saying a thing often enough then it becomes true, as noted by Lewis Carroll?

> "Just the place for a Snark!" the Bellman cried,
>
> As he landed his crew with care;
>
> Supporting each man on the top of the tide
>
> By a finger entwined in his hair.
>
> "Just the place for a Snark! I have said it twice:
>
> That alone should encourage the crew.
>
> Just the place for a Snark! I have said it thrice:
>
> What I tell you three times is true."

It is certainly true that, amongst many other things, you can find the remnants of lipoproteins inside plaques. Please note that I did not say LDL, I said lipoproteins. Perhaps I should say it thrice, for thence it shalt be true.

Whilst it is almost universally believed that these remnants must have been LDL molecules at one time, this is not the case. Once again, as with cholesterol crystals, the obvious assumption has been rapidly jumped to. The thinking has been fast, not slow. But all that glitters is not gold. All that looks like a low-density lipoprotein is not LDL.

Because, shock horror, LDL comes in two different versions. Version one is LDL. This is the one that everyone has heard of, and with supreme and world beating inaccuracy, calls 'bad cholesterol'. Repeat after me, LDL is not, and has never been, cholesterol. This is like saying a car is a human being, because cars contain human beings. Just because LDL molecules contain cholesterol, does not mean they are 'cholesterol'. Sigh, thud.

Version two is Lipoprotein(a) (Lp(a)), spoken as "ell pee ay." Hardly anyone has heard of this version, and therefore it is rarely called anything at all... at least it isn't called cholesterol.

The number of 'ell pee ay' molecules in the bloodstream is usually about a quarter to a fifth that of LDL, although a few unusual individuals have more Lp(a) than LDL. The level is genetically determined, and tends to remain fixed. No drugs have been found to lower it by much, if at all. Therefore, there is no money to be made from lowering it, therefore there has been an almost deafening silence about Lp(a).

This has been a major error, and I shall now attempt to explain why this is so. And why the existence of Lp(a) fully supports the thrombogenic hypothesis. Which is a somewhat complex journey. Sorry.

To begin.

LDL and Lp(a) are very similar. In fact, they are not very similar, they are exactly the same. Apart from one single, yet crucial difference, as shown in Figure 8. Which is that Lp(a) has an additional protein attached to it. This protein is called apolipoprotein(a). I shall call this apo(a) from now on. It is the attachment of this additional protein to LDL that transforms LDL into Lp(a). You can think of Lp(a) as LDL, with a scarf wrapped round its neck. That scarf is the apo(a) molecule.

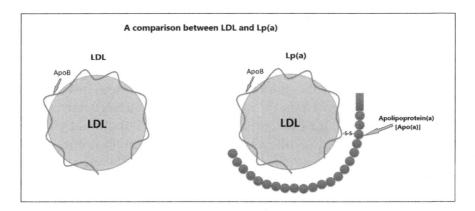

Figure 8

This raises an immediate question. If you are studying a plaque and you see LDL molecules, or what you believe to be the remnants of LDL molecules, how can you possibly know? You could just as easily be observing the remnants of Lp(a).

In fact, there is only one way to sort this out. Which is to specifically search for apo(a) molecules in the plaque. Having said this, you would only try to find apo(a) if you had ever heard of it, or believed it was important in causing heart disease. An unusual thing indeed in cardiovascular research.

This means that plaques have very rarely been examined for Lp(a). Or to be more accurate, they have rarely been examined for the presence of the apo(a) protein. Researchers – who are almost always entirely supportive of the LDL/cholesterol hypothesis – look for LDL particles. Lo and behold, they announce that they have found LDL particles.

Luckily, there have been a few intrepid souls who have decided to hunt specifically for apo(a) in plaques, and they have found it. As in this study "*Detection and Quantification of Lipoprotein(a) in the Arterial Wall of 107 Coronary Bypass Patients.*"

"The aim of this study was to determine the extent of accumulation of lipoprotein (a) (Lp(a)) In human arterial wall and to define Its potential role in atherogenesis... A significant positive correlation was established between serum Lp(a) and arterial wall apolipoprotein [apo (a)]...

"High serum Lp(a) also led to a significant increase of apo B In the arterial wall. This Initial study showed that Lp(a) accumulates in the arterial wall,

partly in the form of lipoprotein-like particles, therefore contributing to plaque formation and coronary heart disease." [40]

As always, a little more explanation is required here, particularly with regard to the passage: '*High serum Lp(a) also led to a significant increase of apo B In the arterial wall.*' Apo B is shorthand for apolipoprotein B. This is another protein that is attached to all LDL molecules. It allows LDL to be recognised by LDL receptors.

However, finding apo B does *not* mean you have found LDL. It could equally mean that you have found Lp(a). Because Lp(a) also has Apo B stuck to the side. In fact, if you find apo(a) and apo B at the same place (co-localised) this means you, absolutely must have found Lp(a), not LDL, because LDL has no apo(a) protein attached.

As made clear(ish) in the same paper:

*"In conclusion, this is **the first study showing a positive correlation of Lp(a) serum levels with apo(a) and apo B accumulation in the arterial wall**. Also, the presence of intact apo(a) and Lp(a)-like particles in human arterial wall was demonstrated for the first time. **We assume that in earlier studies on LDL-like particles in the arterial wall, the apo(a) might have been missed and, at least partly, Lp(a)-like particles might have been isolated**. Our studies imply that Lp(a) enters the arterial wall and accumulates extracellularly, **where apo(a) and apo B can be co-localized** with immunohistochemistry."*

This, like almost all scientific papers, has been written in a most confusing way. In large part because the authors are trying to be careful not to criticise the work of other researchers.

When they say "***We assume that in earlier studies on LDL-like particles in the arterial wall, the apo(a) might have been missed and, at least partly, Lp(a)-like particles might have been isolated***" what this actually means is that previous researchers were either incompetent, or ignorant.

Either they saw lipoproteins in plaques and assumed they were LDL – without bothering to try to find out if they were actually Lp(a) (incompetent). Or they didn't even know Lp(a) existed (ignorant).

The critical importance of searching specifically for apo(a) was further highlighted in another study: *"Quantification of apo(a) and apo B in human atherosclerotic lesions."*

67

*"These results suggest that Lp(a) **accumulates preferentially to LDL in plaques**, and that plaque apo(a) is directly associated with plasma apo(a) levels and is in a form that is **less easily removable than most of the apo B**. This preferential accumulation of apo(a) as a tightly bound fraction in lesions, could be responsible for **the independent association of Lp(a) with cardiovascular disease in humans.**"* [41]

For more detailed information on Lp(a) and CVD see the paper *"Lipoprotein (a) as a cause of cardiovascular disease: insights from epidemiology, genetics, and biology."* [42] Good luck reading that jargon filled belter.

Gathering all of this together, what it means is that, in the same way as with cholesterol crystals, something was found to be present plaques, in this case it was lipoprotein particles. It was immediately decreed that these must be LDL molecules aka 'bad cholesterol' and therefore fully supported the cholesterol (LDL) hypothesis.

However, as with cholesterol crystals, what we have here is another case of mistaken identity. It is not LDL it is Lp(a) you are looking at. In the last few years, the role of Lp(a) in CVD has started to enter mainstream consciousness again... finally. Here is an article from the New York Times.

"To millions of Americans, Bob Harper was the picture of health, a celebrity fitness trainer who whipped people into shape each week on the hit TV show 'The Biggest Loser.'

"But last February, Mr. Harper, 52, suffered a massive heart attack at a New York City gym and went into cardiac arrest. He was saved by a bystander who administered CPR and a team of paramedics who rushed him to a hospital, where he spent two days in a coma.

"When he awoke, Mr. Harper was baffled, as were his doctors. His annual medical checkups had indicated he was in excellent health. How could this have happened to someone seemingly so healthy?

*"The culprit, it turned out, was a fatty particle in the blood called lipoprotein(a). While doctors routinely test for other lipoproteins like HDL and LDL cholesterol, few test for lipoprotein(a), also known as Lp(a), high levels of **which triple the risk** of having a heart attack or stroke at an early age."* [43]

You can, if you wish, search for Lp(a) and CVD, and you can find hundreds, nay thousands of papers on the subject.

At this point you may be thinking, well what does this matter? If LDL and Lp(a) are virtually the same thing, it still means that raised cholesterol, or LDL, or a version of LDL, causes CVD... doesn't it? Well, it could mean that, but it does not, not even remotely.

To explain. As is the case in much of human biology, and physiology, things that look virtually identical can have very different effects in the body. A small tweak here, a small tweak there, and you are heading down a completely different route. Sometimes in the exact opposite direction. This is certainly true with LDL and Lp(a).

The primary function of LDL is to carry cholesterol around the body, and deposit it in cells crying out for more. On the other hand, Lp(a), although it does contain the same concentration of cholesterol, and cholesterol esters, plays a completely different role. It is *not* a cholesterol transporter, instead it has a key role in blood clotting.

You can think of it this way. Lp(a) is an LDL molecule that has been hijacked to transport apo(a) about.

Please bear with me here as I try to explain what Lp(a) does, and why it does what it does. This is a tale which has a few steps in it. It begins with vitamin C and ends with fibrinolysis. Or maybe the other way around. At this point in the narrative, have a cup of coffee and stretch. This bit does become complicated. I need you fresh, and alert. So, Sophia and Chloe, please put down your mobile phones for just one second *please*, and pay attention at the back...

Vitamin C to fibrinolysis – a journey

The first thing I need to do here is to explain what fibrinolysis means. It is literally the 'lysis' or slicing apart of fibrin. Fibrin is a critical component of all blood clots. It can be thought of as long strands of protein (like the silk of a spider's web) that wrap themselves around blood clots as they form, binding them tightly together, and making them extremely difficult to break down.

I should add that you don't have long strands of fibrin floating about free in the bloodstream, it would just get tangled with everything it came across and jam up the works. Instead, you have short strands of a protein called fibrinogen. When a blood clot starts to form, small strands of fibrinogen are stuck together, end-to-end, to form fibrin – the long sticky strand.

Whilst fibrin is required to bind clots tightly together, it is essential to be able to break it apart again. If you didn't have a mechanism for doing this, then blood clots would be almost impossible to remove. If not impossible, then the process may take years, decades, a lifetime even. Bruises would turn into permanent blood clots, hanging around almost forever. A clot in a blood vessel would take years to dissolve. If, indeed, it ever did.

Luckily, evolution did what evolution does, and a solution was devised to chop fibrin apart. This allows blood clots/thrombi, once they have stemmed the bleeding, to be 'lysed' and removed.

The system works as follows. Every blood clot, whilst coming together, has a protein drawn into it called plasminogen. Plasminogen then lurks within the clot, doing nothing at all, unless it is activated.

Activation occurs when the active site of *Tissue Plasminogen Activator* (tPA) locks onto plasminogen and transforms plasminogen into plasmin. It is then *plasmin*, the activated enzyme, that chops fibrin apart. And that is how you shave blood clots down.

Plasminogen + tissue plasminogen activator → plasmin → fibrinolysis (breakdown of a blood clot)

Tissue plasminogen activator was discovered some years ago, and is now manufactured as a drug, known colloquially as a 'clotbuster.' If you are having a stroke, or a heart attack, you may be given tissue plasminogen activator to 'bust' apart the blood clot and open up the artery again.

However, it is not tissue plasminogen activator that actually busts the clot. It is plasmin, and plasmin is derived from plasminogen. Please remember this point, it is mission critical.

Time to change direction slightly, and move onto vitamin C.

Almost all animals can synthesize their own vitamin C. Humans, however, along with a very few other mammals, including guinea pigs (for some reason this always amuses me), cannot. We cast aside this ability about 40 million years ago, so I am informed. Why? It seems a bit careless. But there you go; evolution sometimes acts in mysterious ways.

Now, because we cannot make our own vitamin C, we must eat it, and it's vital that we eat enough. Because vitamin C has many different, critical, functions in the body. One of the most vital is that is used in the manufacture of collagen.

Collagen is the single most important support molecule in the human body. Think of collagen like the steel bars in reinforced concrete. Without collagen, your body begins to disintegrate.

One of the first things that start to disintegrate are your blood vessels. Without enough collagen they begin to crack and leak. Which is why the first visible sign of scurvy (severe lack of vitamin C), is bleeding gums. Followed by bleeding everything else, followed by death – usually from bleeding to death.

Yes, we humans have a serious design flaw. We cannot manufacture our own vitamin C, without which we die, slowly and horribly. So, suck that lemon. Or in the case of the British, suck that lime.

Americans have been known to call British people 'limeys.' This is because British sailors used to carry a large supply of limes on board ships to prevent scurvy. I hope they had sufficient gin and tonic supplies to temper the taste. For those who didn't have access to limes, other vitamin C containing foods were widely available.

However, if you were to find yourself unable to get sufficient vitamin C, nature came up with a patch to help keep you alive until you could get hold of it again. That patch is – you may have seen this coming – Lp(a).

If cracks do start to develop in blood vessels, then Lp(a) is attracted to the areas of damage. It binds with exposed proteins in the blood vessel wall and creates a strong 'plug' to prevent blood loss. Effectively, it becomes a key part of the innermost section of the thrombus, the part which is stuck directly to the artery wall.

What it then does, and here is where the story starts to come together, is that it blocks the action of tissue plasminogen activator. Or, to put it another way, it stops plasminogen being converted to plasmin. Which means that the fibrin holding the thrombus together, in that section of the clot, cannot be easily lysed, or broken down. This makes the clot far more difficult to chop into small pieces, and remove.

This is clearly a good thing, if your blood vessels are splitting open due to vitamin C deficiency. However, it is a bad thing if you don't want extremely resilient thrombi stuck to your artery walls. Or, extremely difficult to break down thrombi drawn into your artery walls.

How does Lp(a) block fibrinolysis?

Lp(a) blocks fibrinolysis because apo(a) and plasminogen are virtually identical in structure, apart from a different 'fold' at one end. How proteins are folded is critical to their function. You may have heard of prions, that can cause mad-cow disease. Prions are simply mis-folded proteins that get into the brain, are multiplied, and create mayhem.

Because of this different fold, apo(a) blocks the action of tissue plasminogen activator. It is the wrong piece in a complex machine, jamming up the works. For those of a technical bent, you could read the paper. *"Inhibition of plasminogen activation by apo(a): role of carboxyl-terminal lysines and identification of inhibitory domains in apo(a)."* [44]

Then again, you may not feel up to it. Even I, self-appointed cardiovascular research geek of the year, found that one exceedingly tough going. The jargon reaches high into the sky. Anyway, whatever the exact and complex biochemical processes by which Lp(a) prevents fibrinolysis, the simple message is as follows. If you have Lp(a) in a blood clot, it makes that clot far more difficult to get rid of.

This difficulty is highlighted in the following passage, where the authors use the phrase '*extremely unfavourable clot properties*':

*"We here provide the first evidence that elevated plasma **Lp(a) levels correlate with decreased fibrin clot permeation and impaired susceptibility to fibrinolysis** both in apparently healthy subjects and patients with advanced coronary artery disease. The relationship between Lp(a) and clots ...are associated with **extremely unfavourable clot properties.**"* [45]

I think I need to stop here before things get too technical, so I shall attempt to summarize the findings on Lp(a):

- Humans have Lp(a) in the blood stream, in some cases at higher levels than LDL (although it is normally about a quarter of the LDL level)

- LDL and Lp(a) are identical in structure, other than the attachment of the protein apo(a) to Lp(a)

- Lp(a) is designed to protect against the arterial damage caused by vitamin C deficiency (and other forms of arterial damage)

- Lp(a) is incorporated into blood clots that form on damaged artery walls

- Lp(a) makes blood clots far more difficult to remove

- Lp(a) can be found in high concentrations in atherosclerotic plaques

- A raised Lp(a) level can, at least, triple the risk of cardiovascular disease

Relating this back to the discussion as to whether or not there is LDL in plaques, I hope it is now clear that when you see what you believe to be the remnants of LDL it is far more likely that you are looking at Lp(a) than LDL.

Does this mean there is no LDL in atherosclerotic plaques? No, I am certain that there is some LDL in there as well. When blood clots form, almost everything in the bloodstream gets dragged in, including LDL. In addition, 'lipid surfaces' are where clots/fibrin are constructed, and LDL provides a good lipid surface for this to happen.

This is a very technical area indeed. If you want to know more, you can read the paper "*Lipid–protein interactions in blood coagulation.*" Again, not a page turner.[46]

One of the great frustrations is that so little new research is being done in this area. Lp(a) was starting to become an object of great interest in the late 1980s, and early 1990s. Then, along came statins, and alternative research came to a juddering halt. I should highlight the fact that statins have very little impact on Lp(a). A fact from which you can draw your own conclusions.

This sudden, screeching to a halt, was discussed in a review paper from 2016:

*"... there remains considerable evidence that Lp(a) may contribute to atherothrombotic disease, both through promotion of atherosclerosis and promotion of thrombosis/inhibition of fibrinolysis. **It cannot have escaped the attention of the reader that many of the basic science and clinical/ epidemiological studies cited in this review are more than 20 years old. This reflects, in part, a long fallow period in Lp(a) research prior to the publication of large genetic studies that pointed to a causal role for Lp(a) in the development of CAD.** The time is now ripe to revisit the prothrombotic/ antifibrinolytic potential of Lp(a) with a view toward understanding its mechanistic contribution to atherothrombotic events."[47]*

Yes, science most definitely has its trends. Once billions and billions of dollars were rolling in from statins, the trend was most certainly to run at high speed, and in the exact opposite direction, from any research that did not support the LDL hypothesis. The world became a very unfriendly place for anyone with alternative views.

I may remind you of the tale of Kilmer McCulley. He was not looking at blood clotting, at least not directly, but he was pursuing a line of research that directly contradicted the cholesterol hypothesis. Then, suddenly, that door was firmly slammed shut.

As you can imagine, attacks on him, and others – such as the book burning suffered by Uffe Ravnskov – brought alternative hypotheses to a screeching halt. Including any work into the role of Lp(a) in CVD. Anyone wishing to move up the research ladder took careful note of McCulley's tale. Word travels exceedingly fast in this community.

Which is why Lp(a) is now, pretty much a *ghost in the machine.* It was too damaging to the LDL hypothesis to be researched, or supported, but the evidence is still there, waiting to be discovered by anyone who chooses to look.

Anyway, getting back to plaques again. The thing I wanted to make clear here is that, as with cholesterol crystals, we are told that plaques are full of LDL – thus LDL must be the cause of heart disease.

Once again, as with cholesterol crystals, when you look at plaques more closely, this seemingly cast-iron fact can simply be turned around through 180 degrees. When you do so, it supports the thrombogenic hypothesis instead.

And this, my friends, is science. It is not super-simple, and problems are not solved by fast thinking, or jumping to conclusions:

- Finding fatty streaks in arteries, and assuming they turn into the type of plaque that causes CVD. Wrong

- Finding cholesterol crystals in plaques and assuming they must have come from LDL. Wrong

- Finding lipoproteins in plaques, and assuming they must be LDL molecules. Wrong

However, if you have decided from the very beginning, that LDL causes CVD, you can see how these 'facts' must have looked like extremely powerful support for the cholesterol hypothesis. Simple. Simple but wrong. Simplicity is always terribly seductive. The siren song capable of dragging all researchers to their doom. In this case, it did.

CHAPTER 2

Can plaques really be the remains of blood clots?

Moving away from cholesterol almost entirely, it is now time to dive into the heart of the matter. Can plaques truly be the remnants of blood clots. Does the evidence fit?

Perhaps a good place to start this discussion is by returning to the very earliest years of research into CVD once more. Here we are back in the mid-nineteenth century. A time of serious and unsmiling men wearing heavy dark coats, with impressive beards and hats. Often very tall hats. Even this far back, right at the beginning, there were those who believed that plaques were the remains of blood clots.

Men such as Karl von Rokitansky, the contemporary of Virchow mentioned a few times so far. He was one of the very first researchers to study plaques in detail, and he was convinced that they were the result of repeated deposition of blood clots.

"Rokitansky proposed that the disease is the result of an excessive intimal deposition of blood components (blood clots) including fibrin. He maintained that localized thickening, atheromatous changes and calcification of the arterial wall are due to the repeated deposition of blood elements and their subsequent metamorphosis and degeneration on the lining membrane of the vascular wall." [48]

I am pretty certain that this must make Rokitansky the very first person to propose the thrombogenic hypothesis. He actually called it, as mentioned earlier, the 'encrustation hypothesis'. In truth, it wasn't really a hypothesis, he was just stating what he saw. Namely, thrombi in various stages of growth and repair. As far as I know, he did not propose any underlying process.

At this point I would like to focus your attention on what I consider to be Rokitansky's key observation. Which is that, right from the start, with no other theories to muddy his thinking, he noted the presence of fibrin... in all plaques. Frankly, I am impressed that he knew what fibrin was, but he did.

Just to remind you that fibrin is the long sticky strand of protein that binds all clots together. Fibrin is created as the rest of a blood clot forms. Which leads to the obvious question. How does fibrin end up, wrapped around a plaque, within an artery wall?

It is true that clots, with associated fibrin, can develop spontaneously in the bloodstream, without any damage to blood vessel walls. This is what we call a deep vein thrombosis (DVT). In this condition, a clot starts off within a vein which can grow large enough to cause a complete blockage.

DVTs are often caused by immobility, with sufficient pressure on a vein to stop the blood flow. At which point a clot can spontaneously spring into life. The sort of things that can make this happen are, lying stationary on a bed in hospital. Or having to wear a cast after a fracture, then lying in bed. This is probably the most powerful trigger of all.

Before the medical profession became more aware of DVTs, many people lying in hospital beds simply died of the resultant pulmonary embolism. This is where the DVT breaks free and travels into the lungs, where it gets stuck. Bad news.

This is no minor problem.

For decades patients were strictly commanded to lie immobile in bed for six weeks following a heart attack. Many of them, possibly tens of millions over the years, died of the resultant pulmonary embolism.

Prolonged immobility is not always needed to trigger a DVT. A long-haul flight can be enough. Sitting in the same position for hours on end, putting pressure on a vein and stopping blood flow, along with a degree of dehydration. For some people, that is all that is required.

I am forever telling elderly patients not to cross their legs, filling them with tales of DVT terror. They all immediately uncross their legs then, inevitably, 30 seconds later, cross them again. I can't blame them, it's exactly what I do. In addition to immobility, some people have pro-thrombotic conditions that can make spontaneous blood clots much more likely.

However, DVTs develop *within* the vein, and not inside the vein wall, and no fibrin ends up in any blood vessel wall when this happens*. In fact, it is difficult to think of any way you can get fibrin inside an artery wall, unless it arrived there as a part of a blood clot.

More tellingly, you can even find fibrin in an artery wall when there is nothing else of a plaque to be seen:

"...in apparently healthy human subjects there appears to be a significant amount of fibrin deposited within arteries, and this should give pause for thought about the possible relationship between clotting and atherosclerosis." [49]

How did the fibrin get there? Well, it most certainly did not spontaneously generate. The only possible answer is that it arrived as part of a thrombus, which was then gradually broken down and removed. The bits that remained were fibrin. A very tough protein to dissolve – without enough plasmin.

To my mind, finding fibrin in an otherwise healthy artery wall is like finding bones in the ground. All that remains of a dead body after the rest has rotted and been stripped away by the worms.

If we look beyond the normal artery wall, it becomes clear that fibrin is a key component of all plaques. Right from the start, then through all stages of development (hyper-jargon alert):

*"**Fibrin appears to be a multi-potential component of atherogenesis, intervening at virtually all stages of lesion development.** Fibrin also provides a continuing source of fibrin degradation products (FDP), and these have mitogenic activity which will sustain SMC proliferation in growing plaques, and act as chemo attractants for blood leucocytes. **Accumulation of the lipid core in fibrous plaques may also be influenced by fibrin which appears to bind the lipoprotein Lp(a) with high affinity, thereby immobilizing its lipid moiety within the lesion.**"* [50]

- Lesion = a damaged or abnormal 'thing' (Not a word I like)

- Mitogenic = causes cells to divide and grow

- Fibrin degradation products = bits of fibrin left, after it has been chopped up a bit

- SMC = smooth muscle cell

---

* There is a significant proviso to this, which I will deal with later.

- Leucocytes = (in this case) macrophages

- Chemoattractant = a chemical that attracts other things to it

- Moiety = A smaller part of a bigger thing

- Jargon = The dead language of the expert

This short jargon filled passage describes a series of key facts about fibrin. Not only is it present in all plaques. It also stimulates further growth and attracts many of the other substances found within. Fibrin degradation products also drive smooth muscle cells to divide and multiply. Smooth muscle cells, mentioned earlier, are another important component of all plaques.

In addition to all this, fibrin degradation products draw macrophages into the area, and fibrin itself remains tightly bound to Lp(a), trapping the 'fats' contained within the Lp(a), providing the building blocks for the lipid core of the plaque to develop. Finally, fibrin binds to red blood cells which, in turn, provide the 'free' cholesterol that is the building block for cholesterol crystals.

What of platelets, another key component of all blood clots?

*"Abundant evidence published from the 1960s and onwards supports the essential role of platelets in the initial stages of atherosclerosis, as recently reviewed. Governed by disturbed flow, **platelets adhere to the arterial wall in vivo, even in the absence of endothelial cell denudation, initiating lesion formation.**"* [51]

Which means that platelets too, can initiate plaque formation by sticking tightly to the artery wall. This can happen even if endothelial cells have only been damaged, not stripped off. Then, like fibrin, they attract all the other players into the game of plaques.

Taking stock at this point, we now know that plaques contain fibrin, platelets, macrophages, red blood cells, Lp(a), and cholesterol crystals (with the cholesterol coming from red blood cells). All of which can be found in blood clots. Does this mean that plaques are clots? In my world, if it looks like a duck, and quacks like a duck – it is most likely a duck.

Moving that thought along, if plaques consist of blood clot after blood clot, shaved down, then all piled on top of another then, at least in theory, some plaques could be multi-layered. Or at least, there might well be visible layers inside those plaques that have not turned into indistinguishable mush.

In the midst of the *American Heart Association* document mentioned earlier, they made this statement:

*"The architecture of some multi-layered fibroatheromas could also be explained by **repeated disruptions of the lesion surface, hematomas, and thrombotic deposits.**"* [52]

Yes, if you managed to get that far before being overtaken by sleep, the AHA states that many plaques are, indeed, multi-layered. To the untrained eye they look a bit like tree rings, with layer upon layer, one on top of the other. How could you achieve such an appearance? Clot after clot, after clot? This seems the only possible explanation.

The idea of repeated thrombus formation causing plaque growth, is reinforced by a quote that I used earlier, from the journal *Atherosclerosis*.

*"In addition, **plaque rupture and subsequent healing is recognized to be a major cause of further rapid plaque progression.**"* [53]

This concept is strongly supported by another article in the Journal *Heart*.

*"**Subclinical** [no symptoms] **episodes of plaque disruption followed by healing are a stimulus to plaque growth that occurs suddenly** and is a major factor in causing chronic high grade coronary stenosis [narrowed coronary arteries]. This mechanism would explain the **phasic rather than linear** progression of coronary disease observed in angiograms carried out annually in patients with chronic ischaemic heart disease."* [54]

Phasic, rather than linear. A somewhat convoluted way of stating that plaques do not gradually enlarge. Instead, they suddenly jump in size. How does this occur? Because a clot has formed on top of an already existing plaque. It has then been incorporated, causing the plaque to enlarge.

An episode like this may well cause no symptoms, because the thrombus was not big enough to fully block the artery. However, the incorporation of this new thrombus into the artery wall will cause a 'phasic' jump in size.

So yes, plaques do not slowly enlarge as LDL accumulates one molecule every four seconds, or so. This, as I pointed out earlier, is a completely ridiculous concept anyway. They grow in sudden spurts.

My favourite publication covering all these observations cannot be referenced, because I think I have the only copy of the document that remains in existence. It was a short booklet entitled *"Pathologic triggers – new insights into cardiovascular risk."* It was produced by a company called Medi Cine Inc. based in London and New York. It was written on behalf of a pharmaceutical company in 1992.

On page four there is this section *"platelets and atherosclerosis progression."* Platelets are the small blood cells that I have not discussed in any detail up to now. However, they are the single most important player in blood clotting. They are sometimes called the conductors of the clotting orchestra. They bring together fibrin, and red blood cells, and many clotting factors, they are complicated wee buggers.

They also stick together (aggregate) and become part of every clot. Which means that they create the initial 'plug' to stem bleeding. Without platelets you would bleed to death after the smallest cut.

In fact, if you learn nothing more about clotting system, remember fibrin and platelets. Platelets get the clot started, then drag in everything else that makes up a clot. Fibrin then finishes the thrombus off, by wrapping it all up, nice and tight. Anyway, back to the document.

*"Several features of mature plaques, such as their **multi-layered pattern**, suggest that **platelet aggregation and thrombus formation** are key elements in the progression of atherosclerosis. **Platelets** are also known to provide a rich source of growth factors, which **can stimulate plaque development**."*

That could not be any much clearer, could it. Plaques grow through repeated episodes of clot deposition. Then platelets, along with fibrin, stimulate further plaque enlargement. Perhaps you can guess which pharmaceutical company paid for this document to be produced? A document which placed blood clotting very firmly at the very heart of CVD.

A company that then went on to complete a hostile takeover of Warner Lambert, thus acquiring the rights to Lipitor (atorvastatin). The statin which went on to become the world's largest selling drug – ever. From then on it was cholesterol, cholesterol, all the way.

Yes, once upon a time, before they had a cholesterol lowering drug, Pfizer had decided to progress down the thrombogenic route. Why did they change their mind? I think money might be a possible answer.

Statins had started to make vast sums of money; the cholesterol hypothesis was being ruthlessly and highly successfully promoted by their main rival – Merck. Pfizer didn't have a statin, so they simply took over a company that did.

They then marketed the bejesus out of it, and they never mentioned that idiotic thrombogenic theory ever again. Who knows, they may even be slightly embarrassed to be reminded of their earlier dalliance. Although, given my previous experiences with that industry, I suspect not.

I particularly liked the fact that an important section of the Pfizer document covered fibrinolysis. It also discussed my old favourites: tissue plasminogen activator, plasmin, and plasminogen. It finished thus:

"If fibrinolysis is incomplete, thrombus may become incorporated into the plaque, and may cause severe stenosis." [narrowing of the artery].

Yes, oh yes, they knew. Of course, they knew – they probably still do. They are not daft. They employ some of the finest scientific minds in the world. Unfortunately, the finest scientific minds in the world are very clearly directed to make money – not to explore the true causes of disease. Perish the very thought. Imagine how much money they would lose if we could actually prevent, or even cure, CVD.

(BTW, the document is photographed, and available to view on my blog).

Just before moving on from this area, I would like to mention someone very important in my thinking and knowledge – a former teacher of mine – and that is Elspeth Smith. It is now clear to me that she had explored and developed the thrombogenic theory further than anyone else.

In one small group teaching session at Aberdeen University, she informed a group of fresh-faced medical students, including me, that LDL cannot cross the endothelium. This was my first real exposure to a crack in the façade of conventional thinking. That comment, I have since come to realise, triggered the itch that I have spent several decades trying to scratch. It is a great regret that I never had the opportunity to discuss ideas with her. I was but a minion, she was far too senior, and I was an idiot. Still am, but I have learned to disguise it better.

Sadly, she never got the recognition that she deserved. I hope that the publication of this book may go some way towards rectifying that injustice. Over the years I have read almost everything she ever wrote on the subject. Including this, succinct, passage from nearly 40 years ago:

"After many years of neglect, the role of thrombosis in myocardial infarction is being reassessed. It is increasingly clear that all aspects of the haemostatic [blood clotting] system are involved: not only in the acute occlusive event, but also in all stages of atherosclerotic plaque development from the initiation of atherogenesis to the expansion and growth of large plaques." [55]

Goodness me, there it is, in one paragraph. But recognition was never to be hers, for she suffered the terrible scientific misfortune, as did Kilmer McCully, to find herself researching alternative ideas that were in direct contradiction to the dreaded, almighty, cholesterol hypothesis.

Even worse, it was at a time when statins were arriving on the scene. Ready to rule the world with their trillion dollars' worth of sales. Against that commercial behemoth, she was never going to get anywhere. Nor, frankly, was anyone else.

Just to remind you of the environment in which any researcher critical of the cholesterol hypothesis had to operate.

"...It was worse than that, you couldn't get ideas funded that went in other directions than cholesterol," he says. "You were intentionally discouraged from pursuing alternative questions. I've never dealt with a subject in my life that elicited such an immediate hostile response."

In case you are wondering, things have not got any better. Here is the title of an article published in the Annals of Internal Medicine in 2017 by Steven Nissen. He is one of the most influential cardiologists in the world.

"Statin Denial: An Internet-Driven Cult With Deadly Consequences." [56]

Yes, that was the actual title of an actual article written in a journal that purports to be scientific. The attack was enthusiastically taken up a little later by the *Mail on Sunday* in 2019 entitled:

"The deadly propaganda of the statin deniers: The drugs DO protect you from heart attacks but as this devastating investigation reveals thousands are refusing them...

"Dr Malcolm Kendrick, Dr Zoë Harcombe and Dr Aseem Malhotra are all deniers." [57]

Look mum, I made the front page of the *Mail on Sunday*. I think she was hoping for the Nobel Prize. Sorry. Still, she doesn't read the *Mail on*

Sunday, so she may have missed it. At least I certainly hope she doesn't read the *Mail on Sunday*.

Yes, from time to time, people have accused me of being a conspiracy theorist. A loon who thinks that the world of heart disease research is being directed and controlled by huge companies, and academic institutions, with vested interests in keeping the cholesterol hypothesis alive.

I now reply that I am **an** evidence-**b**ased **c**onspiracy **d**iscoverer (ABCD). I am not a theorist at all. I am simply reporting facts. Heart disease research *is* being directed and controlled by huge companies, publishing companies, academic institutions, all with vested interests in keeping the cholesterol hypothesis alive. Which make me **an** evidence-**b**ased **c**onspiracy **d**iscoverer using **e**stablished **f**acts (ABCDEF) – catchy acronym? Ok, yes, it's rubbish.

People argue that statins have now gone off patent, and so they make only a fraction of the money they used to, so who is bothering to protect statins. The reality is that new LDL lowering agents are being developed all the time. The cholesterol lowering market is not shrinking, it is growing. It is massive, and will remain so for many, many, years to come.

Therefore, any criticism of statins is seen to undermine the cholesterol hypothesis itself, so it is ruthlessly attacked by the powers that be. Cholesterol must be lowered – by order of the management (of the world).

The reason why you have not heard of alternatives to the cholesterol hypothesis is not that they fail to make sense, at least from a scientific perspective. Nor that there is a lack of data to support them. There is pile towering high into the sky. I have only quoted a miniscule fraction of the evidence in support of the thrombogenic hypothesis.

The reality is that the reason why you have not heard of the thrombogenic hypothesis is almost entirely because of money. A substance that can move research in any direction it wishes. A substance that can effectively purchase silence. A substance that has had the power to turn cholesterol into gold.

Statins have now achieved the remarkable feat of registering around $1,000,000,000,000.00 in sales (at the time of writing). That is a trillion dollars. I have no idea of the value of cholesterol lowering foods, or low-fat foods designed to 'lower cholesterol.' But it must be getting close to a trillion – maybe more. Anyone threatening that highly lucrative market is not going to be welcomed with open arms.

But that is enough of this, or you might begin to believe that I am not a fully-fledged cheerleader for the pharmaceutical industry. In truth, they have developed some cracking drugs, and driven equally brilliant innovations, but they most certainly have a darker side.

Moving away from such gloomy thoughts, my main aim up to now is to convince you that the thrombogenic hypothesis does not represent some fringe, lunatic idea. Nor should you think that I am a lonely kook, sitting in a shed at the bottom of the garden, banging at my keyboard in a deranged manner. The only person in the world to believe that blood clots, or blood clotting, may be the underlying cause of cardiovascular disease.

There have been others, there was Elspeth Smith – my heart disease heroine. Her quote is so important that it bears repeating.

"After many years of neglect, the role of thrombosis in myocardial infarction is being reassessed. It is increasingly clear that all aspects of the haemostatic [blood clotting] system are involved: not only in the acute occlusive event, but also in all stages of atherosclerotic plaque development from the initiation of atherogenesis to the expansion and growth of large plaques."

Amen.

Now, I shall move on to describe the actual process in more detail. Then I shall bring all the key risk factors together to create a working model of CVD. One that puts everything in place. I shall finish by explaining what you can do to avoid CVD. Although, once you understand exactly what causes CVD, you can probably work it all out for yourself.

CHAPTER 3

The thrombogenic process – the players

At this point I need to introduce you more formally to the key players in the game:

- The arteries and atherosclerosis
- The endothelium – endothelial cells
- The glycocalyx
- The blood clot/thrombus
- Endothelial progenitor cells
- Nitric oxide

I shall try to explain the role they all play in plaque formation, and plaque growth/rupture. This, you will be glad to hear, is the super-simplified version. Listen, I can bore people for days on this subject.

The arteries and atherosclerosis

There are many different types of blood vessel in the body ranging from pretty darned big, to minuscule. The largest blood vessel is the aorta which can be a good three centimetres in diameter. The smallest are capillaries, which are no wider than a single red blood cell. Slightly less than a hundredth of a millimetre. Far thinner than a human hair.

Atherosclerosis only, naturally, develops in the large to mid-size arteries in the body. It never, ever, naturally, develops in the veins. Despite veins being exposed to exactly the same level of LDL as the arteries – thought I would just pop that in.

In the section above I used the word 'body' deliberately. As mentioned earlier, there are also arteries and veins in the lungs. This means that, in effect, we have two separate circulation systems.

There is the 'systemic' circulation. Which is the word used to describe the blood vessels supplying every part of the body, apart from the lungs. Then there is the 'pulmonary' circulation, a term that includes all the blood vessels in the lungs.

The right side of the heart pumps the blood through the lungs, then it heads back to the heart, where the left side then pumps it around the rest of the body. Round and round it goes.

It's important to draw this distinction, because it is exceptionally rare for atherosclerosis to develop in any blood vessel in the lungs. Neither the arteries, nor the veins, no matter what size. Indeed, if you do find atherosclerosis in the lungs then you are looking at something very important – an almost certain cause.

Getting back to the systemic circulation. Yes, it is possible to get plaques in a vein, but only if you artificially turn a vein into an artery. An example of this is when you use a vein to create a coronary artery bypass graft (CABG). During this operation a section of vein is stripped out of the leg, then stitched onto a coronary artery either side of the blockage to bypass it. Vein grafts can then rapidly jam up with atherosclerosis.

Moving back to arteries, they have three main sections (and so do veins, although vein walls are much thinner):

- Externa

- Media

- Endothelium (sometimes called intima)

The externa consists of tough fibrous material that binds the artery together.

The media, middle part of the artery, is mainly made up of smooth muscle cells (SMCs). These can contract, to narrow the artery; or relax, to dilate the artery. This helps to regulate the blood pressure and can direct blood flow to different parts of the body – and suchlike. The media is not nearly as simple as this of course, nothing ever is, but that will do for now.

The endothelium is the inner layer that faces the bloodstream.

Atherosclerosis, or atherosclerotic plaques, develop underneath the endothelium and grow down into the media. A big plaque would be about the size of a petit pois, maybe a bit smaller, a proper sized pea perhaps – depending on the artery where it forms (Figure 9).

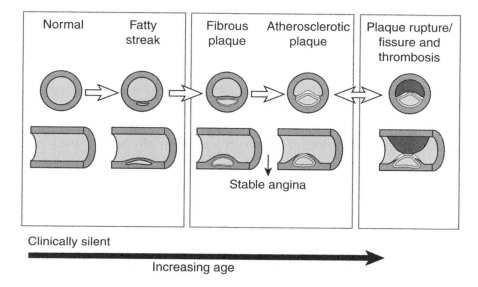

Figure 9

To give you further idea of the scale we are talking about here, a thrombus, which is as small as the size of a grain of rice, can block an artery in the brain, or heart, leading to significant damage.

A final point that I need to mention is that larger arteries, and veins, are supplied with nutrients, and oxygen, by their own blood vessels. These are called *vasa vasorum*. Literally, blood vessels of the blood vessels. This is important to bear in mind when we look at the process of atherosclerosis and what can, and what cannot, cause it.

The endothelium

The endothelium lines all blood vessels, including arteries. It is made up of two thin layers. Layer one is the endothelial cells themselves. These face the bloodstream, usually in a single layer, a bit like wall tiles. Underneath the endothelial cells lies the supportive 'sub-endothelial' layer. This consists of a bit of 'interstitial liquid' some elastic fibres, some collagen, a few white blood cells, some more supportive tissue.

Taken together, the two layers have been called many, many, different things. Endothelium, epithelium, endothelial layer, intima, intimal layer... no two papers call it the same thing. Which makes reading clinical papers in the area tricky – as always.

To try to keep confusion to the minimum, in this book I will be sticking, as far as possible, to the term 'endothelium'. Although I am mostly talking about endothelial cells themselves because this is where the main action takes place.

The total surface area of endothelial cells is around the size of a football pitch, and they are amongst the most complex and active cells in the body. In fact, I consider the endothelium to be a separate organ of the body. This is because it is so critical to our physiology, and it has so very many functions. It is an exceedingly thin organ.

I also need to make it clear that in the arteries, big enough for plaques to develop, endothelial cells form an absolute barrier to the movement of substances from the bloodstream into the artery wall beneath. As discussed in Part One.

Or, to put this another way, a healthy and undamaged endothelium is all that is needed to prevent harmful substances, or non-harmful substances, entering the artery wall. On the other hand, once you damage the endothelium, all hell can break loose. Albeit in an area that is generally the size of a grain of rice, or a small petit pois. Cry havoc and let loose the (teeny-weeny) dogs of war.

However, important caveat warning, all endothelium is not the same. When blood vessels become very small, for example the arterioles and capillaries, the endothelium here alters dramatically. It now has gaps in it called 'fenestrations.' In addition, the tight junctions between the cells open up a bit, and the basement membrane – a tough layer lying just under endothelial cells – loosens.

This is because substances have to move in and out of the bloodstream once they reach their destination. There would be no point in the blood reaching, say, the Bowman's capsule* in the kidneys, then passing straight through, without various waste products leaking out – to be disposed of.

Which means that, at the very smallest 'micro' level, blood vessels become leaky. One of the reasons for mentioning this is because the vasa vasorum are also leaky, as they must be. Which means that LDL can move in and out of arterioles and capillaries, and straight into the artery wall – and also any vein wall.

---

* Bowman's capsule is a cup-like structure at the beginning of a nephron in the kidney where the first step in the filtration of blood to form urine happens.

This, in turn, means that the endothelium, lining the artery, is not actually a barrier to LDL at all. Any LDL that wishes to enter the artery wall, can simply get in through the back door – using the vasa vasorum.

Think upon that, dear reader. And whilst you're thinking on that, think on the fact that large veins have more vasa vasorum than arteries. Then ask yourself why LDL does not build up in veins to create plaques. Then see if you can come up with an answer to that question. Because I never could.

The glycocalyx

Here is something which I would roughly estimate that 99.8% of doctors have never heard of. Which is quite frankly amazing. My very accurate estimate is based on asking ten doctors if they had ever heard of it, and they all said no. Actually, they didn't say no, because doctors hate to admit they don't know something, including me[*]. But none of them could explain what it was.

The glycocalyx is the thing that makes many fish slippery, very slippery indeed. It is a layer of proteins and sugars (glycoproteins) which looks like a miniature meadow under a microscope. It is the super Teflon of the natural world (Figure 10).

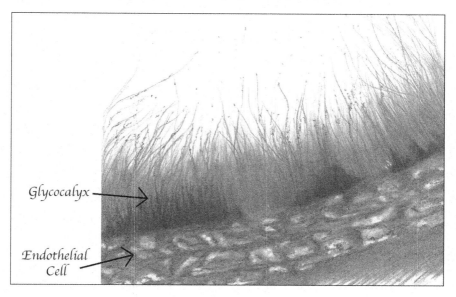

Figure 10

---

[*] Especially me, in truth.

However, it is not just fish that have a glycocalyx to make them slippery, and protect them from infections, and suchlike. Our endothelial cells are also covered (on one side) by this amazing and complicated layer that protects the endothelium from damage. It also contains a whole series of enzymes and other chemicals.

Perhaps the most important of these molecules are powerful anti-coagulants (things that prevent blood clotting), such as: tissue factor inhibitor, antithrombin, protein C and nitric oxide (NO). So, not only is the glycocalyx 'non-stick' it actively resists the formation of blood clots.

Below is a more complete list of its functions. You can skip this list if you want, or read it, and wonder once again, as I do, at how complex the human body is. You would almost think it had been designed... ☺

The glycocalyx:

- Forms the interface between the vessel wall and moving blood

- Acts as the exclusion zone between blood cells and the endothelium

- Acts as a barrier against leakage of fluid, proteins and lipids across the vascular wall

- Interacts dynamically with blood constituents

- Acts as the "molecular sieve" for plasma proteins

- Modulates adhesion of inflammatory cells and platelets to the endothelial surface

- Functions as a sensor and mechano-transducer of the fluid shear forces to which the endothelium is exposed; thus, the glycocalyx mediates shear-stress-dependent nitric oxide production

- Retains protective enzymes (e.g. superoxide dismutase)

- Retains anticoagulation factors, e.g.: tissue factor inhibitor, protein C, nitric oxide (NO), antithrombin[58]

The presence of the glycocalyx is another of the reasons why, when people tell me that LDL can leak past the endothelium and into the vessel wall behind, I just look at them as I would a young and innocent child, who has as yet learned little, and wonder if they have any idea of how ridiculous that sounds.

Do they even remotely understand the enormous complexity of the endothelial barrier, tight junctions, ion channels and suchlike? Have they ever heard of the glycocalyx that lines all endothelial cells? No, is pretty much the answer to all that.

Just to focus briefly on one item on that list above, where it states that the glycocalyx ... "*acts as a barrier against leakage of fluid, proteins **and lipids** across the vascular wall.*" (For lipid read LDL).

The truth is that if you have a healthy glycocalyx, then you have a major protective barrier against endothelial damage, and also the formation of blood clots, and therefore CVD. Just to give you one golly gee whizz fact about the glycocalyx – and also the endothelium.

If a white blood cell e.g., a macrophage wants to get through the endothelium, messages are passed from one to the other. The endothelial cells will then release the tight junctions between them, move apart, allow the macrophage to pass, and then seal themselves back together again. When this happens, the glycocalyx is stripped off.

It can be completely repaired and replenished within less than a second.

"The glycocalyx is fragile but self-repairing. The passage of a white cell through a tight-fitting capillary can shred it completely, and yet it will restore itself in less than one second by absorbing plasma constituents." [59]

Pay attention to that bit, *absorbing plasma constituents*. What does that mean? It means it is possible to nurture the glycocalyx with various proteins, and suchlike. This will come up later under – what you can do to prevent CVD.

Anyway, anyone who thinks the heart is a pump, and the blood vessels are simply pipes through which the blood passes, is missing something in the order of 100% of the complexity of the vascular system. Here, you are getting about 0.1%. I know about 1% – max. Everywhere you look, it all becomes more and more incredibly complicated.

I feel the need to add that the enormous complexity of the endothelium, and the very existence of the glycocalyx, was completely unknown when people were coming up with the cholesterol hypothesis.

'Here is my theory about heart disease. Unfortunately, I know the square root of bugger all about the cardiovascular system, but I am sure it is true anyway.'

A. N. Idiot.

The blood clot/thrombus

I have been reading about blood clotting for 30 years and I still do not fully understand exactly what the hell is going on. I am not certain if this is worrying or reassuring. It is beyond mind-bogglingly complicated. I think it is the most sophisticated self-regulating system in the body.

It must be so complex, I think, because the clotting system must prevent us from bleeding to death whilst, at the same time, ensuring that we do not clot to death. We need to live in the Goldilocks' zone. Not too bleedy, not too clotty, just right.

- Too bleedy is called haemophilia (love of bleeding)

- Too clotty is called thrombophilia (love of clotting)

Thrombophilia also has about a hundred other names. Pro-thrombotic, pro-coagulant, hyper-coagulant, etc. etc. Diseases that make your blood more likely to clot are called coagulopathies. Listen, I didn't make up this stupid medical terminology, I just have to live with it, and the endless different ways used to describe exactly the same thing.

As for the blood clot itself, what do you need to know? First, when a blood clot forms, almost everything in the blood gets dragged in, or has some role in blood clotting. There are many things closely involved in blood clotting, whose day job is to do something else completely different. For example, red blood cells.

Their primary role is to transport oxygen and carbon dioxide around the body, but they also have a fundamental role in thrombosis formation. They make up a great deal of the bulk of a thrombus. They also bind powerfully to fibrin, and once they have bound on, they actually then contract down, tightening the fibrin strands to make the thrombus more densely packed, and stronger. Really? Yes really.

Leaving aside such ancillary clotting factors, there are about 20 factors whose entire purpose in life is to stimulate/activate blood clot formation. On the flip side of this coin, we have another 20 that are involved in stopping the clot forming in the first place or breaking it apart once it has formed. Twenty on either side, at least, battling it out.

But I am going to try to keep it simple. The key players in creating a thrombus are:

- Platelets

- Fibrin

- Red blood cells

I am leaving Lp(a) out of the discussion at this point.

Platelets are small cells, without a nucleus, that float about in the blood. They live, they die about a month later, and are removed. Or maybe they are removed and then they die.

If a red blood cell were the size of the Earth, a platelet would be about the size of the moon. If there is damage to a blood vessel, platelets fling themselves into the damaged area to form the initial plug.

Platelets have also been described as the conductors of the clotting system. Whilst acting like a finger in the dyke, they also release hundreds of different chemicals and clotting factors and suchlike. They stick to other platelets, they stick to other things in the blood, such as red blood cells. They drive the 'clotting cascade' which you have probably heard of. This consists of things such as factor VIII, IX, X, XI etc.

The clotting cascade is a kind of self-reinforcing chain reaction, or maybe an avalanche. The end result of which is to turn prothrombin into thrombin. Thrombin, once it has been made, has the job of sticking short strands of fibrinogen together to make fibrin. Why so damnably complex? Not sure.

Fibrin, once it has been constructed, acts as long strong sticky strands of super-tough protein that binds clots tightly together. The creation of fibrin also drags in more red blood cells, which link themselves on to the fibrin. And that, my friends, is a blood clot, all wrapped up nice and tight.

Another important factor that I feel I need to mention is a substance called tissue factor (TF). This does not float about free in the bloodstream. Because if it did, your bloodstream would consist of one great big blood clot, and you would be dead.

Instead, tissue factor sits in various tissues. Let us say, for the sake of simplicity, that it only sits inside the walls of the larger blood vessels – hidden away under the endothelium. If a large vessel is damaged, then tissue factor is exposed to the bloodstream and this activates blood clotting *warp drive* – for those familiar with Star Trek and Star Wars.

Warp drive occurs because tissue factor bypasses most of the stages in the clotting cascade, and forces almost instant fibrin formation.

You may have noticed that if you get a paper cut on a finger it can bleed for an annoyingly long time. This is because you have damaged very small blood vessels, with no tissue factor in them. Which means that the clot forms slowly, sluggishly even.

However, if a bigger blood vessel is damaged the clotting process hits warp speed, as it must. You can't have sluggish blood clot formation when you are, potentially, losing a pint a minute. Or 0.75 litres a minute, to be fully European.

Which means that when there is damage to a larger blood vessel, blood clots develop very quickly. In turn this means that if you damage the endothelium in larger arteries and expose the blood to the underlying artery wall, and the tissue factor lying within, this 'warp drives' the formation a blood clot.

This has all been known for a long, long, time. Here for example is a paper from as far back as 1959,

> *"...any intimal injury can very easily precipitate a local process of coagulation, platelet agglutination and fibrin deposition."* [a.k.a. a blood clot].[60]

Yes, they used the word intima, not endothelium. Of course. Sigh.

What else do you need to know about blood clots... Well, I have already discussed plasminogen, plasmin and tissue plasminogen activator and Lp(a). I think a couple of final things that are of interest here are aspirin and warfarin.

Aspirin can be used to protect people from strokes and heart attacks, because it stops platelets sticking together, it is an 'anti-platelet' medication. There are other 'anti-platelet' agents around today, such as clopidogrel (expensive aspirin).

Now that you know what platelets do, you should be able to see how aspirin, by stopping platelets sticking together, will reduce blood clot formation after endothelial damage, and can reduce the risk of a big clot developing,

Warfarin, on the other hand, is a far more potent anti-coagulant agent than aspirin. In that, if you take too much, there is a real risk of bleeding to death (not so with aspirin). It is prescribed to prevent deep vein thrombosis, and it can also stop clots forming in atrial fibrillation.

Warfarin, though, works in a completely different way to aspirin. It blocks the production of various clotting factors in the liver, and this impairs the clotting cascade and the final step of thrombin generation.

However, if tissue factor is activated, this pretty much bypasses all these clotting factors anyway. So, theoretically, warfarin would not significantly hamper the clot formation that follows endothelial damage, and it doesn't – or at least the effect is very small.

Here is what NICE has to say in the UK in guidance they provide to doctors on various treatments.

"For patients who have had a myocardial infarction (MI), high-intensity warfarin should not be considered as an alternative to aspirin in first-line treatment." [61]

Which is interesting? Well, I think it is interesting anyway. In fact, I love this stuff. I hope that it also gives you an insight into how, once you can understand more clearly how a process in the body works, you can establish how something that seems completely contradictory makes perfect sense.

In this case, for many years, the medical profession tried to use warfarin to reduce the risk of CVD and were unable to understand why it didn't really work when aspirin, a far less 'potent' anticoagulant, did. Now you know why. It may also give you more insight into how flipping complicated this all is.

Endothelial Progenitor Cells

Where do new endothelial cells come from? This an important question which had no answer for the first 140 years of cardiovascular research. Had Karl von Rokitansky known the answer, I believe that the thrombogenic hypothesis would have become utterly dominant, and no-one would even have heard of cholesterol, apart from a few obscure research scientists.

Unfortunately, although Rokitansky was getting some traction with his encrustation hypothesis, Virchow floored him early on with this killer question. *'Karl, me old mate, me old mucker, how can a blood clot form underneath the endothelium? Because, if I may be so bold this, of course, this is where plaques are found. Is it, ahem, not?'*

Rokitansky, it appears, had no real answer. So, gentle reader, the thrombogenic theory suffered a serious hole beneath the water line. Despite bailing madly, it struggled to stay afloat.

What Rokitansky could have said, had he known about endothelial progenitor cells (EPCs) was the following. *'Rudolf, my great and close friend, when the blood clot forms the endothelium is not there. It grows back on top.'* (Thinks) *'So, stick that where the sun don't shine... You complete....'*

Looking back in time, I find it fascinating that no-one seemed to give much thought to the endothelium in the early days. Where does it come from, what does it do, how incredibly complicated it is? For many years, the endothelium was viewed as an inactive lining. A bit like wall tiles, or the dead skin cells, that cover your body. Endothelial cells were passive observers, whilst the real action was going on elsewhere.

Indeed, I have found it exquisitely frustrating to look into the history of CVD and read about researchers gazing at a new layer of endothelium forming, without having a clue what it was, or what it was made of, or even where it came from. *'Guys, guys, where do you think the new endothelium comes from... think!'*

For example, a study was done in 1967, on pigs (ironically funded by a tobacco company). The researchers artificially damaged the endothelium, you don't really want to know how they did this, then waited for a few days before killing the pigs and studying the area of damage to their aortas – the big blood vessel that comes straight out of your heart, down into your abdomen.

Different pigs were killed on different days. Some, a few days after endothelial stripping, others were given a couple of weeks, or more. The idea was to find out what happened during different stages of repair.

This group of researchers reported that after you damage the endothelium a blood clot forms over the area – no surprise. The clot then starts to shrink in size – no surprise. Then, strange cells begin to appear on top of the blood clot....

*"One of the most interesting features was the presence of flattened cells with darkly staining elongated nuclei and spindle shaped cytoplasm lying on the surface of these thrombi and in some areas appeared to form a continuous layer. Judged by the relatively crude criteria of light microscopy **these cells bore a close resemblance to endothelial cells**.*

"As they lay a very considerable distance from the uninjured aortic intima with its viable endothelium, it seems unlikely that all of these covering cells were derived from spreading inwards of new endothelium from the edges of the traumatized site." [62]

In retrospect it is clear as day that they were looking at a new layer of endothelial cells, in the process of covering over a blood clot. Their explanation:

"It seems probable that they (these new cells) were instead derived from mononuclear cells forming part of the thrombus and modified in some way by their new environment."

So close. Why didn't they ask the follow up question – where could these cells possibly have come from?

At that time, it was assumed that new endothelial must grow in from the side of any damaged area. But they don't, they can't, or it is very difficult for them to do so. A mature endothelial cell cannot easily replicate itself – if at all. Personally, I think 'not at all', but the research in this area is sometimes conflicting – to say the least.

Nor can endothelial cells be replaced by new ones growing up from underneath, as happens with damage to your skin. Unlike the skin, there is no new layer of cells gradually creeping up from below, to take over from those that grow old and die and fall off. In arteries there is a single layer of endothelial cells, nothing beneath, and that's that.

So, they cannot grow in from the side, they cannot rise to the surface. Where do they come from?

They come from the only place that they can possibly come from, which is that they are floating about in the bloodstream, having been manufactured in the bone marrow. They have been given the name endothelial *progenitor* cells (EPCs) because they are not fully mature endothelial cells. They are attracted to areas of arterial damage, then stick to the thrombus that has formed on top. They then grow into a new layer of endothelium.

"EPCs migrate toward injured endothelial regions, after they have been mobilized into the circulation. At these places they home or adhere and start to proliferate beginning vascular repair." [63]

The other fascinating thing about endothelial progenitor cells is that they bear a very close relationship to white blood cells, called monocytes.

Because they are relatively immature, endothelial progenitor cells retain the potential to go off in several different directions. One of those directions is to become a monocyte. See *"Will the real EPC please stand up?"* [64]

Monocytes, in turn, can further mature into macrophages – a type of cell that I have mentioned a few times earlier. Thus, an endothelial progenitor cell can become a brand spanking new endothelial cell, or it can turn into a macrophage. At least I am pretty sure that this is the correct version of events. Papers in this area are as close to incomprehensible as it gets.

Macrophages are found in and around all plaques, often in high concentrations. They can also get tangled up and immobilised within the plaque itself. Often being turned into 'foam cells' in the process. This raises the distinct possibility that they arrived, not as macrophages, but as endothelial progenitor cells/monocytes, which were then transformed into macrophages.

I find all this amazing, and mind-boggling. The body has this repair system, endothelial progenitor cells, which are designed to create a new layer of endothelium. But that is not the half of what they can do. The very same cells can turn into macrophages, if needed.

Macrophages, in turn, are the 'clear up' cells that can get rid of any residual blood clot that has been drawn into the artery wall. I think there is also something fascinating about the fact that endothelial cells and macrophages must be very closely related. First cousins.

I am sure that this is important in all sorts of ways. Although I cannot quite work out why. It is probably why they can 'talk' to each other to enable macrophages to move between endothelial cells, if required.

Anyway, pulling this together, the presence of endothelial progenitor cells can fully explain how a thrombus can end up within the artery wall – beneath the endothelium. In fact, it must end up within the artery wall. After all, if any blood clot that formed on an artery were simply allowed to break off and hurtle further down the artery, it would rapidly get stuck and cause mayhem.

Indeed, this is exactly what does happen in most strokes. A thrombus forms on top of an artery in the neck (carotid artery), almost always on top of a pre-existing plaque. It then breaks off and travels up into the brain where it gets stuck, causing a stroke.

Which means that endothelial progenitor cells are therefore critical, not only in forming a new layer of endothelium, to cover over the damage. But also, to protect the body from downstream mayhem.

Given this, you would expect that a reduced production of endothelial progenitor cells would lead to a greatly increased risk of CVD, and it does.

"Endothelial progenitor cells (EPCs) move towards injured endothelium or inflamed tissues and incorporate into foci of neovascularisation, thereby improving blood flow and tissue repair. **Patients with cardiovascular diseases have been shown to exhibit reduced EPC number and function.***"* [65]

The sort of things that can reduce EPC numbers, or function, include:

- Diabetes[66]

- Chronic kidney disease[67]

- Steroids[68]

These factors also, and this is not a coincidence, greatly increase the risk of CVD. Looking at this from another perspective. A lack of endothelial progenitor cells does not cause damage to the endothelium, but severely hampers the repair systems.

Nitric Oxide

My final player on this list is nitric oxide (NO). It is almost impossible to overstate the importance of nitric oxide (NO) on cardiovascular health. It was discovered about the same time as endothelial progenitor cells during the mid-1990s.

For many years it was considered impossible that nitric oxide could exist in the human body. It is a gas – or it would be if you could get enough molecules to gang together. It consists of one oxygen atom and one nitrogen atom. It is chemically written NO^-.

That floating minus sign means it has a free electron, and is a free radical, the free-est of free radicals. It should, in theory, react with anything it comes into contact with. Indeed, in any quantity it should explode, so fast would the reaction be.

Which, in fact, it does. Because one source of nitric oxide is nitro-glycerine, which is one of the most powerful conventional explosives known. Interestingly, if you have angina, and you stick nitro-glycerine under your tongue your angina will disappear. Doctors don't call it nitro-glycerine, they call it glyceryl tri-nitrate (GTN). But it is the same thing.

In fact, it was workers at Alfred Nobel's dynamite factories who first noticed that if they were – extremely carefully – stirring the nitro-glycerine mix, their angina went away. Alfred Nobel, who also had angina, refused to take glyceryl tri-nitrate when it was first developed. Maybe he thought he would explode. Which would have buggered up the Nobel Prize somewhat.

For well over a hundred years, no-one had any idea exactly why glyceryl tri-nitrate got rid of angina – if only temporarily. It was then discovered that it stimulated nitric oxide synthesis.

At one time, nitric oxide used to be called EDRF – endothelium derived relaxation factor. Doctors knew that something unknown, produced by the endothelium, opened up (dilated) blood vessels, they just didn't know what it was. Turns out it was a hyper radical, potentially explosive, gas. Who knew?

However, nitric oxide does far, far, more than to simply dilate narrowed coronary arteries, which is the underlying cause of angina. It also lowers blood pressure by opening up arteries elsewhere in the body. In addition, it stimulates the production of new endothelial progenitor cells in the bone marrow.

If that were not enough, nitric oxide prevents anything sticking to the glycocalyx/endothelium. In fact, it is the most powerful anticoagulant agent known.

I don't think it is an exaggeration to say that nitric oxide is the single most important molecule for cardiovascular health there is. Which means anything that reduces its production will increase the risk of CVD, and vice-versa.

"Adequate levels of endothelial NO are important to preserve normal vascular physiology—in the face of diminished NO bioavailability, there is endothelial dysfunction, leading to increased susceptibility to atherosclerotic disease."[69]

Nitric oxide is also where CVD and erectile dysfunction overlap.

"Nitric oxide (NO) is a physiologic signal essential to penile erection, and disorders that reduce NO synthesis or release in the erectile tissue are commonly associated with erectile dysfunction."[70]

If you have erectile dysfunction, and you rub glyceryl tri-nitrate cream on your penis, it can give you an erection. Glyceryl tri-nitrate cream has been called 'dynamite' cream because, yes, dynamite contains a very high concentration of nitro-glycerine. A little play on words. *'I'm dynamite in bed, baby... ding, dong. Kaboom.'*

Yes, if you increase nitric oxide in the blood vessels of the penis, you will treat erectile dysfunction. Which is how Viagra (sildenafil) works.[71]

The slight irony here is that Viagra was being developed as a drug to treat angina – opening up the arteries in the heart. The volunteers in the early clinical trials did not hand their tablets back, which was unusual. The rest, as they say, is history.

A further thing that you might not expect is that the action of sunlight on the skin creates nitric oxide. This lowers the blood pressure and has major benefits on CVD, outlined in the paper *"Sunlight Has Cardiovascular Benefits Independently of Vitamin D."*

"Skin contains significant stores of nitrogen oxides, which can be converted to NO by UV radiation and exported to the systemic circulation. Human studies show that this pathway can cause arterial vasodilatation and reduced BP." [72]

Which may well be why avoiding the sun can be as bad for you as smoking. A fact described in this Swedish study *"Avoidance of sun exposure as a risk factor for major causes of death: a competing risk analysis of the Melanoma in Southern Sweden cohort"*:

*"**Nonsmokers who avoided sun exposure had a life expectancy similar to smokers** in the highest sun exposure group, indicating that **avoidance of sun exposure is a risk factor for death of a similar magnitude as smoking**. Compared to the highest sun exposure group, life expectancy of avoiders of sun exposure was reduced by 0.6–2.1 years.*

*"**The longer life expectancy amongst women with active sun exposure habits was related to a decrease in CVD.**"* [73]

Here, then, is the power of that little molecule nitric oxide revealed. Which is why I am contemplating having a new line of t-shirts printed. 'Say YES to NO'. Specifically designed to be taken off outdoors.

CHAPTER 4

The thrombogenic process
– the process and the risk factors

Now that you know the key players, it is time to move onto the underlying process in a little more detail. Essentially, it is extremely simple. The first step is that the endothelium is damaged, in some way, by something. After this, a blood clot forms to cover the area. Once the clot has stabilised, it is gradually shaved down in size.

Endothelial progenitor cells then move and cover over the clot. In effect, drawing it into the arterial wall.

At this point, macrophages arrive (or have already arrived as endothelial progenitor cells). They clear up the remnant blood clot, and it is gone. That, anyway, is the normal healthy process.

Problems start to happen, and a plaque will kick-off and continue to grow, if:

- There is an increased rate of endothelial damage

- The blood clot formed is bigger, or more difficult to break down, than normal

- The repair systems are impaired in some way

And that's it really.

Which means that any factor that increases the risk of CVD will be doing one of these three things. Maybe all three. Plaques will also develop more rapidly if several factors are working in unison to plot the destruction of your arteries.

On the plus side, if you have protective factors in operation, then you can slow CVD down. Maybe even reverse it. I shall throw in another analogy here, which is potholes in the road.

Road surfaces are under constant attack from rain, ice, tractor tyres, car tyres, direct sunlight and suchlike. Over time they will start to break down, cracks and potholes will develop. Then the potholes will get bigger and bigger.

If the local council spends money on timely repair, or resurfacing, then roads will remain in good condition. If not, things can get very bad indeed. See under, UK roads, currently.

Essentially, what we have with roads is an on-going battle between damage and repair. If repair is going on faster than damage, then all is well. If damage is overwhelming repair, then things will end badly. Cyclists will disappear into huge potholes and suchlike. Car tyres will blow up – I speak from bitter experience here.

The same thing is happening in arteries. If the repair systems can keep pace with damage, then all is well. But if damage outstrips repair all hell can break loose. Which is why, jumping ahead of myself slightly, age is such an important risk factor for CVD. As we age, the rate of damage may not increase. However, the repair systems start to fall apart, in several different ways.

For example:

"Age decreases endothelial progenitor cell recruitment." [74]

"Experimental models suggest that endothelium-derived nitric oxide is reduced with aging, and this reduction is implicated in atherogenesis." [75]

As with most things, if you are young, gambolling through life like an innocent lamb, you can get away with all sorts of nonsense, and the repair systems will, mostly, take care of you. Unfortunately, as you get older, you need to reduce damage as much as possible, because the repair systems will begin to stumble.

Which is why age is simple to explain as a risk for CVD. But can the hypothesis explain everything else? By everything, I mean everything. I have no interest in a hypothesis that explains several things, even most things. Its everything, or nothing. No adaptations or ad-hoc hypothesis for me. Gulp, major hostage to fortune.

But where to start in looking at all of this in greater detail. Today, well over a thousand different factors have been identified as having some role in causing CVD or protecting against CVD. As mentioned before, the number had already reached 246 by 1981.[76] Clearly, it would be impossible to go through them all. Well, maybe not impossible, but somewhat tedious for both you, dear reader, and me... frazzled writer.

As a compromise, I thought I would use the risk factors that make up the Qrisk3 calculator as a basis for the discussion. In some ways this is not ideal, because Qrisk3 includes several things that do not, indeed cannot, directly cause CVD. They can only be associations.

Therefore, before moving on I think this 'associations' point needs to be further explained, because it is very important to understanding.

Association not causation

There is a common saying in epidemiology which is that correlation (association) does not mean causation. One example that is used to explain this point, is the association between yellow fingers and lung cancer.

It has long been known that people with yellow fingers are much more likely to die from lung cancer. True. However, the reason for this association is that people who smoke have yellow fingers. Ergo, smoking leads to both the yellow fingers and the lung cancer. In short, although yellow fingers are closely associated with lung cancer, they are not the cause. Indeed, cannot be the cause.

There would be little point in scrubbing people's fingers with bleach to try to prevent lung cancer. Well, you could try. It would probably stop them smoking for a bit, as they would be unable to hold the cigarette due to pain. What you really need to do, is persuade them to stop smoking.

In the same way, there are many factors that are strongly associated with cardiovascular disease, but they are not a cause – cannot be a cause. Unfortunately, Qrisk3 makes no real distinction between association, and causation. It just lists 20 things that are, currently, very strongly associated with CVD... in the UK, in this decade. Some of which are causal...

Just to remind you of the list

- Age

- Sex

- Smoking

- Diabetes

- Total cholesterol/HDL ratio
- Raised blood pressure
- Variation in two blood pressure readings
- High BMI
- Chronic kidney disease
- Rheumatoid arthritis
- Systemic lupus erythematosus (SLE)
- History of migraines
- Severe mental illness
- On atypical antipsychotic medication
- Using steroid tablets
- Atrial fibrillation
- Diagnosis of erectile dysfunction
- Angina, or heart attack in first degree relative under the age of 60
- Ethnicity
- Postcode

Focussing for a moment or two on the last item on the list which is postcode – in the US the term is Zip code. It is certainly true that people living in certain postcodes are far more likely to die of CVD, but there is no way that your exact geographical location on the planet can lead to a heart attack. Unless, I suppose, your location is standing very close to the edge of a cliff with someone threatening to push you off.

So, why is it included in Qrisk3? Why does it increase your risk? The explanation is that postcode is shorthand for – living in an area of a town, or city, that is socially and economically deprived.

To no-one's great surprise, poor people living in central Liverpool, or Glasgow, or the ghettos of Baltimore, or Detroit, are far more likely to die of CVD than rich people living in leafy suburbia. Therefore, postcode doesn't really mean your exact geographical location. Instead, it is shorthand for *'social deprivation'* or *'low socio-economic status.'*

The impact of social deprivation on health was highlighted in a review by Michael Marmot who, in this case, looked at two areas of Glasgow. Lenzie, which was rich, and Calton, which was poor (socially deprived). Rich man, poor man. The findings were stark:

"...we can see this in Glasgow. When we published the report of the WHO Commission on Social Determinants of Health (CSDH) in 2008, I drew attention to stark inequalities in mortality between local areas of Glasgow: life expectancy of 54 for men in Calton, compared with 82 in Lenzie." [77]

A difference in life expectancy of 28 years for men, living only a few miles apart. Stick that in your Qrisk3 and see what happens. Of course, not all the difference was due to CVD, but a great deal of it was.

The next issue here is that social deprivation, although it is more directly associated with CVD than postcode, still can't kill you, at least not directly. A huge finger does not point down from the sky in Calton, Glasgow, whilst a god-like voice intones from above, *'because thou livest in Calton, thou are poor, and I shall strike thee down with a heart attack... Whereas, those living in Lenzie shalt be spared my wrath. For they are terribly nice people, with well mowed lawns, good credit scores, and reasonable sized TVs – considering the size of their living rooms.'* Crackle of thunder and lightning etc.

Which means that you must move down a layer or two to reach the point where this association becomes something closer to causation. When you do this, it becomes obvious that living in deprived areas makes people far more likely to suffer from such things as: psychosocial stress, loneliness, depression, or severe mental illness.

They are also more likely to smoke and drink, become obese and take drugs, and suchlike.[78] These are the things that kill them.

Moving on from postcode. Other factors on the Qrisk3 list, that are only associated with CVD, include:

- Diagnosis of erectile dysfunction

- Angina, or heart attack in first degree relative under the age of 60

- High BMI

- Atrial fibrillation

- Total cholesterol/HDL ratio

- Sex

Erectile dysfunction (ED) (as mentioned earlier) is caused by endothelial damage, and low nitric oxide. Therefore, it is not a cause of CVD. Instead, it is a result of CVD.

Angina, or heart attack in first degree relative under the age of 60 is not a cause. Again, a big finger does not point down from the sky, striking down people who are related to other people with CVD. There must be some mechanism of action. At least, in part, this will be related to such things as postcode and social deprivation, and smoking.

High BMI (body mass index) is associated with diabetes, and diabetes causes CVD. Which means that BMI is simply a marker for other causal factors. Yellow fingers once more.

Atrial fibrillation increases the risk of strokes by causing blood clots to form within the atrium – upper chamber of the heart – before being ejected and getting stuck in an artery in the brain. The mechanism is completely different to atherosclerotic plaque formation and arterial blockage. It should not really be on this list. It should be on another list completely. But we are currently stuck with it. I suppose this is because a stroke is an important a form of CVD, whatever the underlying cause.

Total cholesterol/HDL ratio is a metabolic sign of underlying insulin resistance. This, in turn, is a sign of diabetes, and it is the diabetes that causes CVD. Yellow fingers again.

Sex... different. Vastly complicated. Why do men suffer more CVD than women? The cause(s) are difficult to disentangle, but the difference is not due to sex hormones, nor watching '*Say yes to the dress*.' Sorry, a pet hate of mine. Sorry, darling daughter, but it really is...

Anyway, in my rather vain attempt to keep things as short as possible I turned to Qrisk3. But, as you can see, even with such a relatively modest list, the complexity multiplies rapidly. We have causes, and associations, and things that are caused *by* CVD, and things that have nothing much to do with CVD, at least not directly, and on and on.

However, lying within the Qrisk3 'pile of stones' there are several and important causes of CVD, and these are the ones I am going to focus on. Although teasing them apart remains tricky as they are, once again, often closely related. For example, '*severe mental illness*' and, '*on atypical antipsychotic medicine*'. You might well struggle to find one, without the other.

Real 'causes' of CVD

Given all these provisos, and codicils, and sub-clauses, here they are, the Qrisk3 causes that I am going to focus on are:

- Smoking

- Diabetes

- Raised blood pressure

- Chronic kidney disease

- Rheumatoid arthritis

- Severe mental illness

- Systemic lupus erythematosus (SLE)

- On atypical antipsychotic medication

- Using steroid tablets

- History of migraines

I know that there are items on this list that most people will not be remotely familiar with. For example, chronic kidney disease and systemic lupus erythematosus. But there you go. I didn't create this list, but I will be explaining everything in more detail as we go along.

Now, having stripped down Qrisk3 to its component parts, we are left with 10 factors on Qrisk3 that can directly cause CVD. Your mission, should you wish to accept it, is to work out how they do it, and establish how they all fit within the thrombogenic hypothesis. Alternatively, I will do it for you.

Smoking – and other smoky things

Let us begin, at the top, with perhaps the easiest of them all. Smoking. However, if I am going to talk about smoking, I think it is critical to include other 'smoky' things. Which means that I am bringing in other factors such as:

- Diesel particles/car exhaust fumes

- Air pollution

- Wood fires

- Coal mining

- Lead (the heavy metal)

Essentially, what we're looking at here are toxic and very small particles floating in the air than can be inhaled into your lungs. Once in your lungs, they can get into bloodstream, where they create havoc.

I suppose you may be wondering how something you inhale can get into the bloodstream. Did I not say earlier that substances cannot simply leak past endothelial cells, and endothelial cells line your lungs, both on the atmospheric side, and the bloodstream side.

True, however, also remember that in very small blood vessels (and airway vessels) the endothelium becomes porous, or leaky – on both sides, as in a capillary. At the very far end of every airway in your lungs are little sacks, called alveoli. Here is where the exchange of gases takes place. This is also the place where many substances, other than oxygen and carbon dioxide – can freely move from one side to the other. If, that is, they are small enough.

To give you a few examples of molecules that can leak in an out. If you eat garlic, the next day your breath smells of garlic (sort of). If you go on a 'keto' diet, your breath will smell of ketones – small molecules that can escape from the bloodstream and are then exhaled.

Moving in the other direction, nicotine can easily enter your bloodstream after smoking a cigarette. As can viruses, as can many other drugs. Crack cocaine, heroin etc. At one time there was an attempt to launch inhaled insulin – because insulin can be absorbed from your lungs into your bloodstream. This failed, because the amount of insulin that was absorbed was far too variable to establish good blood sugar control.

However, despite the inhaled insulin failure, the message here is that your lungs do not provide anything like a perfect barrier. Things you breathe in, if they are of a sufficiently small size – often called nanoparticles – can cross the endothelium and enter the bloodstream. At which point they can bang up against the glycocalyx and endothelium, with the potential to wreak havoc.

Let's start by looking at cigarettes.

When you light up, a large number of nanoparticles find their way into the bloodstream and attack the endothelium. This damage does not take years to build up, it is virtually instantaneous.

A healthy volunteer, smoking a single cigarette, can kill so many endothelial cells that their remnants can be measured in a blood test. Endothelial cell remnants are called microparticles (MPs). A sudden increase in microparticles indicates that endothelial cells have been obliterated.

The good news for cigarette smokers is that the death of endothelial cells simultaneously triggers the production of brand spanking new endothelial progenitor cells (EPCs) in the bone marrow. So, the repair system kicks in immediately.

For example, a study in volunteers found that:

*"Brief active smoking of one cigarette generated an **acute release of EPC and MPs** (microparticles), of which the latter contained nuclear matter. Together, these results demonstrate acute effects of cigarette smoke on **endothelial, platelet and leukocyte function as well as injury to the vascular wall.**"* [79]

Another study demonstrated that:

*"Vascular dysfunction induced by smoking is initiated by **reduced nitric oxide (NO) bioavailability** and further by the increased expression of adhesion molecules and subsequent **endothelial dysfunction**. Smoking-induced **increased adherence of platelets and macrophages provokes the development of a procoagulant** and inflammatory environment."* [80]

In short, smoking one cigarette instantly triggers at least two of the three 'thrombogenic' processes'. Endothelial damage, and the stimulation of blood clots. Luckily, smoking also stimulates endothelial progenitor cell production (probably due to distress messages released by the damaged and dying endothelial cells). Which means that the repair systems are simultaneously activated.

Obviously, there must come a point where the damage done by heavy smoking starts to overwhelm the repair systems. Where is the point? Unknown, but it is more likely to be reached if a smoker is doing other things that may be toxic to the endothelium.

Unfortunately, smoking is far from alone in wreaking havoc on the endothelium. Vehicle exhaust fumes, wood smoke, or any other very small particles that hang about in the air can have the same impact:

*"There is a **proven link between exposure to traffic-derived particulate air pollution and the incidence of platelet-driven cardiovascular***

diseases. It is suggested that inhalation of small, nanosized particles increases cardiovascular risk via toxicological and inflammatory processes and **translocation of nanoparticles into the bloodstream has been shown in experimental models.**"

As this paper goes on to say: "*This study provides a potential mechanism for the* **increased thrombotic risk** *associated with exposure to ambient particulate air pollution.*"[81]

It is clear that smoking, and inhaling vehicle exhaust fumes, cause CVD through the exact same mechanisms. So does – and I almost hate to say this – wood smoke. I speak as someone with a wood burning stove, and I do love the gentle flames, and the comforting smell, and the malt whisky cradled in my hand, rugby on the television...

Unfortunately, this is also a signal for my endothelial cells to drop dead, whilst my blood gets ready to form a nasty little blood clot somewhere deep inside in a coronary artery. Oh well.

"*Exposure to smoke from wildfires was associated with increased rates of emergency room visits for heart- and stroke-related illness, especially among adults age 65 and older.*"[82]

As is my wont, when I find something that causes CVD, I start to look for other things that are likely to do the same thing, in much the same way. Which is why I decided to look at coal dust inhalation, and coal miners. I found that yes, coal miners are at far greater risk of CVD.[83]

The data here are more complex to analyse, because coal dust particles can often be too large to get into the blood stream, and they get trapped in the lung tissue instead. This leads to pneumoconiosis (chronic lung damage due to coal dust inhalation). Which means that you need to focus on the coal dust '*nanoparticles*'. These are sometimes designated as '*particulate matter 10*' the ones that are small enough slip past the endothelium.

Looking at particles of this size, researchers have induced atherosclerosis in rats, using coal dust inhalation: "Subchronic inhalation of **'particulate matter 10' coal dust induces atherosclerosis in the aorta of diabetic and nondiabetic rats.**"[84]

The relationship between inhaling nanoparticles, and CVD, is almost certainly the reason why a group of UK researchers found that chronic obstructive airways disease (COPD) was the number one risk factor for CVD.

Quick diversion. A short time ago, a group of researchers in the UK decided to study data gathered on 378,256 patients from UK general practices. They were trying to establish which factors were most important in predicting future risk. As you may note, there was only about a 60% overlap with Qrisk3.

The paper was called *"Can machine-learning improve cardiovascular risk prediction using routine clinical data?"* [85]

Here is what they found to be the top 10 risk factors, in order. With number one being highest risk, and number 10 lowest risk:

1. Chronic obstructive pulmonary disease

2. Oral corticosteroid prescribed

3. Age

4. Severe mental illness

5. Ethnicity South Asian

6. Immunosuppressant prescribed

7. Socio-economic-status quintile 3

8. Socio-economic status quintile 4

9. Chronic kidney disease

10. Socio-economic status quintile 2

Prior to reading their paper I had never come across the chronic obstructive pulmonary disease (COPD) association before, and for a while it rather stumped me.

How can chronic lung disease possibly cause CVD, I thought to myself? Then, in one of my regular forehead slapping moments, the answer became blindingly obvious. Chronic lung disease represents long term lung damage.

Chronic = developing or going on for a long time.

Obstructive = the lungs are damaged, thickened, full of 'lesions' and the airways are narrowed and obstructed.

Pulmonary Disease = disease of the lungs.

If you have long term lung damage, it is a sign that your lungs have

113

been under constant attack by unpleasant and damaging substances for years. Many of these substances will inevitably have been entering the bloodstream, attacking the endothelium – for years.

Which means that the relationship here is not that chronic lung disease causes CVD, not directly. What we have here, once more, is an association. By which I mean that inhaling toxic substances for decades will cause both chronic lung disease and CVD.

Looked at in this light, chronic obstructive pulmonary disease is the 'yellow fingers' of smoking. Although, in this case, chronic lung disease is a serious disease in its own right.

Then, just to make things even more confusing. If your lungs have become damaged, they are likely to become considerably more 'leaky.' This will result in more toxic substances being able to enter the bloodstream. In this way chronic lung disease, in its later stages, can also become a more potent cause of CVD.

In retrospect I should not have been remotely surprised that chronic lung disease is one of the most potent risk factors for CVD. Once you think about it, it would only have been surprising if it hadn't.

The final item I am going to look at here, with regard to inhaled nanoparticles, is lead – the heavy metal. Lead, like most heavy metals, is highly toxic stuff. It also tends to linger in the body for years, decades even. Usually hiding in the bones, and gradually being released from bones into the bloodstream. Our bodies are not very efficient at clearing out heavy metals. Although in time they will go. Mostly.

Years ago, people had a wide variety of sources from which to get lead into their bodies. Water from lead pipes, lead paint, lead pencils, toy soldiers (of which I had many), other children's toys – great for sucking... Over the years, lead has been slowly been removed from the environment. However, for more than half a century, one of most important routes into the body was through inhalation.

"[Lead] Exposure occurs through various ways like inhalation, ingestion or skin contact. Direct contact of lead or lead-based compounds through the mouth, nose, eyes and through cracks of the skin may also increase lead levels. **In adults, about 35–40% of inhaled lead dust is deposited in the lungs and about 95% goes into the bloodstream."** [86]

At one time, car exhausts pumped out hundreds of thousands of tons of lead into the atmosphere, and we all happily breathed it in.

Unhappily, it helped to kill hundreds of thousands of people. As highlighted in this Lancet study *"Low-level lead exposure and mortality in US adults: a population-based cohort study."*

*"Our findings suggest that, of 2-3 million deaths every year in the USA, about **400,000 are attributable to lead exposure**, an estimate that is about ten times larger than the current one."* [87]

Four hundred thousand deaths in the US, each year! That definitely deserves the first exclamation mark in this book. I read somewhere that exclamation marks are a bit passé, so I try to avoid them.

Which means that all those smiling happy oil executives, who informed us for decades that putting lead in fuel was not a health problem, may not have been telling us the truth, the whole truth, and nothing but the truth. They may, indeed, have been lying little shits!!! Yes, I know!

Most of those deaths were from CVD. Around 250,000 per year. I must admit that when I first looked at these figures, I thought... can this possibly be right? One sixth of all deaths attributable to lead... blimey. Quarter of a million CVD deaths a year due to lead. Blimey, again, as they say.

You would imagine this to have made headlines around the world. Lead toxicity causes more deaths, per year than, say, 1,000 plane crashes, and that's in the US alone. Hold the front page. How much noise did this 2018 study make? Silence was the stern reply.

This was not just a one-off, outlier. Other studies have confirmed that lead toxicity can increase the risk of CVD death by more than 700%. Once you reach this level of increased risk, even in an observational study, you are looking directly at a cause. [88]

How does lead cause CVD? Yes, it's the same old culprits as before. Reduced nitric oxide production, and increased blood clotting:

*"Lead causes endothelial dysfunction by binding and inhibiting endothelial nitric oxide synthase and **decreasing nitric oxide production**."* [89]

*"These results suggest that **lead exposure can provoke procoagulant activity in erythrocytes...contributing to enhanced clot formation**."* [90]

So, although they may seem completely unrelated, cigarettes and lead can both lead to CVD through precisely the same basic mechanism. As can inhaling diesel/exhaust fumes, or woodsmoke.

Of course, other heavy metals and other pollutants, can cause the same problems, but few have had the ubiquity of lead. Everyone ingested, and breathed in lead, from childhood to adulthood. The land close to roads remains saturated with it. Today, it is beginning to clear from bones and blood, and brains and, to keep the 'b' theme going, roadside bushes.

Yet, despite the obvious damage that it causes, have you ever heard it mentioned in relation to CVD, even in passing? Does it appear on any of the risk calculators? The short answer is no. The long answer is also... no.

Yet, ironically, it is one of the risk factors – a true direct *causal* risk factor – that you can do something about. Sorry for jumping ahead of myself a little here. Later, I will discuss a treatment that can reduce the risk of dying of CVD by around 50% (relative risk), simply by reducing the amount of lead in your body. As proven in a randomised controlled clinical trial. Gold standard stuff.

At this point I feel the need to fly a kite, which is the following: Could lead have been a highly significant, yet hidden factor, responsible for some of the unexplained patterns of CVD?

For example, the US was the first country to fill the atmosphere, and the wider environment, with lead from fuel. It was also the first country to suffer a sharp increase in CVD. Other countries such as the UK, Australia, and Western Europe then followed.

Now that lead has been removed from toys, and lead-pipes, and paint, and most households, and more recently has been completely removed from fuel, the rate of CVD is falling, and falling.

I am not suggesting that lead can explain every pattern of CVD in every country. Not by any manner of means. After all CVD rates began to fall in the US almost two decades before lead was removed from fuel – although it was being removed from lead pipes, children's toys, paint and suchlike long before then.

However, I strongly believe that lead, and other pollutants, must have played a significant role in the rise or fall of CVD in many countries. A role that is never mentioned.

As a post note, whether vaping will prove to cause the same problems as smoking is not yet known. My own belief that inhaling any microparticles into the lungs – via smoke or not – may well prove to be a problem.

Despite this, my general view of vaping remains, at present, that inhaling vapour has got to be better than sucking on a burning stick and drawing the result of that combustion into your lungs. But you never know, maybe, from a heart disease perspective, it will turn out to be worse.

Diabetes

As with smoking, and other smoky things, diabetes is a major player in the CVD game. Mainly because so many people have diabetes, and the numbers appear to be inexorably rising. At the time of writing, there are around 5 million people with diabetes in the UK, and 35 million in the US.

The reality is that diabetes harms far more people than this. Because the increased risk is not restricted to those who have received a formal diagnosis. The damage starts long before that point is ever reached.

With diabetes you are not perfectly well on Monday, and then suddenly ill and diagnosed with diabetes on Friday. Diabetes (type 2 diabetes) is a condition of slow progression. Moving from completely normal, through various stages, to the final diagnosis. Something that can take years, decades even.

To explain how this progression works, it is perhaps easiest to think of diabetes as a condition of gradually worsening insulin resistance. By insulin resistance I mean a state in which – for various reasons – the insulin you produce begins to work less and less effectively, due to 'resistance' to its actions.

Why does this happen? This is far too complicated to get into in this book, but a triad of 'stress', high carbohydrate intake, and abdominal obesity are very much to the fore.

Whatever the underlying cause, as insulin resistance gets worse the beta-cells in the pancreas (the cells that synthesise insulin) need to produce ever more insulin to keep the blood sugar under control. Eventually, the resistance becomes too great, and the sugar level breaks free.

Which means that the direction of travel towards diabetes is, broadly, as follows.

- **Stage one**: Blood sugar levels are normal all the time, insulin levels are higher after a meal – as insulin is having to battle harder to keep sugar levels down.

- **Stage two**: Blood sugar levels are somewhat raised, but only after a meal. Insulin levels are now higher all the time – as insulin is battling even harder and starting to fail at mealtimes.

117

- **Stage three**: Blood sugar level peak after a meal and are now also raised (somewhat) between meals, insulin levels even higher.

- **Stage four**: Type 2 diabetes is diagnosed as the blood sugar level breaks free. Insulin levels can often fall at this time, as insulin gives up the fight, the term 'burnt-out' insulin secretion is sometimes used.

However, because insulin is never routinely measured, the first two stages are not normally picked up. It is only when the sugar levels begin to climb that the underlying problem is finally revealed.

All of which means that, long before type 2 diabetes is formally diagnosed, you will have been suffering from raised blood sugar levels. The levels will have been spiking after a meal, and this will have been going on for years.

This state is increasingly referred to as 'prediabetes'. A disease concept now heavily promoted by the pharmaceutical industry who, quelle surprise, have a drug for that. Actually many, very expensive drugs for that. Kerrching!

In this case, maybe they have a point.

Because people with prediabetes have a greatly increased risk of CVD, which is very nearly as bad as people with overt type 2 diabetes. Unfortunately, they will almost certainly be blissfully unaware that they have a problem.

This means that the total number of people 'at risk' is far higher than the number of people formally diagnosed. There are at least as many people with prediabetes, as diabetes. Possibly more.

How does diabetes/prediabetes cause CVD? (I will just call everything diabetes from now on). Here are some of the mechanisms. You will have begun to recognise them by now:

- Reduced nitric oxide synthesis.[91]

- Endothelial damage.[92]

- Increased blood coagulation.[93]

- A reduction in circulating endothelial progenitor cells.[94]

Unfortunately, with diabetes, the damage does not end here. A high blood sugar (hyperglycaemia) can create a whole series of additional, major health problems. This is because it damages the glycocalyx. The slippery protective layer, covering your endothelium.

This effect was highlighted in the paper with the catchy title: *"Loss of endothelial glycocalyx during acute hyperglycemia coincides with endothelial dysfunction and coagulation activation in vivo."* (In vivo means in a real live person, not just in vitro – in a test tube).

"Hyperglycemia is associated with increased susceptibility to atherothrombotic stimuli. The glycocalyx, a layer of proteoglycans covering the endothelium, is involved in the protective capacity of the vessel wall. We therefore evaluated whether hyperglycemia affects the glycocalyx, thereby increasing vascular vulnerability...

*"In the present study, we showed that the glycocalyx constitutes a large intravascular compartment in healthy volunteers that can be estimated in a reproducible fashion in vivo. More importantly, we showed that **hyperglycemic clamping elicits a profound reduction in glycocalyx volume** that coincides with **increased circulating plasma levels of glycocalyx constituents like hyaluronan**, an observation that is consistent with the release of glycocalyx constituents into the circulation."* [95]

When the blood sugar level spikes, the glycocalyx is stripped off. So much so that fragments of it e.g., *hyaluronan* can be found floating about in the blood.

This is bad news for the larger arteries, leading to atherosclerosis. However, it is even worse for the small blood vessels such as the arterioles and the capillaries, as these are also lined with glycocalyx.

Damage to these blood vessels is called microvascular disease (MVD). Micro vessel disease looks nothing like large vessel disease, primarily because there is no room for an atherosclerotic plaque to develop. It would be like a snake swallowing an elephant.

Instead, you get other types of blood vessel destruction. This can be seen most clearly when looking into the back of the eyes. Here the blood vessels are laid out for inspection – on the retina.

Visible problems include:

- Microaneurysms (capillary wall dilation/ballooning)

- Haemorrhages (rupture of arterioles and capillaries)

- Hard exudates (deposits of various materials as a result of leakage)

119

- Cotton-wool spots (accumulations of axoplasmic* debris caused by poor capillary blood flow).[96]

Essentially, with microvascular disease, the micro vessels block up, balloon, leak, then burst apart. This severely reduces blood flow to key parts of organs, where it is most needed. Such as the Bowman's capsule in the kidney, or nerve cells in the arms and legs, or the blood vessels in the eyes.

Which is why micro vessel disease drives a whole series of additional major complications. which include:

- Neuropathy – damaged neurones, leading to loss of feeling in hands and feet etc. (Also, cognitive problems, including Alzheimer's/depression etc)

- Nephropathy – damage to the kidneys

- Retinopathy – damage to eyes and loss of eyesight

This combination of large and small vessel disease also has a major impact on reducing blood flow in the limbs, especially the feet. This means that small abrasions can turn into ulcers, which are at risk of breaking down and becoming infected. Small cuts can also fail to heal, becoming another site for infections.

In the end, micro vessel disease can lead to tissue breakdown, necrosis and gangrene. In the most extreme cases limbs may have to be amputated. Indeed, diabetes is by far the most common reason for limb amputations.

If that wasn't bad enough, a further problem is that, because there are fewer 'micro' channels for the blood to flow through, the overall 'peripheral resistance' to blood flow increases. This, in turn, means that the blood pressure must rise to force the blood through those arterioles and capillaries that remain. The hypertension that results then goes on to multiply all the other problems associated with diabetes.[97]

This deadly combination of large and small blood vessel disease, with all the downstream health problems, means that diabetes is leading to a major health disaster. The cost of managing diabetes is

---

* Axoplasm refers to the material inside neurones. If you find axoplasmic debris, it means that neurones are dying, or dead.

now estimated at £14 bn in the UK, and $300 bn in the US. Yes, the US pays far too much for healthcare.

The good news is that there are simple ways to bring your blood sugar under control – that have nothing to do with taking drugs.

Raised blood pressure

Just to start by giving you a quick refresher on blood pressure. In arteries the blood pressure is primarily created by the pumping of the heart. The highest pressure occurs when the heart is contracting. Then, when the squeezing stops, the blood pressure falls. It does not reach zero before the heart contracts again. Which means that the blood pressure oscillates up and down like a wave.

The highest pressure reached is called the systolic blood pressure (systole = contraction of the heart). The lowest pressure, as the heart refills, is called the diastolic blood pressure (diastole = relaxation of the heart).

Which is why the blood pressure is reported as two figures. Highest (systolic) and lowest (diastolic). Normal adult blood pressure is around 120/70 mmHg. By which I mean it rises to a max of 120 mmHg and falls back down to a minimum of 70 mmHg.

The measurement used is calibrated in mmHg = millimetres of mercury, which is a very arcane thing indeed. It means the height that a column of mercury that can be pushed up inside a glass tube, by the pressure of blood in the artery. Hg is the chemical symbol for mercury by the way, in case you were wondering.

One hundred and twenty millimetres of mercury is equivalent to about nine feet of blood. Which is the height to which the blood would spurt, if you punctured a large artery and nothing got in the way. You can perhaps see why mercury, a very dense liquid compared to water, was used. A nine-foot-long sphygmomanometer would have been a bit cumbersome to cart around.

Moving away from the systemic arterial blood pressure. The blood pressure in the lungs, the pulmonary circulation, is much lower. It is around 20/8 mmHg – max.

The pressure in the veins is lower still, at around 6 mmHg on average, although it can be much higher in your ankles when you are standing upright. There is only one figure used here, because the pressure in the veins does not go up and down with the beating of the heart.

That's the basics.

When it comes to CVD these are the key points that follow on:

- Atherosclerosis never (naturally) develops in any vein

- Atherosclerosis only very occasionally develops in the pulmonary circulation (usually only if the blood pressure is raised, a condition known as 'pulmonary hypertension')

- Atherosclerosis regularly develops in the systemic arteries

It is also important to mention that the most common places for plaques to develop are where the arteries branch and divide. These points are called bifurcations, like branches on a tree.

Knowing this I think it can be confidently stated that for plaques to develop, you need a sufficiently high blood pressure, and the impact of this 'sufficiently high' blood pressure will be magnified at the bifurcation points. The branch points.

In my mind's eye I view an artery as white-water river, rampaging down a mountainside. Then hitting a fork in the river. Boulders getting turned over by the sheer force of the water as it hurtles past.

Whereas I think of a vein as being the same river as it turns into a delta, approaching the sea. Meandering, slow moving, oozing gently through flower-covered flatlands. In a vein, the endothelium is sitting on a boardwalk by the riverside, leaning back on a comfy chair, fishing rod in hand, a bottle of Jack Daniels nearby. No stress, just nice and relaxed. A tune plays on the radio.

Sittin' in the mornin' sun

I'll be sittin' when the evenin' comes

Watchin' the ships roll in

Then I watch 'em roll away again

I'm sittin' on the dock of the bay

Watchin' the tide, roll away

I'm sittin' on the dock of the bay

Wastin' time...

Meanwhile, upstream, in the artery, a plucky endothelial cell is gritting its teeth, clinging on, arms burning with the effort, as a maelstrom crashes over it, trying to strip it off.

In the background an orchestra sits, determinedly head down, hammering through the Ride of the Valkyrie. Above, bolts of lightning shatter across a darkening sky. The conductor stands high on a craggy peak, manically thrashing his arms in a desperate attempt to keep the orchestra under control.

Perhaps a little overdramatic? A touch too Gothic. Well, if you sit too long at a computer, writing about CVD, the laser focus begins to waver at times. Anyway, the general point stands. Endothelial cells in the arteries are under immense 'biomechanical stress.' Endothelial cells in veins… are not.

Thinking such things, my mind tends to wander off and ask questions such as. Where in the body would you find the greatest biomechanical stress on the endothelium? *The* point of absolute maximum battering.

Well, my thoughts turned to heart itself, then I considered the valves in the heart. Then my attention turned to the heart valve that sits at the top of the left ventricle. This is called the aortic valve, because it forms the one-way barrier between the left ventricle and the aorta (Figure 11).

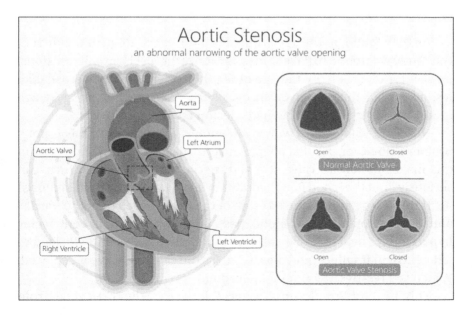

Figure 11

The left ventricle is by far the most powerful of all the chambers in the heart. When it contracts, it blasts open the aortic valve and blood hammers past. Then, when it relaxes, the aortic valve slams violently shut. This valve is certainly 'Under pressure' – to quote Freddie Mercury. And the endothelium sitting on top is also under pressure.

I cannot think of any place in the body where the biomechanical forces will be greater. Nor where the stresses on the endothelium could be exceeded. So, I had a look to see what goes on here.

I need to mention that the three 'cusps' that make up the aortic valve are so thin that you are never going to develop a conventional atherosclerotic plaque here, because there is simply no room for it. However, you could/should see signs of things that look pretty much like atherosclerosis. And, indeed, you do.

Here, from a study called "*Atherosclerosis-like lesions of the aortic valve are common in adults of all ages: a necropsy study.*" (Necropsy means, after death. It is kind of difficult to study the aortic valve in life. It just won't stay still for long enough).

"Conclusions: Atherosclerosis-like lesions in the aortic valve are prevalent in adults of all age groups, including young subjects aged 20–40 years, suggesting that the disease process leading to aortic stenosis is common, often beginning in early adulthood." [98]

As they found, in the age group 41 to 60, every single individual in this study was found to have some degree of atherosclerotic-like lesions, on at least one cusp. By the age of 60, there were atherosclerosis-like lesions on all three cusps... in everyone. Even in the youngest age group, 20-40-years old, 80% had a lesion on at least one cusp.

Not that I want this to worry you unduly. For most of us this is not a problem. However, in some people, severe calcification can build up, and this makes the entire valve stiff and rigid (stenotic). This, in turn, can seriously limit the blood flow, a condition known as 'aortic valve stenosis'.

If this does happen, the left side of the heart needs to pump harder and harder to force the blood past. This leads to left ventricular hypertrophy (heart muscle enlargement) which will eventually lead to left ventricular failure, and death. Unless the calcified valve is replaced. Which is a relatively common operation.

This inexorable build-up of 'atherosclerosis' on the aortic valve, from an early age, provides inarguable evidence that biomechanical stress is probably the most important factor required for atherosclerotic plaques to develop. Without it, as in the veins, nothing happens, no matter how many other risk factors are present. With it, as on the aortic valve, atherosclerosis – or a version thereof – always develops, in everyone.

Now, that all seems very nice and simple. Raised blood pressure (hypertension) increases the risk of CVD by creating biomechanical stress, leading to endothelial damage. Therefore, if we lower the blood pressure, all will be well...

I would like to say that the story is that simple and ends there. Unfortunately, it does not. There is a nagging problem here, which is as follows. Whilst it is easy to see how high blood pressure can increase the risk of CVD, it is rather more difficult to work out what causes the blood pressure to rise in the first place.

Unremarked by almost everyone in the medical profession, a very large elephant exists in the room of high blood pressure. Which is the fact that, in over 90% of cases, the cause of hypertension is unknown.[99] There is also no known cure. All that you can do is to take drugs to lower the blood pressure. (Well, you can do other things, such as lose weight and take exercise, but the medical profession likes drugs best).

Hypertension of no known cause often has the fancy title 'essential hypertension'. This may sound like an impressive diagnosis, and it does a good job of camouflaging the elephant. However, if you translate essential hypertension into plain English, it simply means... 'raised blood pressure of no known cause.' Elephant now in full view.

Which means that, with hypertension, we have a 'disease' with no known cause, or cure. In the UK nearly 13 million adults have been diagnosed with hypertension.[100] That would be around 100 million in the US. In the whole wide world – probably a billion. I may be guessing a bit about the entire world, but I don't think I can be that far out.

You would hope that with a condition affecting more than a billion people, a little more effort would be made to find out what causes it. It would also be nice to know how to cure it, not simply find ever more complex ways to lower it.

So, what is going on here?

What's going on here is that we have, yet again, a complicated situation. Which is that one of the primary underlying causes of hypertension is often... CVD itself.

How on earth can CVD cause hypertension you may ask? Well, as I mentioned in the section about diabetes, if the micro vessels start to block, and break, the total peripheral resistance increases – this is the resistance in the smaller blood vessels, which goes up when the blood vessels narrow, or reduce in number. To maintain blood flow, the blood pressure must rise – and it does.

In much the same way, if the larger blood vessels develop plaques, this too will restrict blood flow to the vital organs. To keep blood flow up, the blood pressure must rise, and it does.

Some organs have considerably more influence on the blood pressure than others, and if the blood flow to them drops, they can then act. The kidneys, for example, pretty much boss the blood pressure. If blood flow to a kidney falls, this will be immediately noted at kidney HQ central, and the kidney will start to release hormones specifically designed to force the blood pressure back up.

The main hormones involved in this process are renin, aldosterone and angiotensin. They make up the renin aldosterone angiotensin system (RAAS). When this system is triggered, it constricts the blood vessels, the kidneys also keep a tight hold of water and sodium, which increases the blood volume. These actions, and many others, drive the blood pressure up.

This adaptive mechanism can be seen very clearly in a condition called renal artery stenosis. Here, an artery supplying blood to a kidney (renal artery), is narrowed (stenosed). The kidney will object mightily to the lack of blood flow. It activates the RAAS system, and the blood pressure rises throughout the body.

If the artery is opened up again, the kidney stops objecting, the hormones are no longer released, and the blood pressure drops back to normal. In short, here we have a perfect model where a narrowed artery causes the blood pressure to rise, by reducing flow to an organ. Open up the artery, and the blood pressure falls.

A similar process can be seen in the pulmonary circulation. There are times when deep vein thromboses (DVTs) can form in your legs, then break off and travel up into your lungs, passing through the right side of the heart – yes straight through the valves. Which always sounds a bit horrible. They can also, occasionally get stuck – which is even more horrible.

Unfortunately, just to confuse things, when they hit the lungs, these thrombi change their name and become pulmonary emboli a.k.a. blood clots in the lungs.

Question: When is a thrombus not a thrombus?

Answer: When it becomes an embolus.

Assuming the thrombus/embolus doesn't kill you, it is now stuck in the lungs, where it can significantly reduce blood flow. Some people develop multiple thrombi, which further restricts blood supply. At which point the control systems force the right side of the heart to pump harder, to overcome the resistance.

To begin with, the right side of the heart will cope, in large part due to the heart muscle getting thicker and stronger, a condition known as right ventricular hypertrophy (RVH) – as opposed to the left ventricular failure caused by aortic stenosis. With the heart pumping more forcefully, the blood pressure in the lungs rises, leading to pulmonary hypertension.

"Chronic thromboembolic pulmonary hypertension (CTEPH) is the end result of persistent obstruction of the pulmonary arteries by acute or recurrent pulmonary emboli... In a recent prospective study, 3.8% of 314 consecutive patients who presented with acute pulmonary emboli developed symptomatic pulmonary hypertension within 2 years." [101]

So, not that common. However, it happens often enough to provide further proof of concept. Block a renal artery and the pressure rises. Block enough arteries in the lung and the pressure rises. Clear away the blockages, and the blood pressure immediately drops.

Which means, in turn, that atherosclerotic plaques/narrowed arteries are almost certainly one of the most important causes of hypertension. Of course, as with everything in this world, complications to this simple model then immediately set in. Primarily because the high blood pressure caused by plaques can then go on to accelerate the development of more plaques, which creates a self-reinforcing loop. A positive-negative feedback loop.

Sorry, if you wanted nice simple answers and straightforward causal chains, they are not to be found here. What can you do about essential hypertension? I will come to that.

Chronic Kidney Disease

Moving on to the next item on the list, we come across chronic kidney disease (CKD). You've probably never heard of it, but it is the bane of most doctor's lives in the UK. We must search for it, monitor it – and then find that there is bugger all we can do about it.

Diagnosing chronic kidney disease sometimes seems about as useful as saying to someone that, I have diagnosed that you are getting older, and you are therefore going to die rather sooner than someone who is younger. Next! This is because kidney function gradually worsens, in everyone, as they age.

However, as it currently stands, we have a situation whereby around about seven million people in the UK have been formally diagnosed with chronic kidney disease, and 40 million in the US. Which makes it difficult to ignore.

At this point you may be wondering if there is anyone alive without high blood pressure, high LDL levels, diabetes, prediabetes, or chronic kidney disease or something else equally scary.

The answer is no, not really, and if the 'experts' keep lowering the targets required to make a diagnosis of these conditions then the answer will soon be... no-one at all. But never mind, there are drugs you can take – forever – to control these conditions... Kerching!

So, what exactly is chronic kidney disease? Here is the definition from Kidney Care UK

"Chronic kidney disease is a very general term used by healthcare professionals to indicate that our kidneys are damaged, diseased or not functioning correctly, and have been that way for a while."

Well, what do you know? Chronic kidney disease is a condition where there is long standing disease of, or damage to, the kidneys. Really. Or, to quote my daughter. Reeeeeely. Thanks Einstein.

Moving on from that rather pointless circular definition. What is the underlying problem in chronic kidney disease? It is primarily a loss of nephrons, which are the functional unit of the kidneys.

You have about one million nephrons per kidney, and it is generally stated that once half of the nephrons have died, chronic kidney disease will be diagnosed. This doesn't make much sense to me, because you can live perfectly well with only one kidney – but we will let that go for now.

Outside of ageing, what else causes long term damage to the kidneys? Diabetes, both type 1 and type 2, are major culprits. I recently saw a 20-year-old girl with very badly controlled type I diabetes. She had severe chronic kidney disease and was remorselessly heading for dialysis. Not good. It must be said that diabetes, and the teenage years, often do not make for a great combination.

*'Mum. Why do I have to monitor my blood sugar all the time and take insulin... it's not **fair**.'*

'Because, darling, if you do not, you will die.'

I suppose it should be no great surprise to find that diabetes causes chronic kidney disease. Because, as already mentioned, it strips away at the glycocalyx, which leads to micro vessel disease. This destroys the small vessels providing blood supply to the nephrons, so they die.

In addition to diabetes, there are several drugs that can damage your kidneys. Painkillers, such as codeine and morphine are regular offenders. Anti-inflammatory drugs such as ibuprofen and naproxen are the most common suspects. Diuretics (water tablets) may also lead to problems. Dehydration, in the elderly, is a major issue.

Just to complicate things further, hypertension will also accelerate chronic kidney disease. Possibly this is the other way around. In truth, as with CVD and hypertension, chronic kidney disease and hypertension feed off each other.

Indeed, with chronic kidney disease, a whole series of factors are swirling around. Diabetes, CVD, hypertension... chronic kidney disease itself. Which makes the entire area very difficult to disentangle. Can it ever be fully possible to know which is causing what? If one of these factors gets worse, it tends to drag the others down with it.

Having said this, it does seem to be the case that, once it has developed, chronic kidney disease can accelerate CVD independently. This is almost certainly because people with chronic kidney disease have seriously impaired nitric oxide synthesis:

"Chronic kidney disease (CKD) represents a world-wide public health problem. CKD is associated with an increased prevalence of cardiovascular (CVD) disease and the relationship between renal dysfunction and adverse CVD events is now well established.

"Earlier studies have reported that NO production is decreased in CKD and multiple mechanisms were found to be involved in causing NO deficiency in these patients.

"Decreased production or reduced bioavailability of nitric oxide (NO) can result in endothelial dysfunction (ED)." [102]

Closely related to this, there is a significant reduction in endothelial progenitor cell production:

"In conclusion, patients with CKD have reduced numbers of circulating CD34+ EPCs [Another, fancier, term for EPCs], *which decrease progressively with advancing disease severity and increasing serum urea levels. EPC dysfunction results in a functional impairment in cell adherence and endothelial outgrowth formation* [endothelial dysfunction]". [103]

This dual attack on nitric oxide and endothelial progenitor cells is why chronic kidney disease can, and does, accelerate plaque development – all by itself.

Rheumatoid arthritis (RA) and systemic lupus erythematosus (SLE) – and other forms of vasculitis

I must admit that I do find it slightly strange that rheumatoid arthritis and SLE are included in Qrisk3. These are both pretty uncommon conditions, affecting around 1 in 100 people each, probably rather less.

In addition, people with either disease will be fully aware of their diagnosis, and they will be in regular contact with specialist doctors. They will also be more than familiar with the health problems that result. Which means that putting them on Qrisk3 seems a bit redundant for the average Joe.

Having said that, for the purposes of this discussion I am delighted that they are on the list. Because the way they trigger CVD can only really be explained through the thrombogenic hypothesis.

Let me start this discussion by introducing you to the term *vasculitis*.

Vasculitis means damage and inflammation to the blood vessels. Vascular = blood vessels; *'itis'* = inflammation. As in tonsill*itis* = inflammation of the tonsils, or appendic*itis* = inflammation of the appendix.

There are many, many different sorts of vasculitis, and they all have impossible to remember names. However, I do love them, as they are so evocative of a bygone era in medicine. Here are several of them, not including systemic lupus erythematosus or rheumatoid arthritis:

- Polyarteritis nodosa

- Waldenström's macroglobulinemia (my favorite)

- Sjögren's disease

130

- Giant cell arteritis

- Behçet's disease

- Buerger's disease

- Churg-Strauss syndrome

- Cryoglobulinemia

- Granulomatosis with polyangiitis

- Henoch-Schonlein purpura

- Kawasaki disease

- Takayasu's arteritis

This is Harry Potter stuff. Wave your wand about and exclaim... *'Vasculitis obliterans!'* Actually, that *is* another form of vasculitis. The reason why they don't all appear on Qrisk3 is because many of them are considerably rarer than hen's teeth. In addition, they are not widely recognised to increase CVD risk – although they all do, if you choose to look.

Apart from increasing the risk of CVD, another characteristic they have in common is that they are also, what are termed as auto-immune conditions. 'Autoimmune' describes the situation whereby the body decides to attack itself.

Besides the vasculitides – what is the real plural of vasculitis anyway? – there are a wide range of different autoimmune conditions. For example: inflammatory bowel disease, asthma, multiple sclerosis, type I diabetes, psoriasis, Hashimoto's thyroiditis etc.

Why does the body decide to attack itself? Well, if you can answer that, you can get a Nobel prize. Probably two, with an additional knighthood, and a few 'hip, hip, hoorahs' thrown in for good measure.

At present all I can say is that, for reasons unknown, the immune system decides that some parts of the body are now 'alien' and must be destroyed. This is what leads to the damage, and resultant inflammation.

If the immune system decides to attack the endothelium, then you get a vasculitis.

A good example of how destructive this can be is with Kawasaki's disease. Kawasaki's normally affects young children, creating a sudden and potent vasculitis that lasts only a few weeks. If it is identified in time, one form of treatment used is antibiotics. So, you would assume it is caused by a bacterial infection. If so, no-one has yet identified the bug. The other mainstay of treatment is steroids – which can damp down the immune attack.

If it is not treated, Kawasaki's can tear away at the blood vessels, causing terrible damage. This includes the formation of major aneurysms (balloon like swellings in an artery). These can then burst, and cause heart attacks. Not quite the same thing as a myocardial infarction, but the effect is pretty much the same – sudden loss of blood supply to heart muscle.

Heart attacks following Kawasaki's can kill children as young as four. Yes, a heart attack... aged four. Or to put this another way. An acute vasculitis can create such severe arterial damage that an aneurysm – normally a very late-stage development in atherosclerosis – can form in weeks. It can then go on to kill a child from a heart attack before they are old enough to go to school.

Moving back to systemic lupus erythematosus (SLE) and rheumatoid arthritis (RA) again. These are not normally grouped under 'vasculitis', although they could be – should be? Because they both cause vasculitis. Systemic lupus far more so than rheumatoid arthritis. (I shall call systemic lupus erythematosus 'lupus' from now on, It saves on the typing fingers).

The condition of vasculitis accompanying rheumatoid arthritis is called *rheumatoid vasculitis*.[104] It doesn't tend to affect the larger arteries – for reasons that are not really understood. Which may be why it only increases the risk of CVD by around 300%.

On the other hand, lupus has a massive impact. Therefore, I am going to focus the discussion here.

"Traditional Framingham cardiovascular risk factors do not account for the entire risk in patients with SLE*, with a shockingly higher risk among patients with SLE after adjusting for the following traditional risk factors: relative risk is 10.1 for nonfatal MI, 17.0 for death due to coronary heart disease (CHD), 7.5 for overall CHD, and 7.9 for stroke."

Presenting them in a more readable way. Here is the increased risk of cardiovascular disease in SLE:

---

* They do not account for any of the risk.

Non-fatal myocardial infarction	= **910%**
Death due to CHD/MI	= **1,600%**
Death from overall CVD	= **650%**
Death due to stroke	= **690%**[105]

If you restrict the analysis to younger women, the problem is astronomical. The increased risk of death from CVD in younger women can reach **4,900%**.[106]

Of course, younger women are not generally at a high risk of CVD, so this relative increase in risk is not as frighteningly dramatic in absolute terms, as it would be in an older male population. However, once you reach 4,900% you are staring straight into the heart of the beast itself.

In this case, the heart of the beast is relatively simple to explain. At least it is, using the thrombogenic hypothesis. Because vasculitis can be seen, most simply, as damage to the endothelium/glycocalyx.

This, in turn, means that blood can become regularly exposed to various clotting factors, such as tissue factor, creating a potential avalanche of blood clots.

'The relationship between inflammation and thrombosis is not a recent concept, but it has been largely investigated only in recent years. **Nowadays inflammation-induced thrombosis is considered to be a feature of systemic autoimmune diseases such as Systemic Lupus Erythematosus (SLE), Rheumatoid Arthritis (RA), or Sjögren Syndrome (SS).** Moreover, both venous and arterial thrombosis represents a well-known manifestation of Behçet syndrome (BS).'[107]

You may notice I threw in a couple of other 'vasculitides' with that quote.

Thus, the greatly increased risk of acute thromboses is the main reason for the very high mortality rate in the younger population with lupus. If you want to know all the potential mechanisms by which lupus can cause blood clots, you can read the article. "*Thrombophilia in Systemic Lupus Erythematosus: A review of multiple mechanisms and resultant clinical outcomes.*" [108]

However, with vasculitis of any cause, not just with lupus, there is more than just acute thrombus formation. There is the greatly accelerated development of atherosclerosis.

"Accelerated atherosclerosis and its long-term sequelae are a major cause of late mortality among patients with systemic lupus erythematosus (SLE)." [109]

Which simply confirms that if you increase the rate of blood clotting on artery walls, you will also accelerate the development of atherosclerosis. Before moving on from vasculitis, there are two more important factors that I want to cover. Hughes' syndrome, and cocaine use.

Hughes' syndrome (antiphospholipid syndrome)

A question that I pondered for some time was the following. Why does lupus cause such terrible problems with CVD – compared to other forms of vasculitis, such as rheumatoid arthritis?

I believe that the answer is because, in lupus, there is often an attack on a specific part of endothelial cell membranes, known as phospholipids. Phospholipids are critically important in keeping the endothelial cell membrane intact. In fact, phospholipids pretty much *are* the cell membrane, the bulk of which is made up of a double layer of phospholipids, back-to-back. There are channels and gates and proteins, and lots of cholesterol as well. As you can see in (Figure 12), where we have a double layer, back to back, of phospholipids with various other structures held within. Gates, channels, proteins etc. Lying in between the double layer is a great deal of cholesterol.

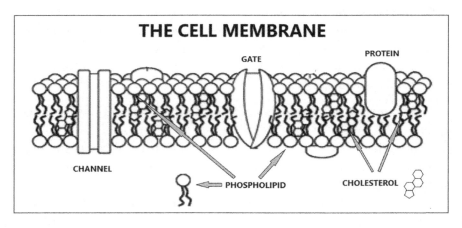

Figure 12

Clearly if you attack the phospholipid membrane, you will damage endothelial cells, and make them leaky, or kill them. This is what

134

happens with a condition known as antiphospholipid syndrome, often called Hughes' syndrome.

Around 50% of people with lupus also have Hughes' syndrome/ antiphospholipid syndrome, and it is this 'double whammy' which makes lupus so damaging.

However, you don't need to have lupus, to suffer from Hughes' syndrome. It can develop all by itself. Even as a stand-alone disease, it greatly increases the risk of strokes, and heart attacks. It is also a common cause of miscarriage. It is often missed in the early stages, and only picked up if someone has a stroke, or heart attack. Or, if a woman has a miscarriage.[110]

"The symptoms of Hughes syndrome are hard to spot, as blood clots aren't something you can easily identify without other health conditions or complications. Sometimes Hughes syndrome causes a lacy red rash or bleeding from your nose and gums. Other signs that you may have Hughes syndrome include:

- Recurring miscarriage or stillbirth

- Blood clots in your legs

- Transient ischemic attack (TIA) (similar to a stroke, but without permanent neurologic effects)

- Stroke, especially if you're under the age of 50

- Low blood platelet count

- Heart attack

"People who have lupus may be more likely to have Hughes' syndrome."[111]

Antiphospholipid syndrome is not listed, as far as I know, as a vasculitis, but in effect, that is what it is. As a footnote, the main medication used in antiphospholipid syndrome is... aspirin (the wonder drug).

Cocaine

Almost the last stop on the vasculitis tour is to look at cocaine.

You may have wondered why cocaine destroys people's noses. The reason is that cocaine is such a powerful inducer of vasculitis that it can obliterate the blood vessels in your nasal septum, which then dies, and disintegrates – vasculitis obliterans indeed.

Unsurprisingly, considering what it can do to the nose, cocaine also causes a major vasculitis throughout the rest of the arterial system.[112] It is most definitely not good stuff to take, as outlined in the paper *"Acute and chronic effects of cocaine on cardiovascular health."*

"Cocaine, compared to other illicit drugs, poses a particular risk for vascular disease and is most involved in emergency room visits, with highest rates for men aged 35–44 years, amounting to a vast social and economic burden. Cocaine-induced damage to the cardiovascular and cerebrovascular systems is widely reported, and is linked with **hypertension, tachycardia, ventricular arrhythmias, myocardial infarction, stroke***, resulting in severe functional impairments or sudden mortality."* [113]

Another paper continues the theme *"Cocaine and coronary artery diseases: a systematic review of the literature"*:

"Moreover, cocaine may promote intracoronary thrombosis, triggered by alterations in the plasma constituents, and platelet aggregation, leading to subsequent myocardial infarction. The long-term use of cocaine may **stimulate atherosclerosis***, probably through* **endothelial cell dysfunction. Significant and severe coronary atherosclerosis is common in young chronic cocaine users** *and there is probably a relationship between the duration and frequency of cocaine use and the extent of coronary disease."* [114]

So, boys and girls, please do not stick cocaine up your nose. First, it destroys your nose, then it destroys your cardiovascular system. You would think that the falling apart of the nose would be sufficient warning of the havoc that cocaine can wreak elsewhere, but hey. Cocaine is cool, man. Unlike dropping dead of a heart attack... man.

However, my main reason for bringing cocaine into the discussion is not as a warning. It is because it is one of those really important things in research. A drug, or agent, that can directly induce CVD/atherosclerosis. This provides direct evidence that if you attack the endothelium, and cause vasculitis, you greatly increase the risk of CVD. Nothing else required.

History of migraines

Migraine, as a risk factor, sits slightly by itself, and the increased risk is so small – in absolute terms – that I considered ignoring it.

However, it forms part of Qrisk3, so talk about it, I shall. In fact, once you start digging down, the links between migraine and CVD are quite fascinating.

As everyone knows, a migraine is a form of headache, often one sided, often very painful, that can be accompanied with an aura – a visual disturbance. Most of us know someone who suffers from migraines, and we know the symptoms can vary greatly from person to person.

The cause? Well, that still remains a matter for considerable debate. However, many researchers believe that the primary underlying cause is vascular. By which I mean irritation/inflammation of the blood vessels in the brain. This can make the vessels dilate, or constrict, leading to the throbbing/pressing pain.

Which means that you could, if you so wished, define migraine as a specific form of vasculitis. To support this idea, here is a short section from a case history on a woman with Crohn's disease (another auto-immune disease), who suffered severe migraines – that were traced back to her vasculitis.

*"A 28-year-old woman with Crohn's disease and known migraine with aura had suffered from daily migraine attacks with recurrent focal neurological deficits for 6 weeks. Cerebral magnetic resonance imaging showed multiple acute, subacute, and chronic ischemic lesions in different vascular territories. Magnetic resonance and computed tomography **angiography demonstrated vessel changes consistent with cerebral vasculitis."* [115]

The paper was called *"Cerebral vasculitis mimicking migraine with aura in a patient with Crohn's disease."*

It has also been found that several other immune diseases can cause a vasculitis and migraine.

Which means that vasculitis can mimic migraine? Or, that it can cause migraine? Perhaps some migraines are caused by vasculitis, whilst others are not, but the association found between migraines and CVD is due to the vasculitis induced migraines? Sorry, I know that is a bit confusing, so read it again if it doesn't make sense. Don't give yourself a migraine doing so.

If you think it is a bit of a stretch to claim that vasculitis causes migraines. Here is a short list of other auto-immune conditions, that are known to cause both vasculitis, and migraines. You may recognise them now:

- Lupus[116]

- Antiphospholipid syndrome[117]

- Sjögren's disease[118]

Looking specifically at antiphospholipid syndrome, migraines are so common in this disease that it has been suggested migraine headaches should be included within the classification of the disease. As discussed in the paper *"Antiphospholipid syndrome (APS) revisited: Would migraine headaches be included in future classification criteria?"*

And so yes, gentle reader, although migraines and the thrombogenic hypothesis may seem a million miles apart. It is actually quite straightforward to bring them together. Here is what an article in the BMJ entitled *"Migraine and risk of cardiovascular diseases: Danish population based matched cohort study"* had to say on the matter:

*"Migraine is associated with ischaemic stroke and ischaemic heart disease, particularly among women and among migraine patients with aura. Potential underlying mechanisms include **endothelial dysfunction, hypercoagulability, platelet aggregation**..."* [119]

The terrible triad emerges, once more.

CHAPTER 5

Sickle cell disease and Avastin (bevacizumab) – a short detour

At this point in the narrative, I am going to take a short detour from Qrisk3 to look at two different stones that I think are extremely important in this tale. In my view, they are potentially the most important stones of all – at least when it comes to the thrombogenic hypothesis.

I searched for them both for a long time. In truth I did not know exactly what I was looking for, but once I found them, I knew. Essentially, I was determined to find *the* disease that was the most potent cause of CVD (I thought I had found it with lupus, but I had not). At the same time, I was looking for *the* drug, the medication, that causes the greatest CVD risk.

I have always believed that it is at the extremes where the answers are most likely to be found. In addition, I reasoned that if two of the most potent causes of CVD could be explained by the thrombogenic hypothesis, then this provided powerful support. Equally, if neither of them was related to the thrombogenic hypothesis, in any way, then what I had on my hands was a dead hypothesis.

I know it may not seem like it, but I have spent considerably more time looking for evidence that contradicts the thrombogenic hypothesis, than I have spent searching for evidence supporting it.

Anyway, the first stone I want to introduce you to here, is a disease that is a direct cause of severe endothelial damage. The second is a drug specifically designed to shut down the endothelial repair processes. Which means that one is damage, the other repair.

Sickle Cell Disease

Whilst looking at pulmonary hypertension in some detail… yes, not the start to a paragraph that gets the pulse racing, but bear with me, I shall start again. Whilst looking at pulmonary hypertension in some detail, I came across a fact so shocking, so unbelievable that it caused my faith in the very nature of science to be shaken to its very core. Better? More gripping?

This fact could upend our very understanding of the nature of the world and everything in it... OK, yes, going over the top now. Start again.

What I found was a disease that can increase the risk of CVD by up to 50,000%. Yes, fifty thousand per cent. And that gets you first prize in *'diseases that are most likely to kill you from CVD'*. Nothing else comes close, not even lupus. Okay, it was just one study that found this astronomical figure, but it still gets first prize from me.

That disease was sickle cell disease.

At this point you might well ask, what on earth sickle cell disease has to do with CVD. If so, perfect, because when you come across a fact like this, one that is able to stop you dead in your tracks, then you know that you are onto something both fascinating and important.

Because it is not just at the extremes where the answers may lie, it is also at the unexpected extremes. Places you never even thought to look. I tripped over the connection between sickle cell disease and CVD whilst looking for something else. Namely, causes of pulmonary hypertension. Sickle cell disease is a cause, by the way.

So, what on earth is going on here, you may think? As did I. Of course, I knew what sickle cell disease was, at least on a superficial level. It is a disease where you have many misshapen 'sickled' red blood cells. They are the shape of a crescent moon, as seen on the flags of Pakistan and Tunisia and Turkey, and suchlike (Figure 13).

Sickle cell disease, in turn, is caused by genetic mutation which, in milder form, can protect against malaria. It makes it more difficult for the malarial parasite to gain entry to red blood cells, which is where the parasite grows and multiplies.

As far as I was concerned, that was about the extent of my knowledge. My excuse for knowing so little is because sickle cell disease is not a major health problem in the UK, certainly not where I trained, Aberdeen in the North East of Scotland. Not too much malaria, and very few migrants up there. A bit too cold for both, I expect. Neither of them would survive a summer before scurrying off to somewhere warmer e.g., the North Pole, in December.

Anyway, why the massive increase in CVD? If I had ever stopped to ponder the matter then I might have asked myself, what is the likely impact of sharp, pointy, sickled cells hammering through arteries at high speed? But I did not. Why not? I suppose, many things are only obvious in retrospect. That's my excuse anyway.

Also, I had no idea that sickle cell disease caused CVD. Neither, it seemed, did almost anyone else. For many years sickle cell disease, in its more severe form, used to be associated with an average life expectancy of around 10 years, even less. Pretty much the last thing anyone was bothered about was death from heart attacks and strokes. No-one with sickle cells disease lived long enough for this to be a problem.

"The life expectancy of patients with sickle cell disease has improved considerably since 1960, when Sir John Dacie described sickle cell disease as 'essentially a disease of childhood.' 'Indeed,' he wrote, 'the mortality is high and relatively few patients reach adult life, even when the standard of medical care is high.' In his 1973 review based on autopsies, Diggs estimated a median survival of 14.3 years, with 20 percent of the deaths occurring in the first 2 years of life, one third occurring before the fifth year of life, half between 5 and 30 years of age, and one sixth after the age of 30." [120]

Average life expectancy is now around 50, maybe even slightly more. Yes, a stunning improvement. Hooray for medicine. However, as people with sickle cell disease have started to live longer, the impact on CVD has become increasingly obvious.

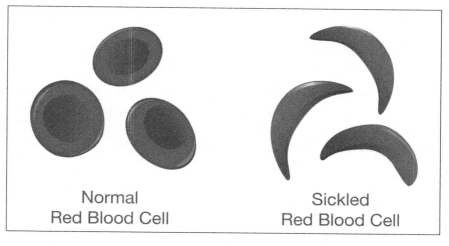

Normal
Red Blood Cell

Sickled
Red Blood Cell

Figure 13

At this point I think it interesting, if tragic, to look a case history of a fourteen-year-old boy with sickle cell disease (SCD).

"A 14 year-old boy was referred to our vascular unit, with gangrene of the right foot. The condition started about 1 year prior to this referral with ulceration of the foot which was treated conservatively. The condition of the foot deteriorated until development of gangrene of most of the foot. The boy is a known patient of SCD. His past medical history revealed right sided stroke when he was 8 years old. His parents have SCD. His brother had also SCD and died suddenly at the age of 5 years."

A stroke aged eight, and his brother died, aged five. This truly is not a nice disease.

As it turned out he had gangrene in the foot because the main arteries in his leg were almost completely blocked by atherosclerosis. Which meant, in turn, that there was not enough blood supply to keep his foot alive.

On further examination, and scans, it was found that almost every single artery in his body was riddled with severe atherosclerosis, with calcification. Calcification, as mentioned a few times before, only occurs at a very late stage in the progression of atherosclerotic plaques.

Which means that we have a 14-year-old boy, with the arteries of a severely diseased 80-year-old. Just in case you were wondering, there were *no* other risk factors for CVD in his case.

*"We report a 14 year-old boy with SCD who developed critical ischemia right foot with **absence** of atherosclerotic risk factors."* [121]

What did the authors themselves think had led to such devastation?

"These lesions were attributed to the rigidity of sickled erythrocytes [red blood cells] causing mechanical injury to the endothelial cells."

There you have it. Rigid, sharp and pointy red blood cells causing mechanical injury to the endothelium. Nothing else needed, no other factor involved.

Others have found much the same thing:

"A recent study of spleens resected from Sickle Cell Disease (SCD) patients... has shown that there were **consistent vascular lesions affecting large arteries**. The*

---

* Spleens are often removed from those with sickle cell disease because they become enlarged and liable to rupture. This means that the arteries in the spleen can be fully examined.

same finding was also shown in studies of brains from SCD patients who developed cerebrovascular accidents (strokes). **These lesions were attributed to the rigidity of sickled erythrocytes causing mechanical injury to the endothelial cells.** *The widespread distribution of the lesions was also suspected in other studies, in which it was suggested that the sickled erythrocyte-endothelial adhesion seen in the microvasculature could be occurring in large arteries and contribute to **large vessel endothelial injury, vascular intimal hyperplasia and thrombosis.***" [122]

Why do I believe that sickle cell disease is so important to the story of CVD? Mainly because, when you are looking at disease causation, the holy grail is to find something that is *'sufficient.'* By sufficient I mean a factor that can cause the disease – all by itself. No need for anything else at all to be present.

In medicine there are very few such factors. Certainly, in the world of CVD, nothing else has ever been found to be 'sufficient'.

However, with sickle cell disease we have one factor, and one only. Sharp, pointy, red blood cells, hammering through the arteries, leading to severe endothelial damage. As you can see, this was sufficient, in the absence of any other risk factor, to destroy the entire arterial system of a 14-year-old boy. In both the systemic and pulmonary circulation… and that is what makes this disease so important.

It is sufficient.

Avastin (bevacizumab)

The other stone I wanted to bring to the table is a drug called Avastin. It has the generic name *bevacizumab*. Avastin was specifically developed to prevent endothelial progenitor cells from being synthesized in the bone marrow, thus blocking the creation of a new layer of endothelium. It also knocks nitric oxide synthesis through the floor.

In short, it pretty much obliterates the endothelial repair systems.

Given what I have written up to now you may be wondering why on earth anyone would be prescribed a drug with such a potentially devastating mechanism of action. Surely Avastin should be banished to the outer darkness?

Not so. It is widely used in cancer treatment. The reason why it is prescribed is that, as solid cancers/tumours grow, they need additional blood supply to provide them with the required nutrients. To achieve this, the tumour hijacks the system specifically designed to create brand spanking new blood vessels.

They do this by manufacturing a hormone called vascular endothelial growth factor (VEGF). This switches on '*angiogenesis*' – literally, the creation of new blood vessels. In this way, cancer cells manage to provide themselves with enough blood, nutrients, and oxygen to keep on growing. The clever little devils.

Clearly, the best way to stop angiogenesis is to block vascular growth factor, and this is where Avastin comes in. It is a vascular endothelial growth factor-inhibitor (VEGF-Inhibitor). By inhibiting vascular growth, it prevents angiogenesis and kills off the tumour. Now you can see why Avastin is used.

Something I found fascinating when researching this area is that Avastin is the offspring of thalidomide. Thalidomide also blocks the formation of new blood vessels. Which is why children born to mothers prescribed thalidomide (at a specific stage in the pregnancy), had such short arms and legs. Without new endothelial cells, the blood vessels could not grow, so the arms and legs could not grow.

Thalidomide is now also used as an anticancer drug, under different names, e.g., Thalomid. I think most patients are blissfully unaware that their cancer drug is actually thalidomide.

Unfortunately, Avastin does not just block the vascular growth factor produced by the cancer cells. It crushes growth factor synthesis throughout the rest of the body. This, in turn, causes a system-wide reduction in both endothelial progenitor cells and nitric oxide.[123]

Anyway, my thinking about Avastin was straightforward. If the thrombogenic hypothesis is correct, Avastin ought to greatly increase the risk of CVD. Mainly by knocking the endothelial repair systems through the floor.

Evidence that this is precisely what happens comes from the paper: *"Cardiovascular Adverse Events in Patients With Cancer Treated With Bevacizumab: A Meta-Analysis of More Than 20 000 Patients."*

"Treatment with bevacizumab increases the risk of arterial adverse events, particularly cardiac and cerebral ischemia, venous adverse events, bleeding, and arterial hypertension. This risk is additionally increased with high doses of bevacizumab." [124]

These risks are not small. If you just focus on strokes and heart attacks, after two years of treatment with Avastin, these were the findings:

Increased risk of stroke = **1,129%**

Increased risk of heart attack = **416%**

At one time, Avastin was nearly withdrawn from the market due to the massive increase in cardiovascular risk. Nowadays an ACE-inhibitor drug (normally prescribed to lower the blood pressure) is prescribed alongside Avastin. ACE-inhibitors stimulate nitric oxide synthesis, and this helps to mitigate some of the worst problems with Avastin.

Anyway, there you have my little detour to look at my two additional stones. Sickle cell disease and Avastin/bevacizumab. I realise that they are of no importance to most people. Sickle cell is rare, and Avastin/bevacizumab is only prescribed to people with specific cancers. However, they both massively increase the risk of CVD, and they can both be linked directly to the thrombogenic hypothesis.

Now, time to move back to the final three items on Qrisk3. At this point everything comes together – I hope.

CHAPTER 6

Steroids, immunosuppressants, antipsychotic medication (and almost everything else) – and cortisol

Here are the last three items on the Qrisk3 list.

- Severe mental illness

- On atypical antipsychotic medication

- Using steroid tablets

In truth I am pretty much ignoring one of them and focussing only on the other two. The one I am virtually ignoring is atypical antipsychotic medication. Because it is, essentially, a subset of severe mental illness and can be dealt with, in passing.

Before getting into greater detail, I want to make it clear that mental illness does not actually need to be that severe. Moderate depression, anxiety, 'stress' (or strain) can be almost as damaging as, say, schizophrenia or bipolar disorder – at least from a CVD perspective.

In addition, because this area can get unbelievably complicated, with many different hormones, and the neurological system all getting involved and swirling about, I am going to concentrate primarily on the actions, and abnormalities, of a single hormone.

Because, in the final analysis, everything I am going to talk about here, from schizophrenia to Australian aboriginals, loneliness, central obesity, diabetes, and social support all circle around this one hormone. Which may seem difficult to believe, but it is pretty much true.

147

The hormone is cortisol. (For those who know their stuff, yes, there is another very closely related hormone called cortis*one* – one converts to the other – I am going to ignore that distinction here).

What is cortisol?

Cortisol is a steroid hormone produced in the *cortex* of the adrenal glands – which sit on top of the kidneys – which is why it is often referred to as a *cortico*steroid. It is called a 'steroid' because it has a steroid backbone. This consists of 17 carbon atoms, arranged in four 'rings'.

This steroid structure acts as a framework for a whole range of other vital substances in our body – including many other hormones, and also cholesterol. The 'rings' are actually three hexagons and a pentagon. A very simplistic steroid structure is shown below in Figure 14.

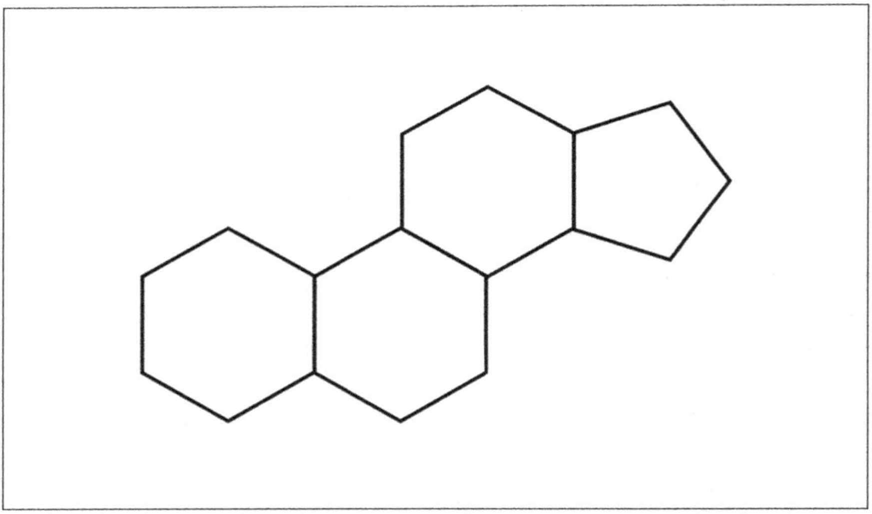

Figure 14

Figure 15 shows the chemical structure of cortisol. You can see that there is a steroid backbone, with oxygen, hydrogen and hydroxyl (OH) groups attached at various points.

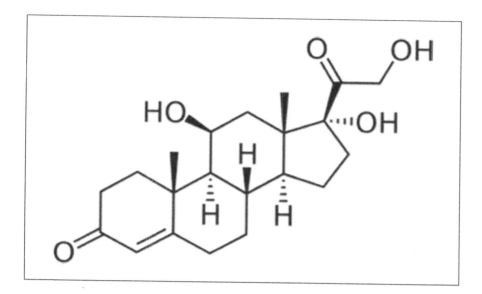

Figure 15

There are many other steroid hormones, but they are usually called something else. For example, oestrogen is another steroid hormone, but it is almost never called that. If the naming system had any logic, oestrogen would be called *ovaro*steroid – or something of the sort. Testosterone is another steroid hormone, made in the testes. But it is not called testo*steroid*, it is called testo*sterone*... sigh.

Leaving the many other steroid hormones to one side, when we talk about the artificial 'steroids' that are used as medications (not the muscle building anabolic 'steroids') they are all variations on the basic cortisol molecule. Which means they can all be called corticosteroids, but mostly they are just called steroids.

(Sometimes, just to increase the complexity, they are called glucocorticoids, because of their effect on raising blood glucose).

The reason for giving you this degree of chemical detail is because I think is important to understand the extremely chemical connection between all steroids and cortisol. As a result of this, they have almost identical adverse effects on the human body.

Just to reinforce how close in structure they truly are, I have included the chemical diagram for a very widely prescribed synthetic steroid called prednisolone (prednisone in the US) (Figure 16). See if you can spot the difference between cortisol and prednisolone... and good luck with that (Clue, look for the different angle).

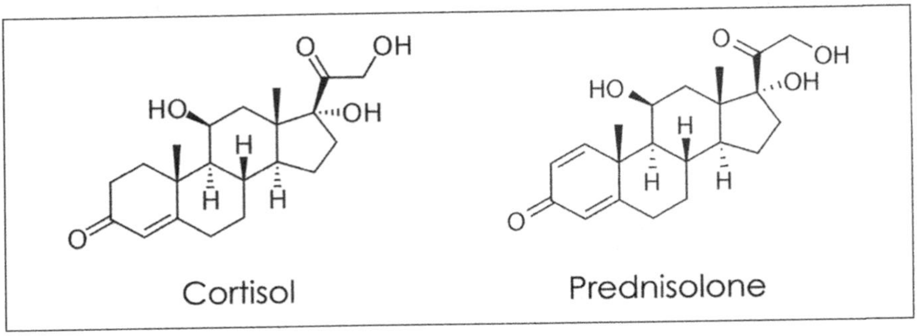

Cortisol   Prednisolone

Figure 16

So, when Qrisk3 lists 'steroid' tablets as a risk factor for CVD this actually means *cortico*steroid tablets. By which they also mean, in essence, cortisol. For the purposes of this discussion, steroids and cortisol are fully interchangeable, and I will be switching between them in a relatively random fashion.

What are the effects of cortisol on the body?

Cortisol has many wide-ranging effects. Looked at from a metabolic perspective, cortisol is the main catabolic hormone. By which I mean that it stimulates the breakdown and release of energy stores. This is the process also known as catabolism.

Cortisol does this, because it is one of the key 'fight or flight' hormones. If you need to run, or fight, then cortisol will make sure you have the energy needed. To achieve this, cortisol stimulates the synthesis and release of glucose from the liver (glucogenesis). It also chops apart proteins, various bits of which are then used to make more glucose for quick energy use.

In addition, cortisol drives the release of 'fat' stores in subcutaneous fat (the fat that lies beneath the skin). This leads to an increase in free fatty acids (FFAs) in the bloodstream. When they reach the liver, FFAs are then further broken down into ketone bodies, which are another easy-to-use energy source.

All of which means that, if you are going to have a fight, where all the released energy stores will be used up, then everything is good.

(A good gym session will work just as well). However, if your cortisol levels stay high for prolonged periods of time, all those extra glucose molecules and FFAs that are now sloshing about in the bloodstream cannot be used. Which means that they must find somewhere else to go, and so they do.

What happens in this metabolic state, is that stored energy is moved from subcutaneous fat, and muscle, and redirected into the fat stores, mainly found within the abdomen. These fat stores are known as visceral fat, or omental fat or... as usual there are many different names used to describe exactly the same thing.

Another less scientific name for this is the beer belly. Thin man, thin arms and legs, big round belly. Less often, thin woman, big round belly. Women usually store fat in different places.

A more scientific description of a beer belly is having a high waist-hip ratio (WHR). This is also called central obesity. Whichever of the many, many, many, names you decide to use to describe a build-up of visceral fat, the hormone that drives this body shape is cortisol.

Put in the simplest possible terms, cortisol sucks energy from the periphery and deposits it centrally.

"Cortisol affects fat distribution by causing fat to be stored centrally – around the organs. Cortisol exposure can increase visceral fat – the fat surrounding the organs – in animals. People with diseases associated with extreme exposure to cortisol, such as severe recurrent depression and Cushing's disease also have excessive amounts of visceral fat." [125]

Cushing's disease, mentioned above, is a condition where the adrenal glands produce too much cortisol, day in, day out – for various reasons. Often due to a cortisol-secreting tumour in the adrenal glands – although there are several other causes.

Not only does cortisol make you fat in the middle, it also makes you insulin resistant, because cortisol is a direct antagonist to insulin, at all sites of action. Which is hardly surprising. Insulin is the main anabolic hormone – anabolism means energy storage. On the other hand, cortisol is the catabolic hormone. Therefore, cortisol and insulin slug it out.

This system wide battle can lead to severe insulin resistance which, as mentioned earlier, is the main underlying cause of type 2 diabetes.

A comprehensive list of the signs and symptoms of excess cortisol, as seen in Cushing's disease, is listed on the National Institute of

Diabetes website:

- Weight gain

- Thin arms and legs

- A round face

- Increased fat around the base of the neck

- A fatty hump between the shoulders (buffalo hump)

- Easy bruising

- Wide purple stretch marks, mainly on the abdomen, breasts, hips, and under the arms

- Weak muscles

- And the main complications…

- Heart attack and stroke

- Blood clots in the legs and lungs

- Infections

- Bone loss and fractures

- High blood pressure

- Unhealthy cholesterol levels (this means total cholesterol to HDL ratio)

- Depression or other mood changes

- Memory loss or trouble concentrating

- Insulin resistance and prediabetes

- Type 2 diabetes [126]

This is far from the end, there are other direct links from Cushing's disease to CVD. Perhaps the most important is that cortisol suppresses nitric oxide synthesis which, as you know, raises blood pressure. It is also highly toxic to the glycocalyx and endothelium.[127] In addition to this, cortisol stimulates the production of clotting factors in the liver, creating a pro-coagulant state.[128]

I could go on, listing more and more problems, but I think you get the general idea. High cortisol levels are extremely bad for you. The most obvious external sign is usually central obesity. A beer belly. A high waist-hip ratio.

Given the metabolic catastrophe that can be caused by excess cortisol, you may wonder why on earth anyone would prescribe steroids to anyone, for anything. The answer is that cortisol – and the many steroids that are based on it – are the most powerful immunosuppressants known.

There are a whole host of auto-immune diseases, some of which I have mentioned before. Crohn's disease, rheumatoid arthritis, asthma, eczema, lupus etc. etc. These are conditions where the body decides to attack itself. Steroids can virtually eliminate this wonky immune response.

Why does cortisol possess this potent action? I don't really know. What are the possible survival advantages to dampening down a system that was designed, in large part, to attack and kill infective agents? I have never seen a satisfactory explanation, and believe me, I have looked. But there must be one. The body does nothing without a reason.

When artificial steroids were first synthesized, they appeared to be miracle drugs for terrible conditions such as rheumatoid arthritis, or Crohn's disease. A few hefty doses, and auto-immune diseases simply melted away. Steroids also became the cornerstone of drug therapies used in organ transplantation. This is because they stopped the host immune system from attacking the transplanted organ.

Hoorah... Nobel prizes all round. But then the iron rule of life took over. *'If it seems too good to be true, it is.'* Over longer periods of time, the massive doses of steroids that were used in the early, heady days, started to cause terrible health problems. Patients became very unwell, and many died.

One of the reasons for this was a massive increase in the risk of all kinds of infections. Small cuts failed to heal and turned into cellulitis and gangrene. Minor chest infections became pneumonia. Urine infections spread through the body causing sepsis – and suchlike. Yes, the immune system does have its uses.

Patients also began flinging blood clots off in all directions, then dying of strokes and heart attacks. In addition, many of them ended up with diabetes. Furthermore, skin, muscle and peripheral fat started to waste away, whilst people developed central obesity and buffalo humps. Blood pressure went through the roof – and suchlike.

Here is a section from a recent *New York Times* article, on steroids, which pretty much sums up most of the downsides.

"In addition to weight gain, side effects may include high blood pressure, deteriorating bones that can result in osteoporosis, diabetes, thinning of the skin, muscle weakness, moon face (caused by increased fat deposits, which may also occur in the stomach, chest and upper back), cataracts, glaucoma, ulcers, easy bruising, increased sweating, acne, arterial deposits that can lead to heart disease and, because of their effect on immunity, delayed healing of wounds and an increased risk of infection that can persist for a year or more after the medication is stopped." [129]

Yes, steroids are very much a double-edged sword. Brilliant, but deadly. I suppose I should mention at this point that there is, at least, a five-fold increase in deaths from CVD with Cushing's. [130]

The increased risk with synthetic steroid use is much the same:

"Patients prescribed systemic glucocorticoids who developed iatrogenic* *Cushing's syndrome had nearly a **three times greater risk of cardiovascular disease**, including coronary heart disease, heart failure, and cerebrovascular disease than patients prescribed glucocorticoids who were not known to have developed a cushingoid appearance. **This risk increased to over fourfold** in comparison with people not prescribed glucocorticoids."* [131]

Despite these very serious downsides, steroids are still very widely prescribed because, in many cases, the benefits outweigh the harms. Hundreds of millions of people use steroid inhalers in asthma, very safely. The dose of inhaled steroids is far too small to create a major problem. Steroids creams rule the world of eczema treatment, just be careful about thinning the skin. Oral steroids remain the backbone of treating many autoimmune diseases. Used with caution or intermittently.

Abnormal cortisol levels and mental illness

So, where have we got to. Well, it should be clear that cortisol/steroids can cause CVD, and exactly how this happens. However, I suppose you

---

* Iatrogenic means, disease caused by the treatment.

could rightly argue that Cushing's, and high dose steroids, represent extreme forms of 'steroid' exposure. These examples can't really tell us much about less severe problems with cortisol.

A good point, which leads to the next step in the discussion. Can less severe disruptions in cortisol secretion also cause CVD? If so, can these disruptions be caused by mental illness? If so...

In fact, I am going to turn these questions around and start again. Can mental illness cause abnormal cortisol levels? If so, how does this happen.

To answer this, we need to look at the system the body uses to deal with stress in a little more detail. Before starting down this path, I want to make it clear that the word stress is not the right one. Instead, what we are talking about is strain.

- Stress is the external force placed on an object

- Strain is the resultant deformation

Unfortunately, we seem to become trapped using the word stress, now, and forevermore. Which is a pity because the correct word is *strain*. Why is this distinction important? One reason is that we have absolutely no way to measure psychological stress, or stressors. Just to give a quick example of what I mean.

Two people are asked to give a talk to 500 people. The first person is excited, stimulated, and looks forward to it. The second person is filled with fear and dread. Which means that exactly the same stressor – giving a talk – can have an entirely different effect.

Just to complicate things even further, both people may say that the idea of giving a talk is stressful. However, for one of them, the experience is positive, exciting; for the other it is negative, anxiety producing, depressing, so you have no idea if what they are experiencing is positive, or negative.

In short, the word stress tells you nothing of any damned use.

What we need to do, instead, is to focus on strain i.e., the resultant deformation. This, in turn, depends on a whole host of different factors, which are unique to each person. Such as their coping skills, their memories of events, their genetics, their upbringing, their overall resilience, what else is going on in their life at the time etc.

Another reason why we need to focus on strain is that it can be measured. Not perfectly, because strain does not exist on an exactly calibrated scale between one and a hundred. However, it is possible to establish whether the 'strain' system itself has become dysfunctional, or damaged. And the easiest way to do this is to measure the cortisol level.

If your 'strain' system is healthy then your cortisol levels will normally peak just before you get up in the morning, and then gradually fall, until you go to bed. They can also rise and fall during the day, depending on things that happen to you. Eating a meal tends to pop the cortisol level up for an hour or so.

Exercise can also increase cortisol levels, as can giving a talk to 500 people. The main point, and the one that I want to really focus on here, is that cortisol secretion is flexible. It rises to meet demand, then falls when the demand has gone. If that flexibility disappears, this represents a flashing red warning light. It tells you that the strain system has been badly damaged. In the end it will take the rest of your health down with it.

Before moving on to what can cause damage, I need to describe the 'strain' system in a little more detail – even though no-one ever calls it the strain system. So, somewhat reluctantly, I will switch back to use the word stress.

The 'fight' or 'flight' system

Deep within our brains we have an interconnected network of hormones and nerves which coordinates how we react to sudden threats – real or perceived. It is very primitive. It is not under conscious control, and when it fires off, all hell is let loose.

It also reacts very, very, fast. This is because it was designed to save your life, without interference from slow and deliberate conscious thought. If a twig snaps in the forest you have no time to establish exactly what caused it. You just need to run, or fight, or both. You can work out what caused it later. You can laugh it off later.

The system itself comprises two main, interconnected, parts. There is the unconscious, or autonomic, nervous system. Then there is the hormonal part, which consists of several different hormones: adrenaline, nor-adrenaline, cortisol, growth hormone and glucagon. The entire system is sometimes referred to as the 'neuro-hormonal' system.

The actions of the two separate parts, the hormones and unconscious nervous system, are coordinated by the hypothalamus and the pituitary gland (which sit close together in the brain), and the adrenal glands, which site on top of the kidneys. Together, this triad is known as the hypothalamic, pituitary, adrenal axis. Or the HPA-axis for short.

It works, as follows. Under threat, the hypothalamus sends an alarm message to the pituitary gland, which then releases a series of 'pre-hormones' that travel through the bloodstream, mainly arriving at the adrenal glands. These pre-hormones instruct the adrenal glands (and other glands) to release the 'stress' hormones – adrenaline, cortisol, glucagon and suchlike.

Working closely alongside this hormonal response, the hypothalamus sends messages down the spine through the autonomic nerves. These autonomic nerve fibres leave the spine at various points, and become closely intertwined within all our organs, and muscles, and blood vessels... and skin and bladder and bowels.

I feel I need to mention that there are two opposing parts to the autonomic nervous system. There is the sympathetic part – which activates the 'fight or flight' actions – and there is the parasympathetic, which does the exact opposite. The parasympathetic reduces the heart rate, directs blood to the bowels, slows the breathing rate, lowers the blood pressure and suchlike. Essentially it readies the body for relaxation, eating, digesting, anabolism, sex.

If you want, you can think of them this way. The sympathetic and parasympathetic are yin, and yang. Some have termed these two opposing systems 'Fight and flight' or 'Feed and breed'. Which I rather like.

Getting back to the fight and flight part. The sympathetic nerves have many different actions. They speed up the heart rate, they dilate the pupils, and open blood vessels to the muscles to increase blood supply. The respiratory rate increases, the liver produces more clotting factors, the pancreas kicks out more glucagon (to raise blood sugar) and so on and so forth. You are now, to quote the WWE, 'ready to rumble'.

This is all healthy, and normal. Indeed, putting your HPA-axis under extreme stress from time to time can be fun, and exhilarating. It is why people go on roller-coaster rides, and head for the ghost train, or watch scary movies. It is why young men, and to a lesser extent young woman, box, and play rugby, and base jump and – in some cases – climb enormously high vertical rock faces without ropes. Bonkers.

Some people call these things an adrenaline rush, although increasing the adrenaline level is only a small part of what happens when you kick the entire neuro-hormonal system into life. It could be called a cortisol rush, or a glucagon rush, or a sympathetic nervous system rush.

Unfortunately, this can all be far from positive. Activation can be extraordinarily unpleasant. Because sudden HPA-axis activation is the physiological basis of a panic attack. An overwhelming sensation of fear and dread, sweating, cold, clammy, cramping in the pit of the stomach, heart racing, rapid breathing.

It is called a panic attack because the HPA-axis suddenly activates when there is nothing obvious to panic about… no clear danger. Essentially it could be said to trigger itself. This '*HPA-axis hypersensitivity*' is one of the major problems seen in post-traumatic stress disorder (PTSD). A condition whereby the 'fight' or 'flight' system hits high alert at the drop of a hat. Not pleasant.

Anyway, that is a very quick run through the neurohormonal stem system, the HPA-axis, the 'fight or flight' system, the stress system – choose your preferred label. Next, what makes it go wrong?

Mental illness and damage to the hypothalamic pituitary adrenal axis (HPA-axis)

Perhaps the most powerful driver of HPA-axis dysfunction is severe mental illness, and this can be seen very clearly in depression.

"Upwards of 40-60% of depressed patients experience hypercortisolemia [high blood cortisol levels] *or other disturbances of the HPA system."* [132]

This, in turn, leads on to severe insulin resistance, as described in the paper: "*Cortisol dysregulation: the bidirectional link between stress, depression, and type 2 diabetes mellitus.*"

*"Depression is associated with cross-sectional and **longitudinal alterations in the diurnal cortisol curve**, including **a blunted cortisol awakening response** and flattening of the diurnal cortisol curve. Flattening of the diurnal cortisol curve is also associated with **insulin resistance and type 2 diabetes mellitus**. In this article, we review and summarize the **evidence supporting hypothalamic–pituitary–adrenal axis dysregulation as an important biological link between stress, depression, and type 2 diabetes mellitus**."* [133]

Yes, severe depression can actually drive type 2 diabetes. Not a lot of doctors know this, and when I tell them they often don't believe me. Even though the association between mental illness and diabetes was first written about in 1919.

"Kooy noted in 1919 that 'it is a remarkable fact that some persons, who are in

a state of agitation, especially those of a neuropathic condition, show a temporary excretion of sugar.' This condition was referred to at the time as "nervous glycosuria." [134]

Glycosuria = glucose in the urine. You only excrete sugar in the urine when you blood sugar is very high. A condition otherwise known as... diabetes.

Just to cover off the final step in this causal chain. Can depression also cause CVD? Here is an article from Medical News Today on the subject. I chose this quote because I felt that it said it best:

"Heart disease is now the leading cause of death both in the United States and worldwide. Depression, meanwhile, is the 'leading cause of disability worldwide,' as well as one of the most common mental health conditions in the U.S. A significant body of research has established a connection between the two conditions.

"For example, reviews of existing studies have shown that people with cardiovascular disease are more likely to have depression, and people with depression have a higher risk of developing cardiovascular disease.

"Also, those with depression and heart disease are more likely to die from the latter than those who only have heart disease. This relationship is also proportional, meaning that the more severe the depression, the more likely it is that a person will develop heart disease or die from it." [135]

If we move to schizophrenia things get much worse. Schizophrenia is probably the most severe mental illness of all. As with depression, it is closely associated with significant HPA-axis dysfunction. Here, from the review article *"A systematic review of the activity of the hypothalamic–pituitary–adrenal axis in first episode psychosis."*

*"This systematic review highlights that converging evidence exists to suggest that individuals with a first episode of psychosis show **a specific pattern of HPA axis hyperactivity, demonstrated by higher baseline cortisol levels** compared with controls, and a **blunted cortisol awakening response.** Moreover, MRI studies demonstrate that these individuals also exhibit **an enlarged pituitary** in comparison to healthy controls shortly after psychosis onset, supporting HPA axis hyperactivity in this sample."* [136]

I find it fascinating that schizophrenia can cause an actual physical, structural difference within the brain. In this case, the pituitary gland enlarges.

The association between schizophrenia and CVD is also hugely significant.

159

"Although patients with schizophrenia are 10 to 20 times more likely than the general population to commit suicide, more than two thirds of patients with schizophrenia, compared with approximately one-half in the general population, die of coronary heart disease (CHD). The chief risk factors for this excess risk of death are cigarette smoking, obesity leading to dyslipidemia, insulin resistance and diabetes, and hypertension." [137]

You may not think that two thirds, instead of a half, is that much of a difference. However, you must bear in mind that many of those with schizophrenia commit suicide, which accounts for a tragically high proportion of deaths. This then leaves a much smaller population left to die from CVD. Which means that two thirds figure is, actually, extraordinary. It includes almost everyone who does not commit suicide.

At this point I shall take a quick detour to cover atypical antipsychotic medications. These drugs are, essentially, newer generation drugs used (mainly) to help control and treat schizophrenia. So, I think they fit here.

The reason why they add to the increased CVD risk in Schizophrenia (and other serious medical illness) is that they directly worsen insulin resistance. In the article *"Metabolic Syndrome and Mental Illness"* the authors called this 'adverse metabolic effects.'

"Patients with major mental illnesses such as schizophrenia and bipolar disorder have increased risks of morbidity and mortality compared with the general population, with a 25- to 30-year shorter life span due primarily to premature cardiovascular disease (CVD) [e.g., myocardial infarction (MI)], *stroke). Key modifiable risk factors that contribute to excess morbidity and mortality include cardiometabolic factors, such as overweight and obesity, dyslipidemia, diabetes, hypertension, and smoking. Although these risk factors are present within the general population, epidemiologic data suggest that patients with major mental illnesses have an increased prevalence of some or all of these risk factors. Treatment with psychotropic medications, including second-generation, or atypical, antipsychotic medications, can also be associated with adverse metabolic effects."* [138]

By adverse metabolic effects, they mean insulin resistance. This can lead to frighteningly rapid weight gain. Anyway, I think that ties off atypical antipsychotic medications, as found in Qrisk3. They can cause insulin resistance. They can also cause massive weight gain.

160

The last condition I want to look at here at is bipolar disorder. Here is a short passage from the paper: *"The relationship between bipolar disorder and type 2 diabetes: more than just co-morbid disorders."*

*"***Type 2 diabetes mellitus (T2DM) rates are three times higher in patients with bipolar disorder (BD), compared to the general population***. This is a major contributing factor to the elevated risk of cardiovascular mortality, the leading cause of death in bipolar patients... **Patients with BD and T2DM have a more severe course of illness** and are more refractory to treatment. Control of their diabetes is poorer when compared to diabetics without BD... **Physicians need to be aware of the increased risk for T2DM and cardiovascular disease in bipolar patients**, and appropriate prevention, screening, case finding, and treatment is recommended."* [139]

When it comes to severe mental illness, wherever you look, whatever parameters you chose to look at, the process repeats itself. Mental illness causes HPA-axis dysfunction, this leads to abnormal cortisol secretion, followed by insulin resistance/type 2 diabetes – then a greatly increased risk of CVD.

Less severe mental illness – psychosocial strain

At this point I think it is time to step down the severity of mental illness. Although we are now looking at much lower levels of mental 'strain', the increased risk of CVD remains extremely high.

The first condition I want to cover is post-traumatic stress disorder (PTSD). You may not feel that PTSD should be defined as a *less* severe mental illness. It can certainly destroy health and happiness. However, I feel it is not as damaging as, say, schizophrenia, severe depression and bipolar disease.

Leaving that argument aside, can we see the same causal chain in action? The first thing to say is that the evidence linking HPA-axis disruption to PTSD can be conflicting. However, there is no doubt that PTSD can lead to significant structural brain abnormalities.

"There is almost no area of the brain that is not directly or indirectly affected by the stress or trauma impact. The field of neuroimaging has made tremendous advances in the past decade and has contributed greatly to our understanding of post-traumatic stress disorder (PTSD). Recent neuroimaging investigations have shown significant neurobiological changes in PTSD. The areas of the brain that are different in patients with PTSD compared to those in

control subjects appear to be: hippocampus, amygdala, and prefrontal cortex. **The amygdala appears to be hyperreactive to trauma-related stimuli.** *The hallmark symptoms of PTSD may be related to a failure of higher brain regions to dampen the exaggerated symptoms of arousal and distress that are mediated through the amygdala in response to reminders of the traumatic event."* [140]

The amygdala is considered the emotional centre of the brain. It never forgets good experiences. Unfortunately, it never forgets bad experiences either. It is also stimulated by situations of danger and fear. In super-short version, the amygdala is the place in your brain where your emotional responses to various situations are generated – and it retains your responses – seemingly forever.

Following major trauma, the amygdala can become hyper-reactive, and it also sits right next to the hypothalamus, and it cross-talks with it. Often firing threat messages at the hypothalamus. *'Hey, you remember that noise, yes that's the noise you heard just before you were ambushed in Iraq and half your mates were killed.'* Panic! Now!

In PTSD the hypothalamic pituitary adrenal-axis itself may not necessarily be damaged, or dysfunctional. Instead, the amygdala has become 'hyperreactive', sending fear and threat messages directly to the hypothalamus.

Which may be why research into HPA-axis dysfunction and PTSD has been mixed. It is not the axis that has been damaged, it is just being constantly triggered into action by the amygdala.

Having said this, many studies have seen a clear connection, such as this one *"Bouncing back – trauma and the HPA-axis in healthy adults."*

"Dysregulation of the hypothalamic–pituitary–adrenal (HPA)-axis is thought to underlie stress-related psychiatric disorders such as posttraumatic stress disorder (PTSD). Some studies have reported HPA-axis dysregulation in trauma-exposed (TE) adults in the absence of psychiatric morbidity." [141]

On the other hand, there is certainly no argument that PTSD can increase insulin resistance.

"...insulin resistance was 'significantly higher' in participants with PTSD vs controls, including elevated fasting glucose and fasting insulin... Participants with PTSD also had a significantly higher frequency of **metabolic syndrome** **(21.3% vs 1.3%; P <.005)."** [142]

A 15-fold increase in metabolic syndrome with PTSD... Metabolic syndrome is a term I have not really talked about so far, but I cannot avoid it forever. Sorry, yet another explanation required.

Perhaps the simplest way to think of metabolic syndrome is as 'prediabetes'. In fact, increasingly it *is* called prediabetes. Although it has been called several other things over the years:

- Insulin resistance syndrome

- Syndrome X

- Reaven's syndrome

Whatever name is used, Metabolic syndrome is, essentially, a less extreme form of Cushing's syndrome. It has been defined in many ways, but I quite like this super-short summary from the paper "*A comprehensive definition for metabolic syndrome.*"

"In summary, the central features of the metabolic syndrome are insulin resistance, visceral adiposity, atherogenic dyslipidemia and endothelial dysfunction." [143]

I hope you will have come to recognise those four features by now. The four horsemen of the CVD apocalypse. Maybe it is best to think about it in the following way. Metabolic syndrome is Cushing's disease *Lite*.

Moving back to PTSD. Apart from causing the metabolic syndrome, it upsets the sympathetic nervous system in many other ways:

"The authors found evidence that PTSD leads to overactive nerve activity, dysfunctional immune response and activation of the hormone system that controls blood pressure [the renin-angiotensin system]. *'These changes ultimately contribute to the culmination of increased cardiovascular disease risk,' the authors wrote."* [144]

All of which means that, even when we step down the severity of mental illness, the impact on CVD is pretty much the same. Terrible.

Cartesian Duality – fibromyalgia

I think it is beyond any reasonable doubt that psychological trauma can, and does, damage the HPA-axis. Indeed, in schizophrenia it is even possible to measure changes in its physical structure, such as an enlarged pituitary gland.

Unfortunately, any discussion of this area runs straight into what is possibly the most formidable, and implacable barrier in medical thinking. I hesitated as to whether or not to mention it, but I felt that it was too important to remain silent. Given the impact it has had on medical thought, and research.

The barrier here is cartesian duality, named after René Descartes. *'I think, therefore I am.'* Yes, that French philosophy chap. A great brain, no doubt, but he inadvertently created a vast iron curtain, which drapes itself across any discussion about how feelings and emotions can be terribly damaging to our physical health.

Cartesian duality is, essentially, the concept that there is the mind, and there is the body, and never the twain shall meet. Although most doctors would deny they perceive illness in this way, it is clear that a great deal of western medical thought has been built upon Cartesian Duality. Especially when it comes to accepting any possible connection between psychology and physiology. The mind and the body.

According to this essentially 'reductionist' medical philosophy, the body is a complex machine made up of millions of interconnected biochemical processes. A billion tiny levers, if you like. Once we can understand how all the levers function, and how their connections fit together, we can understand exactly how the body works. This even includes all mental illnesses.

For example, using cartesian/reductionist thinking, it has been decreed that depression is caused by a lack of a specific neurotransmitter in the brain, called serotonin. Which means that if we want to treat depression, we give a drug to increase serotonin levels, and all is well. Job done. As for bipolar disorder:

"Bipolar disorder is widely believed to be the result of chemical imbalances in the brain. The chemicals responsible for controlling the brain's functions are called neurotransmitters, and include noradrenaline, serotonin and dopamine. There's some evidence that if there's an imbalance in the levels of 1 or more neurotransmitters, a person may develop some symptoms of bipolar disorder.

"For example, there's evidence that episodes of mania may occur when levels of noradrenaline are too high, and episodes of depression may be the result of noradrenaline levels becoming too low." [145]

Of course, it is true that there are biochemical disturbances to be found within the brain, with mental disease – although no-one has really managed to measure this phenomenon to any degree of accuracy. Even if they exist, do these biochemical disturbances come before, or after things went wrong? By which I mean, for example, do chemical imbalances cause depression, or are they caused *by* depression.

In addition, where does the mind itself fit into this? Is our brain simply a biochemical computer? This is certainly what the neuro-psycho-pharmacologists would have us believe. It is also very much what the pharmaceutical companies would wish us to believe. Because, if there is a biochemical pathway, there is usually a drug to influence it in some way. Money, money, money.

But where are our thoughts, our fears, and expectations in all this? Where do we include the interactions we have with others, our social life, love, caring and kindness? Yes, you are quite right, they are nowhere.

Where is the possibility that, for example, someone could die of a broken heart?

If you think that sounds utterly ridiculous, then you may be surprised to know that it is entirely possible to die of a broken heart. The condition where this occurs is called Takotsubo syndrome. It happens when extreme emotional upset leads to severe cardiac damage up to, and including, death.

"Takotsubo cardiomyopathy is a temporary heart condition that is brought on by stress. It has the same symptoms as a heart attack but is not caused by any underlying cardiovascular disease.

"It is also known as stress cardiomyopathy, apical ballooning, or broken heart syndrome. Takotsubo cardiomyopathy most often affects women between the ages of 61 and 76 years. The condition commonly occurs immediately after experiencing extreme emotional or physical stress." [146]

How serious can it get? Bad enough that your heart muscle can tear apart. Here is a short section from a study looking at Takotsubo Cardiomyopathy (TCM).

*"Due to devastating complications of TCM, our case highlights the need for close monitoring of patients with TCM for the first few days. Special consideration should be paid to older female patients as they have higher rates of **cardiac rupture**."* [147]

Cardiac rupture. A heart literally ripped in two. Which means that, when people say they are heartbroken, they can really mean it. The heart can actually... break. Entirely due to serious psychological upset.

I use this example simply to highlight the fact that our physical health can be massively affected by our mental health. I have occasionally argued that our brains are simply too big. If they go wrong, if our thinking goes wrong, this can kill us – actually, physically, kill us. Bang, dead.

It can be sudden, as with Takotsubo cardiomyopathy. Or, it can take years to have an effect. For example, chronic anxiety and depression leading to HPA-axis dysfunction, then the metabolic syndrome, then CVD.

However, the point that I am trying to make here, hopefully with some success, is that there is no such thing as Cartesian duality. It is just a way of compartmentalising thinking about illness. Easy, but wrong. You cannot just separate the mind from the body.

One condition where the mind and body interact in perhaps the most complex and difficult to disentangle way is with fibromyalgia. This is a diagnosis that goes in and out of favour as in – is it a real thing? Or is it a physical, or psychological condition? Or is it simply a form of prolonged mental distress?

The truth is that fibromyalgia is a real thing, even if it is extremely difficult to pin it down. However, there is little point in trying to tease it apart, because it is an entangled physical and a psychological condition. Here is what the Mayo clinic has to say about fibromyalgia.

"Fibromyalgia is a disorder characterized by widespread musculoskeletal pain accompanied by fatigue, sleep, memory and mood issues. Researchers believe that fibromyalgia amplifies painful sensations by affecting the way your brain processes pain signals.

"Symptoms sometimes begin after a physical trauma, surgery, infection or significant psychological stress. In other cases, symptoms gradually accumulate over time with no single triggering event.

"Women are more likely to develop fibromyalgia than are men. Many people who have fibromyalgia also have tension headaches, temporomandibular joint (TMJ) disorders, irritable bowel syndrome, anxiety and depression." [148]

Fibromyalgia often follows a history of childhood physical and sexual abuse, and PTSD. You can look all these things for yourself, they are easy to find. As you might have worked out for yourself, fibromyalgia is also closely associated with HPA-dysfunction and the metabolic syndrome.

It is also linked to abnormal cortisol secretion, as outlined in the paper *"Fibromyalgia syndrome is associated with **hypo**cortisolism"* (low cortisol levels).

"Patients with FMS (fibromyalgia syndrome) had significantly lower cortisol levels during the day, most pronounced in the morning. As expected, FMS patients reported more pain, stress, sleeping problems, anxiety, and depression.

"Conclusion: The results lend support to the hypothesis of a dysfunction in the hypothalamus-pituitary-adrenal axis in FMS (fibromyalgia syndrome) patients, with generally lower cortisol values, most pronounced upon awakening."

In the end it doubles, at least doubles, the risk of CVD.[149]

Unfortunately, the treatments for fibromyalgia are almost entirely used to help with the physical manifestations of the condition. This means painkillers... for the pain. Then anti-anxiety drugs... for the anxiety. Then there is amitriptyline, or duloxetine, or gabapentin... also for the pain. Then sleeping tablets... for the insomnia. Then beta-blockers... also for anxiety. And on and on.

In fact, if I see the diagnosis of fibromyalgia in the notes, I can usually write their drug chart out in my head. Strong painkillers, including some form of opioid, such as morphine, or a fentanyl patch. Paracetamol, codeine/tramadol, then a whole serious of other painkillers for 'neuropathic' pain, diazepam (or some other anxiety drug), propranolol and on, and on.

Indeed, these make up, what I call, my drugs of doom. This is because, any patient on two painkillers (especially tramadol), amitriptyline, diazepam, gabapentin, an anti-depressant, and a sleeping tablet is, frankly, doomed.

They are almost never going to get off them, and any new symptom they complain of is simply battered down with a new, more powerful, addictive drug. Or an increased dose of anti-depressant – probably two combined. Maybe three if you are lucky. Special bonus if you are prescribed venlafaxine – the *'final throw of the dice'* antidepressant.

I was recently looking after a woman with a diagnosis of fibromyalgia. Apart from all her other drugs of doom she was on two grams of a slow-release opioid daily. A normal dose of this powerful painkiller would be 10 milligrams – or 10 one thousandths of a gram.

She was on 200 times that dose, each day. It had been stepped up and stepped up over the years as her tolerance increased. If I gave you, dear reader, two grams of a slow-release opioid then you would be dead within 30 minutes – max.

This is cartesian duality at its most damaging. I know, as far as I can know anything, that the underlying cause of her symptoms was severe psychological strain. I can only speculate as to the cause, because she would not, could not, accept that her problems were anything but physical. *'Are you saying it's all in my mind!'* Outrage, anger, upset. Yes, it's not just doctors that cling desperately to cartesian duality.

This lady was willing to take doses of drugs that would fell an elephant, rather than admit any psychological explanation for her problems. She was also extremely scary, and the nurses usually left her room with their tails firmly between their legs having been angrily shouted out for some terrible crime. Not stirring her tea anti-clockwise, or something.

Over the years her doctor(s) had played along with this increasingly desperate and angry game, treating each symptom as a real, physical thing. Until, inevitably, the treatment had become far worse than the underlying disease. In her case 10 horribly addictive drugs, piled one on top of each other. With an elephant felling dose of opioid to finish things off.

The reality for her, and many others, is that what happens in your mind, if it goes wrong, can destroy you. Often through the pathway of HPA-axis dysfunction, then CVD. Unfortunately, Cartesian duality places a mile-high barrier in thinking about disease in this way. This is just *'Woolly nonsense. Find me a proper, easy to measure biochemical pathway that I can alter with a drug, or please remain silent.'*

When you look at it without any preconceptions, it is clear as day that a high burden of negative psychological 'stressors' can be horribly damaging, often fatal. What are these negative stressors? Here is long, but non-exhaustive list:

- Childhood neglect

- Battlefield trauma

- Bullying boss/general bullying

- Financial collapse/financial worries

- Job insecurity

- Racism

- Lack of social support

- Being at the bottom of the social hierarchy

- Lack of control in work – or in life in general

- Loneliness

- Abusive partner

- Childhood physical or sexual abuse

- Living in a violent neighbourhood

- Forced relocation/migration/immigration

Of course, these things all tend to swirl and interact with each other. Anyone who works in social care, education, the police, or medicine, will know that there is a large, vulnerable underclass in this world. People, even entire extended families, who find life extremely difficult, and who would tick several items on the list above. In some cases, all of them. They are not easy to deal with.

Such people struggle, rage, drink, self-harm, take drugs, and do a hundred unhealthy things a day. They don't tend to respond well to authority – to put it mildly. They don't want life to be this way, but for them – it is. Not fair, a hundred times unfair, but there you go. Who said life was ever fair? Certainly not me.

Politicians talk about initiatives to improve social mobility, and I give a short, hollow, laugh. Have they *any* idea what life is like for those at the bottom of the heap. Have they ever been in a council house where the floorboards have been broken up and used to keep a fire going in the winter? The money saved to be spent on drugs and booze instead?

The baby burned with an iron because he wouldn't stop crying? Children cowering in the corner, battered and broken. I don't suppose many of the children brought up in such environments will make it to Oxford, or Cambridge, or Harvard or Princeton. Many of them are doomed to replay the disastrous childhoods they suffered as children. Some escape, most don't.

I believe that this, the combined burden of 'psychosocial stressors' is the most important single factor in causing CVD. Of course, it is never one factor, it is many factors that can combine and multiply in hundreds of different ways. I suppose you could say that psychosocial strain truly is multifactorial. Or all due to postcode?

I also believe that entire populations, even entire countries, can be scoured by psychosocial strain. For example, Lithuania.

Lithuania social upheaval and CVD

No, I did not stick a pin in a map blindfold and hit Lithuania. That would have been tricky, as Lithuania is extremely small. In fact, there are two main reasons for starting with this country:

- The data are fascinating

- There have been well conducted studies comparing Lithuania with other countries, specifically looking at HPA-axis dysfunction.

It is with some embarrassment I must admit that, at one point, I dismissed the data from Lithuania. This was because the rate of death from CHD went up and down so quickly that I assumed the figures were nonsense. I had never seen such a pattern anywhere else, ever, at least not at that time.

Below, in Figure 17, is the graph of the deaths from CHD in Lithuanian men under the age of 65, from 1981 to 2009 – I stopped at 2009 because nothing much happened after that, and x-axis started automatically doubling the years – which was annoying.

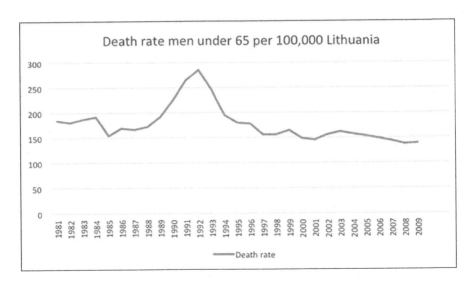

Figure 17

These data come from EuroHeartStats, based on MONICA. I have found them to be fully reliable.

Below, in Figure 18, is another graph, from the same source. This is the death rate for men in the UK, from CHD, under the age of 65.

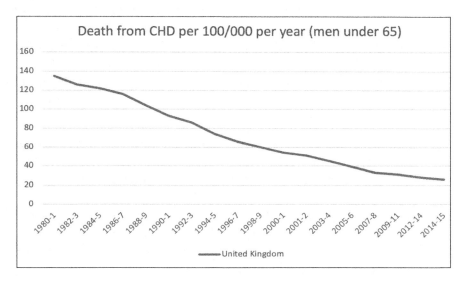

Figure 18

Compare and contrast, as they say. Both countries started in roughly the same place. By 1992 the rate of CHD in Lithuania was nearly four times as high as the UK.

So, what on earth happened in Lithuania, I thought. Then, I slapped my forehead repeatedly. 'Look at the dates, you numbskull'. Yes, as you may have noticed, the rate of CHD took off in 1989, the same year as the Berlin Wall fell.

In my defence, many people, including me, have almost forgotten that there was such a thing as the Soviet Union. The Berlin Wall now consists of a billion tiny fragments, often polished up and displayed on coffee tables as conversation pieces. The whole thing was celebrated by a truly terrible Europop song '*The winds of change.*' Shudder.

Whether or not you remember these events, this was the year when the Lithuanians revolted, the 'singing revolution'. There was massive social upheaval. Jobs were lost, savings trashed, the tanks rolled in from Russia, killed protestors, then rolled out again – along with almost all Soviet investment. Of all the soviet states, Lithuania suffered particularly badly:

"The immediate economic consequences of transformation were significant falls in gross national product. For example, between 1990 and 1993, real GDP had declined in Lithuania – 18%, Ukraine – 10%, Russia – 10.1% and Tajikistan – 12.2%. The first ten years of transformation was a period of great social disruption and chaos. The introduction of a market system of exchange led to a severe decline in gross domestic product, contraction of the labour market, and unemployment leading to social malaise including a rising death and suicide rate." [150]

I am writing this during COVID19, and you may be able to see why I am concerned about trashing the UK economy with lockdown. The economy, and health, are not two separate things. They are extremely closely overlapping and interconnected things.

Anyway, getting back to Lithuania, in a fortunate aligning of the planets a study was done comparing men in Sweden and Lithuania. The researchers were trying to work out why Lithuanian men had four times the CHD death rate of Swedish men.

The study ran from 1993 to 1995. It missed the Lithuanian peak by two years, when the difference would have been nearly seven-fold. Still, they got close to the perfect timing. Whether by luck or good judgement I have no idea.

The study itself was called LiVcordia, looking at men living in **Li**nköping in Sweden and **Vi**lnius in Lithuania. The purpose of the study?

*"In recent decades coronary heart disease (CHD) mortality has declined in Western Europe and increased in Central and Eastern Europe. **A large difference in CHD mortality has developed and the causes are not known.** Lithuania and Sweden had similar CHD mortality rates for middle-aged men twenty years ago but in 1994 this mortality was four times higher in Lithuania than in Sweden. Also within countries **CHD mortality is higher in low socioeconomic groups.**'*

What did they conclude?

*"**Conclusions:** Thus, based on our survey on risk factors for CHD, it can be stated that **traditional risk factors seem not to explain the different***

172

*CHD mortality rates between Lithuania and Sweden. **Possible alternative explanations are psychosocial strain** and oxidative stress. These factors were also found among men in underprivileged groups within the cities. Therefore, the **influence of the risk factors studied may be relevant also for socioeconomic inequalities in CHD mortality within countries.***"

('Seem not' in a scientific paper can be translated as 'do not'. It is a way of not upsetting the other experts too much).

I am happy to report that these researchers also looked specifically at HPA-axis dysfunction, and cortisol secretion. What they found was that men in Lithuania had higher baseline levels of cortisol. However, critically, when they were exposed to a 'stress' test, their cortisol level barely moved. In contrast, Swedish men showed a rapid rise, then fall.

*"Baseline cortisol levels were higher in Vilnius than Linköping. Cortisol rise with stress was **four times higher** for Linköping than Vilnius."*

This lack of response to a 'stress-test' is an extremely powerful signal. It represents a burnt-out HPA-axis. As the researchers themselves put it, Vilnius men demonstrated:

*"An unfavourable pattern of psychosocial risk factors for CHD: **job strain, social isolation, depression and vital exhaustion characterised Vilnius men, who also showed an attenuated cortisol response to the laboratory stress test.** This stress response has earlier been shown in states of chronic stress; loss of dynamic capacity to respond to new demands may be a predisposing factor for disease. **Vilnius men had more peripheral atherosclerosis; thicker intima media, more and larger plaques and greater** (arterial) **stiffness."** [151]*

Which means that, in this study, we have the pathway fully in place.

Psychosocial strain → HPA-axis dysfunction→ a four (to eight) fold increase in the risk of CHD.

These causal connections were further strengthened by research done in Sweden at around the same time by Bjorntorp and Rosmond. These two researchers did a mass of work that connected HPA-axis dysfunction, the metabolic syndrome, and CHD.

They focussed on visceral obesity as the main, visible sign of the underlying cortisol dysfunction, as outlined in their paper *"Visceral Obesity: A 'Civilisation Syndrome.'"*

*"**The syndrome of visceral obesity**, has several features of the unhealthy life-style that has developed in urbanized countries. Positive energy balance, physical inactivity, smoking, alcohol, and stress seem to be important ingredients of the syndrome of visceral obesity. These are the components of what might be labelled a 'Civilization Syndrome.'*

*"It is hypothetically suggested that these life-style factors are closely connected via **neuroendocrine disturbances to prevalent diseases such as NIDDM*, CVD, and stroke** as well as their risk factors, and that visceral accumulation might be a marker for this syndrome."* [152]

Bjorntorp is another of my unsung heroes of CVD research. He had a laser focus on how 'strain' leads to HPA-axis dysfunction, leading to the metabolic syndrome and then CVD. Unfortunately, his work, alongside long-term collaborator Rosmond, now only exists within the deep shadow cast by the cholesterol hypothesis.

Before moving on from Bjorntorp, here is another section from a paper he wrote, along with Rosmond entitled *"Neuroendocrine abnormalities in visceral obesity."*

"It seems likely, based on cross-sectional observations in men and longitudinal studies in animals that a prolonged period of HPA axis stimulation is followed by a continuous degradation of the regulatory mechanisms. An end stage is a rigid cortisol secretion with low morning values. In parallel with this is a diminished function of the feed-back control as well as an inhibition of growth and sex steroid hormones. Evidence also suggests that the sympathetic nervous centers become activated in parallel.

"The net effects of this cascade of neuroendocrine–endocrine perturbations will be insulin resistance as well as visceral accumulation of body fat. These are effects of cortisol in combination with the diminished secretion of growth and sex steroid secretions, which in normal concentrations antagonize the cortisol effects. Blood pressure will also be elevated, which might be a consequence of central stimulation of the sympathetic nervous system, with added effects of insulin. What has developed is a hypothalamic arousal with the Metabolic Syndrome as a consequence." [153]

That one passage outlines all that I have tried to say about how strain causes CVD, and exactly how this happens, all done in a mere 164 words. My excuse is that took me rather longer because I had to explain a mass of jargon on the way.

---

* NIDDM = non-insulin dependent diabetes/type 2 diabetes

174

Anyway, the absolutely key point from that passage, and the takeaway message here is that a rigid system, an inflexible system, is a damaged system. During a 24-hour period, people with HPA-axis dysfunction will produce almost exactly the same amount of cortisol as healthy individuals. But it is unresponsive, fixed, flattened, burnt-out.

Indeed, if you decide to measure the cortisol level in the morning it will be lower in someone with a dysfunctional HPA-axis than in a healthy individual. Which has led many researchers to state that there is no connection between stress and CVD. Because people with low morning cortisol levels are far more likely to die of CVD.

This is, of course, exactly the wrong conclusion. A perfect example of having absolutely no idea what you are talking about. Idiots.

Anyway, that was Lithuania, Sweden, and Bjorntorp. Time to move on and ask the question. Was this sudden explosion in CVD only seen in Lithuania, or did it occur in other Soviet countries at the same time? Time to turn our attention to Russia itself.

Russia – social dislocation and CVD

Although the Soviet Union began its painful disintegration in 1989, Russia limped on within the Union for a couple of years. Then, in August 1991 there was a coup attempt. It fizzled out, but it signalled the final death knell. By December 1991 Gorbachev had gone, Yeltsin – a man known to enjoy his vodka – was now in charge of Russia, and large-scale market reforms to the economy were underway. There was no longer any Soviet Union. It had gone.

What then happened to health was a complete and utter disaster.

"The transition to market economies in many post-communist societies of the former Soviet Union and other former eastern bloc countries in Europe has produced a 'demographic collapse,' a recent report by the United Nations Development Programme has found. Among the most serious findings is a four-year drop in life expectancy among Russian men since 1980, from 62 years to 58.

"The development programme's report also noted significant drops in life expectancy in Armenia, Belarus, Bulgaria, Latvia, Lithuania, and Romania. The immediate cause of the rising mortality, said the report, is the 'rise in self-destructive behaviour, especially among men.' Old problems such as alcoholism have increased; drug misuse a relatively new problem in the former communist bloc has risen dramatically in recent years. The report Transition 1999 stated that suicide rates have climbed steeply too, by 60% in Russia, 80% in Lithuania, and 95% in Latvia since 1989.

*"But behind the self-destructive behaviour, the authors say, are **economic factors, including rising poverty rates, unemployment, financial insecurity, and corruption**. Whereas only 4% of the population of the region had incomes equivalent to $4 (£2.50) a day or less in 1988, that figure had climbed to 32% by 1994. In addition, the transition to a market economy has been accompanied by lower living standards (including poorer diets), a deterioration in social services, and major cutbacks in health spending.*

"'What we are arguing,' said Omar Noman, an economist for the development fund and one of the report's contributors, 'is that the transition to market economies [in the region] is the biggest ... killer we have seen in the 20th century, if you take out famines and wars. The sudden shock and what it did to the system ... has effectively meant that five million [Russian men's] lives have been lost in the 1990s.'" [154]

Five *million* Russian men's lives lost.

Not all the deaths were due to strain and HPA-axis dysfunction, and not all deaths were due to CVD, but the vast majority were.

If you look at CHD deaths, they show the same early pattern as Lithuania (Figure 19). Although the sharp rise only begins a couple of years later. 1991, rather than 1989. Which figures, because this is when Russia imploded – not 1989.

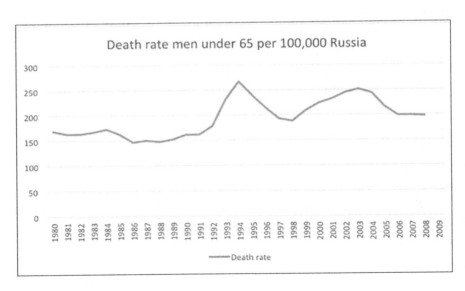

Figure 19

However, as you will no doubt have noticed, after 1998 the deaths rates separate dramatically. In Lithuania deaths dropped back to baseline, then continued their previous slow decline. Deaths in Russia were falling almost as dramatically, but then they took off again.

What could have caused this second deadly rise? The Soviet Union can only break up once, and market reforms can only happen once. You can, however, have more than one economic disaster.

As it turns out, in August 1998 there was a massive banking collapse. It virtually wiped out the stock market and destroyed the value of the rouble. At the same time unemployment skyrocketed and the savings of the common man were obliterated – again. The recovery took years.

"The enormity of Russia's financial collapse on Aug. 17, 1998 only really hit home with me the next day. 'We are so f-cked,' George Kogan, one of Moscow's most famous and longest serving equity salesman, explained to me standing in the apartment of Simon Dunlop, one of Moscow's most famous entrepreneurs. 'The whole system has just crashed. It will take years for Russia to recover.'" [155]

Yes, Russia managed to have not just one financial crash, but two, in rapid succession. Were the CHD deaths that followed all due to the impact on the economy, or did other 'social' factors play a role?

It is almost certain that other factors were important. However, there is strong evidence that financial worries, alone, can be deadly enough to explain the Russian pattern. For example, a study in South Africa found that people with significant money worries were *thirteen* times more likely to die from CHD:

*"People who reported significant **financial stress were 13 times more likely to have a heart attack** than those who had minimal or no stress. Among those who experienced moderate work-related stress levels, the chances of having a heart attack were 5.6 times higher."* [156]

In short, financial hardship, and worries about money, are one of the main drivers of CVD – especially in men. Which is exactly what happened in Russia. Two economic crashes, two spikes in CVD. One spike – perhaps a coincidence. Two spikes…

"As a whole, the Eastern European experience provides unique evidence of the powerful effect of social reforms on both long-term and short-term trends in CHD." [157]

Others tried to explain what happened, using more traditional models. They failed:

"We find no evidence that a reduction in the effectiveness of the medical care system is related to increased mortality. Nor do we find evidence that a change in the composition of the diet is related to increases in Russian mortality." [158]

Of course, alcohol, drugs and suicide also played their part in the rapid changes in overall mortality. However, when those factors explode this is just another manifestation of extreme psychosocial strain. A different side to the same coin that drives HPA-axis dysfunction. A side that contains job strain, social isolation, depression and vital exhaustion.

Knowing such things, my mind tends to wander about the world, looking for the countries, or populations, which I believe have suffered the greatest psychosocial strain. Of course, Russia ranks high up there, along with most of the ex-soviet countries. In fact, last time I looked, here were the top 20 countries in the CHD mortality statistics. [159]

1. **Turkmenistan**

2. **Ukraine**

3. **Kyrgyzstan**

4. **Belarus**

5. **Uzbekistan**

6. **Moldova**

7. Yemen

8. **Azerbaijan**

9. **Russia**

10. **Tajikistan**

11. Afghanistan

12. Syria

13. Pakistan

14. Mongolia

15. **Lithuania**

16. **Georgia**

17. Sudan

18. Egypt

19. Iraq

20. Lebanon

Nine of the top 10 are ex-soviet countries, with Yemen making a completely unsurprising entry at number seven. As for the other countries in the top 20... not terribly surprising really. If, that is, you believe that social disruption and psychosocial stress can drive CVD.

However, leaving entire countries aside, we can move to specific populations within countries. I think it can be confidently stated that the people who have suffered most terribly from psychosocial stress are the indigenous populations. People whose lands were invaded, then taken over by others. Yes, we are talking about Australian aboriginals, Native Americans, the Inuit, the Nepalese, the Maori in New Zealand and suchlike.

Aboriginals, psychosocial strain and CVD

I am not going to look at all aboriginal populations. You can do that yourself if you wish, and you will find that they pretty much all show the same things. Greatly reduced life expectancy, massive problems with drugs and alcohol abuse, and very high rates of CVD. This depressing pattern repeats from indigenous population to indigenous population.

It seems that having your lands invaded, followed by having your entire culture ripped apart, with most of it thrown in the dustbin, does terrible things to an indigenous people. They become lost, dissociated, angry. Perhaps most importantly, they become powerless, invisible, helpless, scrabbling at the bottom of the social pile. It most certainly does their health no good.

"Indigenous Australians have the worst life expectancy rates of any indigenous population in the world, a United Nations report says. But it's not news to Aboriginal health experts. They say it simply confirms what Australian health services have known for years.

"Aboriginal Medical Services Alliance of the Northern Territory (AMSANT) chief executive officer John Paterson said the findings of the report, which examined the indigenous populations of 90 countries, were no surprise. The UN report – State of the World's Indigenous Peoples – showed indigenous people in Australia and Nepal fared the worst, dying up to 20 years earlier than their non-indigenous counterparts. In Guatemala, the life expectancy gap is 13 years and in New Zealand it is 11." [160]

Can this be related to HPA-dysfunction? Do Australian aboriginals, for example, have abnormal cortisol secretion? Of course, they do:

"Stress hormones underlie Indigenous health gap in Australia:

"James Cook University scientists have made a disturbing finding about some young Indigenous people's biological reaction to stress, but one that could help close the health gap for indigenous people.

"The researchers have found young adult Indigenous people they tested show impaired secretion of the stress hormone cortisol and that their biological stress response is linked to the racial discrimination they experience.

"Professor Zoltan Sarnyai led the team of scientists from the Australian Institute of Tropical Health and Medicine at JCU.

"In their study published in the journal Scientific Reports, the team showed for the first time that the biologically important 'morning rise' of cortisol that prepares us to effectively deal with the daily hassles and stresses of life is **missing** *in otherwise healthy Indigenous young adults."* [161]

So, do they also have more type 2 diabetes? Of course, they do:

"Type 2 diabetes is the fastest growing chronic disease in Australia. Aboriginal and Torres Strait Islander people are at higher risk of type 2 diabetes than the general population. It's estimated that the prevalence of type 2 diabetes in Indigenous people is 3 to 4 times that of non-Indigenous Australians." [162]

Do they have more CVD? Of course, they do:

Perhaps the most astonishing individual figure comes from young Australian Aboriginal women. Using the Framingham risk calculator (an antecedent of CVrisk and Qrisk3), it was found that younger aboriginal women had *30 times* the predicted rate of CHD death, taking into account the standard risk factors: smoking, diabetes, raised blood pressure, cholesterol levels etc. [163]

Thirty times. Just let that figure sink in. Two thousand nine hundred per cent (2,900%) higher.

To be frank, if I had a risk calculator that could get things as spectacularly wrong as this, very nearly 3,000% wrong, I would blush madly, before throwing it in the bin. Instead, Framingham has been very slightly adapted, and it is now used as the basis for all CV risk calculators around the world. Mind you, it did work quite well for white men in 1950s America, in Framingham, rear Boston. Whoop-dee-do.

When it comes to the general aboriginal population and CVD.

"CVD death rate much higher at younger ages – 8 times as high at ages 35-44 among Indigenous people."

Eight times as high. Pretty much the difference between Lithuania and Sweden at their peak. With all the additional problems thrown in: alcohol abuse, suicide, depression, drugs...

Unfortunately, Australian aboriginals also have other, disastrous health problems. If they don't die of CVD, they die of diabetes and chronic kidney disease.

*"Indigenous people were 4 times as likely as non-Indigenous people to have diabetes – and 3 times as likely to have CKD – as an underlying or associated cause of death. At age 55-64, **death rates for both diseases were 10 times as high for Indigenous people as those for non-Indigenous people.**"*[164]

Immigration and CVD

Other populations that tend to be at very high risk of CVD, tend to be migrant populations, or immigrant populations. I say, 'tend to be', because there are some spectacular examples that very much buck this trend. A well-known example of this was the Rosetan community in Pennsylvania.

At the start of the twentieth century this community moved, virtually lock stock and barrel, from Roseto in Southern Italy to a new Roseto in the US. Here I quote an article from the Huffington Post, because it covers the issue so well:

"It seemed like a virtual fountain of youth, with a heart attack mortality rate roughly half the rate of every surrounding community. Same water, same neighborhood, same occupational mix, same income level ranges, same races. So, what was the difference and why?

"What made Rosetans die less from heart disease than identical towns elsewhere? Family ties. Another observation: they had traditional and cohesive family and community relationships. It turns out that Roseto was peopled by strongly knit Italian American families who did everything right and lived right and consequently lived longer.

"In short, Rosetans were nourished by people.

"In all ways, this happy result was exactly the opposite expectation of well-proven health laws. The Rosetans broke the following long-life rules, and did so with a noticeable relish: and they lived to tell the tale. They smoked old-style Italian stogie cigars, malodorous and remarkably pungent little nips of a cigar guaranteed to give a nicotine fix of unbelievably strong potency. These were not filtered or adulterated in any way.

"Both sexes drank wine with seeming abandon, a beverage which the 1963 era dietician would find almost prehistoric in health value. In fact, wine was consumed in preference to all-American soft drinks and even milk. Forget the cushy office job, Rosetan men worked in such toxic environs as the nearby slate quarries. Working there was notoriously dangerous, not merely hazardous, with 'industrial accidents' and gruesome illnesses caused by inhaling gases, dusts and other niceties.

"And forget the Mediterranean diets of olive oil, light salads and fat-free foods. No, Rosetans fried their sausages and meatballs in lard. They ate salami, hard and soft cheeses all brimming with cholesterol." [165]

The Rosetans were 'nourished by people'. I like that phrase very much.

Apart from the Rosetans, Chinese migrants tend to fare well when they migrate. They often have significantly lower rates of CVD than the surrounding population. Here from a study published in 2015 called the Chinese immigrant paradox.

"Literature on the incidence, mortality, and prognosis of CHD among Chinese living in Western countries was searched systematically in any language using 6 electronic databases up to December 2014. Based on the meta-analysis, Chinese had lower incidence of CHD compared with whites... and South Asians." [166]

The figures demonstrated that the Chinese has less than a third the rate of the surrounding white population: 29% of the rate, to be exact.

On the other hand, those who migrate from South Asian: India, Pakistan, Bangladesh and Sri Lanka – fare very badly. Almost wherever they go. [167]

What are the stand-out features of this migrant population?

*"A characteristic feature of the South Asian population identified from literature is **central/abdominal obesity or high waist-hip ratio**. For any given weight, the proportion of body fat is high and centrally distributed in South Asians. Propensity toward central obesity is an established risk factor and may lead to a higher incidence of CAD (Coronary Artery Disease) among South Asians through its effects on **blood pressure, diabetes, and insulin resistance.**"*

Yes, it's the usual suspects. Central obesity, the metabolic syndrome... CVD.

A study from the US looked at men of Asian Indian origin vs. US origin men. The key findings are in the table below. This study was done a few years back, so the diabetes figures may be lower than you might expect:

Risk factors for Asian Indian Men vs. US Men (age adjusted)

	Asian Indian	US
MI or angina	**7.5%**	**2.5%**
Type 2 diabetes	**7.6%**	**1%**
Smoking	**1.3%**	**27%**
Obesity	**4.2%**	**22%**
Hypertension	**14.2%**	**19.1%**

Table 1

*"To conclude, immigrant Asian Indian men to the US have high prevalence of CHD, NIDDM, low HDL cholesterol levels and hypertriglyceridemia (VLDL levels). All these have **"insulin resistance"** as a common pathogenetic mechanism and seem to be the most important risk factors."*[168]

What the paper didn't really comment on was that Asian Indians in this study smoked far less, 20 times less, they were far less obese (lower BMI), with much lower rates of hypertension. However, there was more central obesity, insulin resistance and diabetes, and three times the rate of CHD.

At this point I believe it is important to mention that not all South Asians are the same – although most researchers have tended to assume that they are. Therefore, for research purposes, they are lumped together into an amorphous mass.

This should never be done, because there is a major religious difference between these groups. There are three main religions in that part of the world: Sikh, Hindu and Muslim, and when the groups migrate, they suffer very different levels of psychosocial stress, as reported in the study *"Subgroup differences in psychosocial factors relating to coronary heart disease in the UK South Asian population."*

"The findings indicate that profiles of psychosocial adversity vary across South Asian religious groups, and this may signify differing levels of psychosocial CHD risk. The Muslim people in this sample were the most psychosocially disadvantaged, followed by Hindus, and with Sikhs reporting the most favorable profiles of the South Asian subgroups." [169]

Apart from social disadvantage, Muslims also suffer considerably more financial disadvantage:

"Muslim people were more likely to report poor socioeconomic circumstances, in terms of home ownership, income, and social deprivation. Chronic stressors were also higher among Muslims compared with Sikhs and Hindus, in the form of **financial strain, overcrowding, and low levels of social cohesion**. *The South Asian population, in general, still remains the subject of racial discrimination in the UK; however,* **the rise of 'Islamophobia' has led to an intensifying effect against British Muslims, particularly in the current political climate. Racism has been investigated as a risk factor for ill health."***

As you might expect, given what you have read up to now, Muslims suffer a far higher rate of CVD than Hindus, then Sikhs – in that order. This is simply a further illustration of the fact that it is an extremely bad idea to find yourself at the bottom of the social heap, like Australian Aboriginals. It is an even worse idea to be subjected to racism and religious intolerance. Muslims in the West do particularly badly, on all counts.

United States and CVD

I am going to keep this short, and simply reproduce an image of deaths from heart disease in the US (Figure 20).[170] You can draw your own conclusions as to what it means.

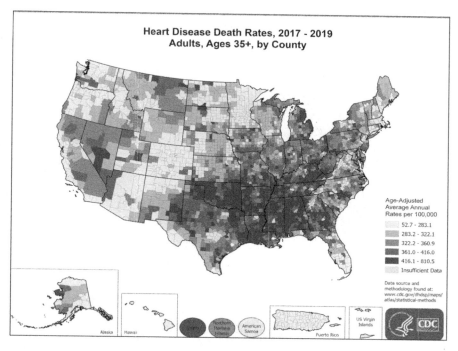

Figure 20

United Kingdom and CVD

Here is an image of the death rate from CVD in the UK (Figure 21).[171]

On this UK map, the very dark areas are, almost without exception, the cities. With the most socially deprived cities, Manchester, Liverpool, Hull, Stoke, Birmingham, Cardiff/Swansea, Glasgow – showing the darkest red. The leafy and wealthy counties of South and East England come off far better than anywhere else.

Below is a map of deprivation in England (not the entire UK) (Figure 22). If you put this over the CVD map of England, it's an almost perfect fit.

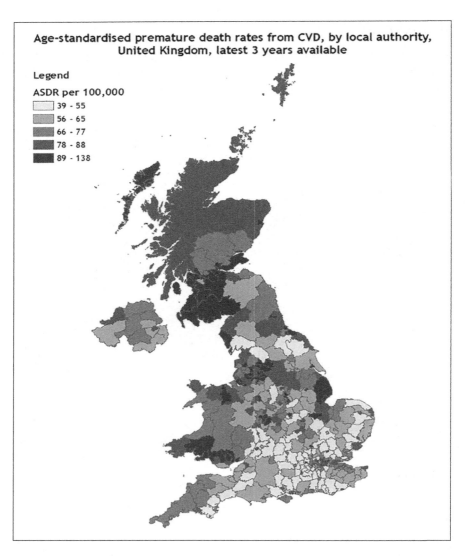

Age-standardised premature death rates from CVD, by local authority, United Kingdom, latest 3 years available

Legend

ASDR per 100,000
- 39 - 55
- 56 - 65
- 66 - 77
- 78 - 88
- 89 - 138

Figure 21

I include London separately below (Figure 23). The darkest bit, the most socially deprived bit, is the East End of London. It is also where EastEnders, the TV program is set. And for anyone who has watched that program you will know that is a gritty drama of working-class life, with all the social issues writ large. Divorce, domestic abuse, drugs, job losses, drinking too much… and suchlike.

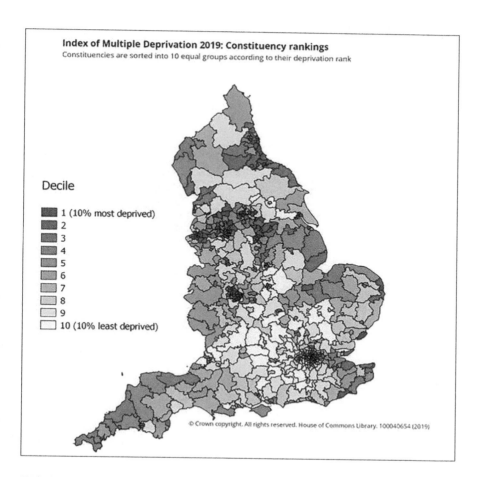

Figure 22

Had the same program been in the South of London, it could have been called *'The Kew Garden Kerrrrazy Gang'* A recurring story line being, how expensive it has become to run a ski chalet in Switzerland, or which artisan bakery has the best Sour Dough culture for baking one's own bread. Or which private school offers the best Pilates classes for darling, sweet, Alfreda, Euripides and Npeter* (the N is silent, I am reliably informed). This program may not be quite so entertaining.

---

* Yes, this a real name. I looked up the most popular upper-class names in England, and simply chose the three most... the three most. The three that made me chuckle most. I had no idea if Euripides is a boy's name, or a girl's name. A boy, I think, on the basis that Euripides was a Greek, male, tragedian. As of course I, ahem, knew.

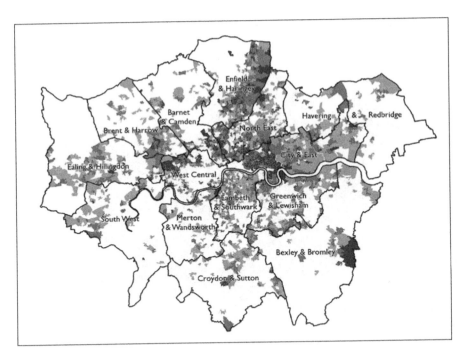

Figure 23

The inescapable fact is that wherever you look, you can see the patterns repeating over, and again. Psychosocial strain, social deprivation, racism, living at the bottom of the heap. These are terrible things for overall health, and especially for CVD. I have often said to anyone, still awake and listening to me by the end of the evening, that health consists of three overlapping parts:

- Physical

- Psychological

- Social

Western medicine deals with the physical pretty well, the psychological... not very well, and the social... not at all. However, if the social side is not addressed it brings everything else down with it.

People cannot achieve anything like full health if they are struggling to bring up a family in a ghetto, surrounded by drug dealers. Or if they live in a tiny, unheated flat with no job, an abusive partner, and five children. I don't imagine anyone is falling over with surprise if I say that 'poverty kills.' Or 'lack of social support kills'. Or that 'people need to be nourished by people.' This is self-evident.

Of course, it is not simply about money. People in poorer countries can live long, healthy and fulfilled lives. It is more about social inequality, living at the bottom of the heap, being treated with disdain, racism, a loss of any sense of community... and suchlike. See under Australian Aboriginals, or Native Americans, or the Maori.

Even the WHO recognises this. This is their first and, in my opinion, their most important statement about health:

"Health is a state of complete physical, mental and social well-being and not merely the absence of disease or infirmity."

I recognise that it is difficult for the medical profession to do a great deal about social health, it is not their area, they are taught little about it. It is far easier to stick to clever things like managing type IV tubular acidosis in chronic renal failure. More difficult to look at the 'soft factors.'

Just to take you back to Roseto again for a moment or two, and an article by Malcolm Gladwell in the *New York Times*. Here he discussed two researchers Bruhn and Wolf who spent years studying the Rosetans in the 1950s/60s – with their very low rate of heart disease.

"When Bruhn and Wolf first presented their findings to the medical community, you can imagine the kind of skepticism they faced. They went to conferences, where their peers were presenting long rows of data, arrayed in complex charts, and referring to this kind of gene or that kind of physiological process, and they talked instead about the mysterious and magical benefits of people stopping to talk to each other on the street and having three generations living under one roof.

"Living a long life, the conventional wisdom said at the time, depended to a great extent on who we were – that is, our genes. It depended on the decisions people made – on what they chose to eat, and how much they chose to exercise, and how effectively they were treated by the medical system. No one was used to thinking about health in terms of a place.

"Wolf and Bruhn had to convince the medical establishment to think about health and heart attacks in an entirely new way: they had to get them to realize that you couldn't understand why someone was healthy if all you did was think about their individual choices or actions in isolation. You had to look beyond the individual. You had to understand what culture they were a part of, and

who their friends and families were, and what town in Italy their family came from. You had to appreciate the idea that community – the values of the world we inhabit and the people we surround ourselves with – has a profound effect on who we are." [172]

This work by Bruhn and Wolf was done 60 years ago and now lies essentially forgotten – another ghost in the machine. Every so often researchers rediscover that, for example, loneliness is an important cause of CVD and premature death. Thud – head hits desk.

Unfortunately, there are no glittering prizes to be won in this area. No lucrative research career studying loneliness. When it comes to lowering LDL levels... now you're talking. I think three Nobel prizes have been won for studying this poor innocuous molecule.

A more recent book *The Blue Zones* covered research done on people who live in places where people live longer than anyone else – zones that just happened to be ringed with a blue pen. Yes, that is why they are called Blue Zones. More prosaic than you might think.

The authors made a significant effort to explain longevity as all being due to a vegetarian diet. However, it is clear – and the authors reluctantly admit it is clear – that the things that stand out in the blue zones are positive social structures, friendship, and strong family ties. The same factors that were found in Roseto – all those many years ago.

Break those ties, disrupt society, create psychosocial stress and you end up with CVD. We all know this intuitively. All I have tried to do, in this part of the book, is to use the paradigm of reductionist Western Cartesian Dualism to explain how living a terrible, lonely, unsupported, bullied, financially stressful life, pulls all those tiny physiological levers that lead to disease. Oh, the terrible irony.

Anyway, kindness, caring, compassion, human touch, friendship, a sense of purpose in life. These things really matter, but they are exceedingly tricky to measure. As Einstein said (in many different formats). *'Most things that matter cannot be measured, and most things that can be measured, don't matter.'*

Those used to be the 16 words that made up the screensaver on my computer. Reductionist thinking can only get you so far in life.

Thus, having dealt with strain, or psychosocial stress, I can now move away from Qrisk3 onto the final two important factors to tie the story off the tale of thrombogenesis. The first is the role of infective agents, the second is pulmonary emboli.

190

CHAPTER 7

Tying off a couple of loose ends (infections and pulmonary emboli)

Infectious agents

Whilst writing this section, I find myself in the midst of the COVID19 pandemic. This is considered as a respiratory virus, so the main problem should be severe pneumonia. Of course, COVID19 can, and does, cause this.

However, it is being discovered, to everyone's apparent amazement, that many people, even most people, are dying as the result of increased blood clotting. Heart attacks, strokes, kidney failure and widespread thrombi in the micro-circulation, known as disseminated intravascular coagulation (DIC).

"Based on recent reports, the most severely ill patients present with coagulopathy, and disseminated intravascular coagulation (DIC)-like massive intravascular clot formation is frequently seen in this cohort." [173]

The reality is that COVID19 is not really a respiratory virus, it is a cardiovascular virus. Or at least, widespread blood clotting is what the majority of people die of, or from.

Then, things appeared to get even stranger. In addition to CVD, another problem started to emerge. Several younger people were found to be developing a delayed immune response following COVID19 infection. In the last few weeks, this phenomenon has been given several different names, such as the one used in the passage below, 'multisystem inflammatory syndrome':

"A mysterious inflammatory syndrome tied to COVID19 that has been reported in children is now also turning up in young adults in their early 20s, according to news reports.

"Symptoms of the syndrom – can vary. But patients tend to have symptoms similar to those found in Kawasaki disease, a rare childhood illness that causes inflammation in blood vessel walls, and in serious cases can cause heart damage, Live Science *previously reported. Symptoms can include fever, abdominal pain, vomiting, diarrhea, neck pain, rash, bloodshot eyes and fatigue, according to the Centers for Disease Control and Prevention."* [174]

In reality this disease is not in the slightest bit mysterious. It is Kawasaki's disease, or a closely related version thereof.

So, how does COVID19, a viral infection, cause both cardiovascular deaths, and Kawasaki's? I would hope by now, that a light bulb has gone off inside your head. Yes, COVID19 is causing a widespread vasculitis.

Any infectious disease that gets into the body, will also get into the bloodstream. With COVID19 the virus gets into cells using an entrance called the ACE2 receptor. These particular receptors are mainly found on endothelial cells. So, these are the cells that are infected.

What then results is damage and destruction to endothelial cells all around the body. What makes things worse is cells that do not die, change their structure and can be seen as alien by the immune system. So, they get attacked, often a few weeks after the initial infection has settled.

"Cardiovascular diseases appear intricately linked with COVID19, with cardiac complications contributing to the elevated morbidity/mortality of COVID19." [175]

The acute vasculitis also helps to explain why diabetes is such a significant risk factor for dying of COVID19. In diabetes, the glycocalyx is already weakened and thinned, and COVID19 doubles down on the damage. It also explains why kidney failure has been another major problem in COVID19. As explained earlier, damage to the glycocalyx causes specific problems with the micro-vessels in the kidney.

In addition, a healthy glycocalyx will almost certainly help to prevent COVID19 from sticking to the ACE2 receptor in the first place, thus making entry into the cells more difficult. The virus almost certainly gets caught up in the glycocalyx micro forest.

I must admit that I have found it slightly surreal to watch the COVID19 saga develop in front of my eyes and note the amazement of researchers in finding that COVID19 can cause both CVD and Kawasaki's. All they needed to do was think endothelial damage/vasculitis. But no-one yet thinks this way. So, it is all considered mysterious.

This slow realisation that COVID19 may be damaging the cardiovascular system has been doubly surprising, because it has been known for years that respiratory viruses can damage the vascular endothelium, and greatly increase the risk of death from blood clots.[176]

Anyway, from the COVID19 saga it becomes pretty clear how viruses can lead to cardiovascular disease, but how do bacteria do it? Bacteria cannot, generally, invade cells. Although there are some that do. More commonly they invade the space around cells (interstitial space), and find their way into damaged tissue, such as a wound.

However, the most serious problems occur if they find their way into the bloodstream. This is because bacteria as they grow, and replicate, produce waste products known as 'exotoxins.' These substances certainly live up to their name, because exotoxins can be extremely toxic, and damaging.

For example, botulism toxin is produced by the clostridium botulinum bacteria, and vanishingly small amounts can be fatal. Although the way this particular exotoxin kills you has nothing to do with CVD. Botulism toxins block nerve transmission, and you die of suffocation – because you can no longer breathe.

Moving back to a CVD perspective. If bacteria get into your bloodstream, the exotoxins can wreak havoc with endothelial cells, as noted in this paper "*Endothelial responses to bacterial toxins in sepsis.*"

*"The endothelium, with its diversity of physiological functions is a **main target of bacterial toxins.**"* [177]

Basically, if you have nasty bacteria in the blood, multiplying at speed, and excreting toxins, this causes a condition known as 'bacterial sepsis', which can be rapidly fatal. In fact, it is one of the most serious medical conditions there is, with a fatality rate close to 50%.

The primary cause of death in bacterial sepsis is disseminated intravascular coagulation (DIC). This is the term for small thrombi springing up in in blood vessels all-round the body – see under COVID19. This causes organs to fail, such as the kidneys and the liver. People who survive can end up losing limbs, because of the catastrophic loss of blood supply to arms and legs, fingers, toes – the tip of the nose.

Sepsis = vasculitis = clots (plus the opening up of tight junctions) and death.

Stepping down the ladder a few rungs, a much less severe and chronic form of 'sepsis' can be caused by periodontal disease (infected gums). Here, long standing infection in the gums can lead to a constant, low-grade leakage of bacteria and exotoxins into the bloodstream day after day. This causes chronic endothelial damage and inflammation.

"A consensus report simultaneously published in the Journal of Periodontology and American Journal of Cardiology recommended periodontists inform patients with periodontal disease (PD) they may have increased risk for cardiovascular disease and that cardiologists recommend patients have oral health checkups.

*"Researchers have found periodontal pathogenic bacteria in atherosclerotic plaque and in the arterial walls. **Periodontal pathogens are associated with endothelial dysfunction.**"* [178]

Indeed, as with almost everything else I have mentioned so far. When you get down to it, the processes causing CVD turn out to be the same. In this case bacterial exotoxins cause CVD in very much the same way as smoking or raised blood sugar levels.

Yes, I know that the agents involved may seem a million miles apart. A stone and a tin of baked beans. However, when you look in greater deal, they simply damage the endothelium – in one way or another.

Just to wrap this section about bacteria a bit more tightly. Another major problem associated with periodontal disease is – surprise, surprise, chronic kidney disease. Well, if you attack the endothelium and the glycocalyx, with exotoxins, that is exactly what you would expect to see.

Here from the paper *"Periodontitis as the risk factor of chronic kidney disease: Mediation analysis"*

"Periodontitis had significant direct effect, and indirect effect through diabetes, on the incidence of CKD. Awareness about systemic morbidities from periodontitis should be emphasized." [179]

Because of these strong and consistent connections between 'infections' and CVD, several researchers, some of whom I know well, believe that the primary cause of CVD is infectious disease. I simply nod and reply that infectious diseases are one of many different causes. They are just another stone with which to build the thrombogenic house.

Pulmonary emboli turning into atherosclerotic plaques

Finally, finally. Hooray you may think, I am going to turn to something that I should maybe have discussed at the start of the section on 'process.' I didn't, because I felt that looking closely at pulmonary emboli was probably the best way to wrap up the entire thrombogenic hypothesis.

I am going to start with a little bit of context.

A major difficulty in studying CVD is that research is severely hampered by three things:

1. Humans are virtually the only species that naturally develop CVD – pigs probably come closest, but there are still many differences.

2. You are not allowed to do experiments on humans whereby the aim is to try to cause CVD. This is, for very good reasons, verboten.

3. It is very difficult to examine arteries, and plaques, in detail until someone has died. Therefore, you cannot watch the same plaque develop over time, at least not in any detail.

Starting with the first problem, which is that studying other species can only tell you so much about a disease that that they don't actually get. Even chimpanzees, our closest relatives, remain almost entirely CVD free.

One group of researchers did look at chimpanzees, living in zoos, who were fed an almost purely vegetarian diet. This is what they found:

*"First, we can see that **the mean total serum cholesterol in this captive chimpanzee population is well above the mean in the human population**, at every decade of life, in both males and females. Second and most intriguingly, we see that unlike the case in humans, **captive chimpanzees have high serum cholesterol levels even in the early decades of life**. Thus, the chimpanzee vasculature is exposed to high cholesterol levels throughout adolescence and adulthood. Indeed the levels in very young chimpanzees fall into a high enough range wherein pharmacological statin therapy would now be seriously considered in children."*[180]

That last sentence seemed rather tongue in cheek to me. A little poke at the cholesterol hypothesis? Just in case you are wondering it is not just total cholesterol, it is also the LDL cholesterol that is higher.

*"... **LDL cholesterol levels of captive chimpanzees were found to be well above matched human levels** and already in a range comparable to the majority of at-risk humans."*

However, despite their higher LDL levels, they simply do not die of acute myocardial infarctions (AMIs). They don't develop significant atherosclerosis either. It is true that they can quite often die of events that are described as heart attacks, but these are not myocardial infarctions.

*"Chimpanzees are our closest evolutionary relatives, with nearly 99% identity of many of our homologous protein sequences. Thus, at first glance it is not surprising that published data about chimpanzees cared for in captivity lists heart failure and/or sudden death due to 'heart attacks' as being among the commonest causes of death. However, closer examination of the clinical and pathological findings indicates that the mechanisms causing heart disease in humans and chimpanzees **are quite different**."*

What chimpanzees die of instead is interstitial myocardial fibrosis (IMF). Which I am not going to explain in any detail here – it is basically a thickening and loss of elasticity of the heart muscle. This is pretty much the same thing that kills young fit athletes from time to time.

However, these chimpanzee 'heart attacks' are never caused by plaque rupture and blockage of an artery.

*"...although mild to moderate atherosclerosis was observed in the aorta and other major blood vessels in some of the chimpanzee necropsies, **no major blockages of the coronary arteries were observed in any case**..."*

So, there you go. Feed our closest relatives an almost purely vegetarian diet, and they end up with far higher LDL levels than us. However, they do not develop any major blockages of their coronary arteries. And whilst they do die of heart attacks, these are not remotely the same thing as a myocardial infarction. Which proves… nothing at all.

If we can't learn a great deal from our nearest living relatives, and you're not allowed to carry out direct, artery damaging experiments on humans, how best to see how plaques start, and grow? The Velicans did their *'snapshot in time series'* by examining people who died in car crashes, and suchlike, at different ages.

This was a good way of getting some idea of what is going on. However, they were unable to study the development of plaques in the same person. This would have been tricky, as their subjects were all dead.

Given all these inherent difficulties, I wanted to know if there were any conditions where you could witness, as clearly as possible, the progression of blood clots into plaques.

I felt this was mission critical. If you have a hypothesis that plaques are the result of blood clots sticking to artery walls, then gradually becoming converted into plaques, it's a good idea to have some strong evidence that this actually happens. Theories are all very well, but physical evidence is much better. Facts beat hypotheses every time. Like rock, paper, scissors.

And so, gentle reader, we turn once more to pulmonary emboli. Which is a condition whereby a blood clot or thrombus arrives in the lungs and gets stuck – at which point it changes its name to an embolism, as in 'pulmonary embolism'.

If the thrombogenic hypothesis is correct, it should be possible to see – at least some of these clots – being converted directly into atherosclerotic plaques.

Which takes us to the article *"Plaque composition in plexogenic and thromboembolic pulmonary hypertension: the critical role of thrombotic material in pultaceous core formation."*

Yes, there's the title from a paper to stop you dead in your tracks and get the pulse racing. '*I really need to read that little beauty.*' Or maybe not.

You may have noticed that we have just stumbled across that word pultaceous again. Suddenly I am tripping over it all over the place. Well, twice anyway. Pultaceous = soft and squidgy. Which also, for the purposes of this discussion, means having a lipid core.

In this paper you also get the special bonus of yet another new word. Which is *plexogenic*. I must admit that was a new one on me as well. Oh well, a day is not lost when you learn something new.

Anyway, what the title of this paper means is that these researchers were studying plaques that develop in the lungs in two main situations. Either, following a pulmonary embolus getting stuck. Or following longer-term raised blood pressure. Technically known as *plexogenic* pulmonary hypertension.

There was actually a third cause here, which is having a ventricular septal defect (hole in the heart between the ventricles). This shunts the blood from the left to the right side of the heart, at very high pressure, from whence it heads off into the lungs – creating pulmonary hypertension. This is known as Eisenmenger's syndrome.

For the sake of this discussion, Einsenmenger's syndrome is basically the same thing as plexogenic pulmonary hypertension. With one important exception – that I will get to.

The first thing to note is that the type of plaques they saw in the two conditions were completely different. In their words

- Chronic thromboembolic pulmonary hypertension is associated with atherosclerotic plaques with **glycophorin-rich pultaceous core**

- Plexogenic pulmonary hypertension (results in) **fibrous plaque**

Oh no, more jargon… glycophorin-rich. What does this mean? Well, glycophorin is a major constituent of red blood cell membranes. So, if you find glycophorin in a plaque, it means you are looking at the remnants of red blood cells.

Now, having beaten the jargon to death with a large stick, or at least half to death, let us move on.

Below is a table of the main features found in the plaques with these two different causes. I should mention that there were 39 subjects with thromboembolic hypertension, and 28 with either plexogenic or Eisenmenger's hypertension:

Feature	Thromboembolic Hypertension	Plexogenic Hypertension	Eisenmenger's syndrome
Subjects	39	9	19
Organising thrombus	34	0	0
Recent thrombotic material	33	0	0
Calcification	18	0	0
Vascular neogenesis	37	0	0

Table 2

As you can see, there were two very different types of plaque. Thromboembolic plaques were full of organising thrombus, recent thrombotic material, and most of them contained cholesterol crystals. There was also calcification in 50% of them. These things were not present in the plaques caused by pulmonary hypertension.

The other critical thing to note with thromboembolic plaques is that almost all of them demonstrated new, micro blood vessels being formed in and around them (vascular neogenesis). In effect, new vasa vasorum were being created around them. Plaque first, new blood vessels second.

That table, if you spend some time pondering it, as I have done, tells you virtually everything you need to know about vulnerable atherosclerotic plaques – the ones that are most likely to rupture and kill you. How they form, and what's in them.

The authors clearly felt this too, as they stated:

"...only chronic thromboembolism significantly predicted the presence of pultaceous material in large pulmonary arteries, with the presence of organised and recent thrombi, calcifications, and cholesterol clefts... **Thromboembolic material is therefore sufficient on its own to induce plaque formation and influence its composition.** *The plaques in the patients with plexogenic pulmonary hypertension consist of fibrous tissue without pultaceous cores."*

In addition, they commented that:

"Furthermore, the angiographically documented absence of coronary atherosclerosis and the pathological confirmation of normal coronary arteries in the hearts of the patients with Eisenmenger's syndrome indirectly confirm the non-atherogenic habitus* of the entire population. **The large pulmonary artery pathology in our patients can therefore be attributed entirely to their thromboembolic or plexogenic hypertension."** [181]

(Just to avoid confusion, these patients were not generally examined post-mortem. Many of them had lung transplants, or major operations to remove obstructive plaques, so their arteries could be examined in great detail, even though they were still alive).

I am just going to repeat what I consider to be the kicker statement in this paper. I have even put it into a box – which may be worse than an exclamation mark.

---

* Non-atherogenic habitus means – a lifestyle and metabolism with none of the currently accepted risk factors for CVD. Basically, they did not have raised cholesterol, they did not have raised blood glucose. In short, they had no risk factors for CVD.

> *Thromboembolic material is therefore **sufficient** on its own to induce plaque formation.*

As you can see, it does seem as if Rokitansky was right, and Elspeth Smith was right. The dangerous plaques, the vulnerable plaques are, indeed, the remnants of blood clots. No other factor needed.

Which means that blood clots are *sufficient*.

Finally, I think I need to add there were three subjects with Einsenmenger's with additional thrombus formation, described as '*ES with thrombus*'. The plaques in these subjects were the same as those seen with thromboembolic hypertension i.e., organising thrombus, with liquid cores, turning into plaque.

This research, fundamental though it is to CVD research, has very rarely been done before, or since. At least not compared to the hundreds of thousands of papers written on cholesterol and/or LDL. In total I managed to find three studies where researchers analysed the conversion of emboli to plaques. There may be more, they are not easy to find.

The first of these studies, and the one that I consider the most important, was done many years ago. It was published in the *Journal of the American Heart Association* as far back as 1955. It looked at children with congenital heart abnormalities which threw blood clots from the heart into the lungs.

The reason why I think it is so powerful, and important, is that they studied children, which means that there can have been no other risk factors – only blood clots.

The other reason why this study was mission critical, is that it can never be done again. At the time, open heart surgery did not exist. There were no heart lung machines to take over blood circulation, so going into the heart to replace a valve or a septal defect was never going to end well. Nowadays the conditions that killed these children, and infants, can be treated. At least in wealthy countries.

With the context explained, we can go back to 1955, and the paper. *"The role of pulmonary hypertension and thromboembolism in the production of pulmonary arteriosclerosis."*

"The idea that pulmonary arteriosclerotic lesions can arise directly from the organization of thrombi is a radical one, *but a great deal of* *supporting evidence has been accumulated in recent years.* **Fibrous intimal thickening of the pulmonary arteries characteristic of pulmonary arteriosclerosis has been produced in experimental animals by repeated intravenous injection of thrombi.**

[In short, one way to produce plaques in the pulmonary circulation, of animals, is to inject thrombi into their veins, which end up as pulmonary emboli – then plaques].

"The stages of development from thrombi to arteriosclerotic lesions have been demonstrated by sacrificing the animals at suitable intervals. In our human cases, we searched for evidence indicating that a similar sequence of events had occurred. **It is quite possible that most thrombi in pulmonary vessels lyse completely leaving no permanent change in the vessel walls.** [they are chopped up by plasmin and disappear].

"It is widely recognized that other thrombi are transformed into fibrous tissue through which pass multiple devious blood channels and we found many such organized, recanalized thrombi in our cases [New small blood vessels had been drilled through the obstructive thrombus, which allowed the blood to flow straight through the blood clot – which had now become fibrous i.e. tough and difficult to shift. Probably would get completely broken down in time]. *However, we found evidence that other,* **less widely recognized forms of organization occurred resulting in fibrous intimal thickening characteristic of arteriosclerosis."** [182]

The discussion section is key:

"...we were able to demonstrate transition stages from clearly recognizable thrombi to arteriosclerotic lesions."

I just love that statement. *"We were able to demonstrate transition stages, from thrombi to arteriosclerotic lesion".* Straight from a blood clot to the vulnerable plaque. Concrete, physical, evidence.

These researchers proved beyond any doubt that clots can, and in fact do, turn into plaques. So, we have the entire process here, start to finish, nothing else required. A sufficient factor. They had already created plaques by injecting thrombi into animals, and they confirmed that this also happened in children.

Unfortunately, they didn't make enough noise about their findings. Unlike the cholesterol zealots, banging their gongs, and chanting their nonsensical slogans. *'Polyunsaturated fats good, saturated fats bad. Statins better.'*

Which means that their work disappeared pretty much without trace. It can now only be found lurking, deep within the machine.

I shall now wrap up this section of the book what is, currently, my single favourite quote:

> *Thromboembolic material is therefore **sufficient** on its own to induce plaque formation.*

Postscript

And so, gentle reader, we come to the end of this section on the process of plaque development and growth. I have introduced you to the players in the game. How plaque formation happens, and what can cause it. I am sorry that I could find no single, simple, answer. The reason for this, is that there isn't one.

One analogy that I like to use when thinking and talking about CVD is one that I have mentioned before. Which is rust on the paintwork of a car. There is no single cause for this, there are many. Whilst they all lead to the same result, factors that can cause it can seem, on first examination, to be a million miles apart. A stone chip, or a tin of baked beans.

You can study these things in isolation, until you are blue in the face. What connects them? They are both made of hard materials, then what? Nothing much, nothing at all really. However, what they *are* is not important. It is what they can do. They can all damage the paintwork.

In the same way, you cannot find answers to CVD by looking at different factors and studying each one in minute detail. Instead, you must ask what can they do? In this way you can bring together a whole world of factors that, at first sight, appear to have nothing in common. For example:

- Smoking

- Lead/other heavy metals

- Exhaust fumes

- Raised blood pressure

- SLE

- Migraines

- Raised blood sugar levels
- Bacterial infection
- Periodontal disease
- Avastin/bevacizumab
- Pulmonary emboli
- Chronic kidney disease
- Sickle cell disease
- Lp(a)
- Hughes' syndrome
- COVID19
- Steroids/cortisol
- Strain/stress
- Scurvy/ Vit C deficiency

Everything on this list increases the risk of CVD because they can all do one of three things. In some cases, all three:

- Damage the glycocalyx/endothelium
- Create bigger, more difficult to shift blood clots
- Interfere with the repair process

In the end it turns out that Paul Rosch was truly a genius. To understand CVD, you must not look at *what* (causes it), you have to look at *how* (it is caused). At which point the windowpane disappears, and you can fly free.

Now we can move on to look at the most effective actions that you can take to slow, or stop, these processes.

PART 2

What can you do to reduce the risk of CVD?

I hope you now have a pretty good idea about the processes that lead to cardiovascular disease. I suppose the next obvious question is, what can you do to stop it happening? In some sort of order, from greatest, to least benefit.

This is tricky. I know that however I approach it, there are actions that have absolutely no relevance to most people. Smoking, for example. Yes, it's highly damaging, but nowadays most people don't smoke. To be perfectly honest, the sort of person who smokes is not likely to be reading this book. Although they might consider buying several copies for friends and relatives.... Just a thought.

In addition, there are a whole series of conditions/diseases/factors that have no impact on the vast majority of people. Because they don't have them, and never will. For instance, rheumatoid arthritis, or a raised Lp(a), or Hughes' disease (antiphospholipid syndrome), or sickle cell disease.

Which means that I am taking a pretty general approach here. Covering the factors that can do the greatest damage to the greatest number people – with a couple of diversions thrown in here and there.

CHAPTER 8

Increase in life expectancy

Before getting started on all that, I want to spend some time looking at an issue that I think is mission critical. Namely, what size of benefit can you get by taking action. By this I mean, essentially, how much longer will you live if you do something that helps. Alternatively, and switching to Eeyore mode, how much earlier will you die if you do something damaging.

Defining benefits in terms of life expectancy gained, or lost, might sound pretty straightforward, but I can assure you that it is not. Indeed, I debated long and hard with myself whether I should even attempt this. In the end I did manage to convince myself, although I did put up a bloody good fight.

Just for starters, I know that every figure I propose can, and undoubtedly will, be hotly contested. By which I mean… attacked. '*How dare you say people will live three months longer, when it is clearly two point eight six*'. In some cases, I am resorting to the scientific technique known as guesswork. Because accurate data simply do not exist.

The main benefit of using life expectancy gained, or lost, is that it does give you a framework where you can compare one action against another. You can then decide whether or not you should be spending time and effort doing something that might gain you a month. When you could add five years by doing something much easier.

To give you one quick example of this – which I will discuss in greater detail later. There is good evidence that it may be possible to increase your lifespan by up to 10 years, simply by going outside, getting into the sun, and sunbathing. Simple, free, and enjoyable. Yes, I know this may be considered somewhat contentious. Possibly the most contentious thing in this book, but it also happens to be true.

On the other hand, you could chew gloomily on statins for 40 years. An activity that will require regular appointments with your GP. Added to this, you will have to pay for a prescription every month. Then you must remember to pick it up from the pharmacy. You will also need blood tests from time to time to check your cholesterol level – and suchlike.

As an added bonus you may well get to suffer adverse effects for the next 40 years. You can then obsess and worry about your cholesterol level. For all this you may gain just under a month. Three days extra for every five years taking the statin.[183]

Sunbathing, or statins. Your choice.

CHAPTER 9

How much longer will you live?

If you're concerned about heart disease and make an appointment to see your doctor about it, they will almost certainly do the following. They will call up all your standard risk factors on the computer: age, sex, blood pressure, family history etc. then plug the results into an on-line risk calculator.

In the US, there are a number of different calculators. The most widely used is probably the ASCVD risk estimator.[184] In the UK we started with Framingham, then moved on to Qrisk1, then Qrisk2 and we now have Qrisk3.[185] At the time of writing Qrisk2 is most commonly used, but Qrisk3 will fully take over at some point. That is, before Qrisk4 is unveiled.

Whichever version the doctor uses, it is designed to work out your risk of a future cardiovascular event. The figure produced will be amazingly precise: 8.2% or 12.6%, or whatever.

As a general rule, figures as seemingly accurate as this should be taken with a large pinch of salt. Seven point two five grams of salt is best. However, the accuracy, or otherwise, of risk calculation is an enormously complex area that I am not going to drown in here.

But what does such a percentage risk actually mean? How much will a 5% risk of a cardiovascular event shave off your lifespan? If you ask your doctor this question, I can absolutely guarantee they will have no idea. None. Zip. Nada.

Doctor: 'Oh my God you have a 10.3% risk of a cardiovascular event.'
Patient: Which means... what? Tell me please doctor. Tell me. I must know.'
Doctor: 'It means you have a 10.3% risk of a cardiovascular event – so you must take a statin every day for the rest of your life. Here is your prescription. Next!'
Patient: 'Oh, all right then, thanks for clearing that up... not.'

Despite the fact that it is very rarely done, it is possible to convert a percentage risk into the common currency of life expectancy – although the end-result always has a bit of wobble room built in. To explain how to do this, I am going to look at a Qrisk3 in more detail.

Using Qrisk3, you input information on 20 different risk factors: blood pressure, age, sex, diabetes etc. That is, assuming you have them all to hand. If you do have all the information available, the in-built algorithm will churn out your risk of having a cardiovascular event (CV event) in the next 10 years. A cardiovascular event, for the sake of simplicity, is a heart attack or a stroke.

I have included an on-screen picture of the Qrisk3 calculator (Figure 24). In this case I inputted figures from an imaginary 70-year-old woman. In this case she has absolutely no modifiable risk factors. She represents *the* perfectly healthy woman. She plays golf and tennis *and* has a personal trainer. There's posh.

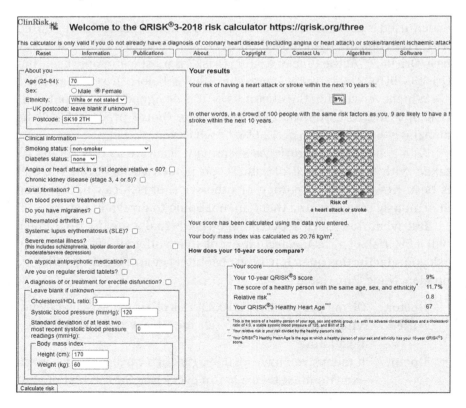

Figure 24

As I hope you can see, from Figure 24, Qrisk3 has established that this woman has a 9% risk. That is, a 9% risk of a cardiovascular event within the next 10 years. Not over her lifetime. This is a key point, to which I shall return.

Now then, pop quiz. Her 9% risk of a CV event in the next 10 years is likely to reduce her life expectancy by:

- One year

- Five years

- One month

- Nine months

- Other

Have you any idea how you go about converting this 9% figure into a reduction in life expectancy? I can pretty much guarantee that you can't – unless you happen to be a passing actuary. In which case '*hellooo!*' and don't be too critical. I'm doing my best.

In order to save you the bother, I am going to work it out for you. In order to do this, I need to input some more information into the Q*Kendrick*3 life-expectancy calculator. Patent pending.

First, I need to know, what are the odds that a cardiovascular event is going to be fatal? Because strokes and heart attacks are not usually fatal. Indeed, they can be pretty minor events. They can occur without any real harm, or residual damage, or even noticeable symptoms. These ones, almost certainly the majority, have no impact on life expectancy.

On the other hand, it has been estimated that around 30% of strokes and heart attacks are actually fatal... combined. This figure can be argued, and doubtless will be. However, I am going to go with it here. It is an amalgam of hundreds of papers I have read over the years.

Moving on, if we use this figure of 30%, it means that her 9% risk of suffering a cardiovascular event, ends up with a 2.7% chance of her dying (9% x 30% = 2.7%).

Unfortunately, we still lack all the information we need. Another critical variable is age. Events that happen when someone is very young will have a far greater impact on life expectancy than when someone is much older.

- A fatal heart attack at the age of 20 reduces life expectancy by (at least) 60 years

- A fatal heart attack at the age of 90, reduces life expectancy by about 3 years*

Onwards and upwards. We now know that there is a 2.7% chance that she will die of a cardiovascular event in the next 10 years. Which, if it does happen, will serve her right for being so terribly smug. Sorry, it will reduce her likely life expectancy by... 20 years? Bong! Sorry, wrong answer.

It is vanishingly unlikely that she will die on the same day that you calculate her risk. The 'event' will most likely occur halfway through the next 10 years i.e., after 5 years. That is, when she is 75. Which means that it will reduce her life expectancy by 15 – not 20 years.

Yes, I do know that the risk of an event increases with every day that she ages. So, it's going to happen somewhat later than five years. Anyway, leaving aside the need for calculus to work this out exactly, we now have sufficient information to establish the impact of her risk on life expectancy.

It goes, as follows. We have a healthy 70-year-old woman, with a 9% risk of suffering an event within 5 years. This will result in a 30% chance of killing her. If so, it will reduce her life expectancy by 15 years. This results in an 'average' reduction in life expectancy of. Drum roll. Almost exactly five months.

15 years life lost (5,475 days) x **2.7%** (chance of this happening) = **149 days** (5 months)

Which, as you may have just worked out, does not match any of the figures in the multiple-choice question I gave you earlier.

1. One year

2. Nine years

3. One month

4. Nine months

5. Other

---

* The older you get, the longer your life expectancy becomes. When you are born, in the UK, it is around 80. If you reach 80 it becomes 90. Once you reach 90 it is about 93. At present, in the UK, my 70-year-old woman can expect to live until she is about 90. In other words, she currently has a 20-year life expectancy.

Apart from 'other', obviously.

The reason for this is that my 70-year-old woman has a 9% chance of nasty things happening... *during the next 10 years*. Not over her lifetime. Which means that we now have to recalculate what is likely to happen between the ages of 80, and 90? (I am ignoring the 2.7% chance that she is already dead from a CV event – or that she has died from something else).

As you can see from Figure 25, as our healthy woman gets older the risk of an event rises dramatically. If this woman does reach 80 – and remains as proportionately healthy as she was at 70 – her risk of a CV event rises to 23%.

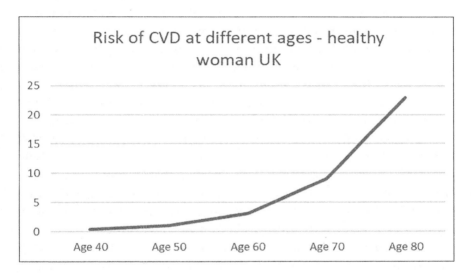

Figure 25

Therefore, the chance of a *fatal* event occurring, in the years from 80 to 90, is:

23% x 30% = **6.9%**

Once again, we are looking at this happening after five years – halfway between 80 and 90. Which means that we now have an additional 6.9% chance that her life expectancy will be reduced by 8 years (at 90 she can be expected to get to 93). Okay, yes, I am brushing over some variables with a devil may care attitude.

213

The additional calculation is as follows:

8 years of life lost (2,920 days) x **6.9%** = **201 days** reduction in life expectancy (~7 months)

Finally, hooray, you may be thinking, although I have taken a few liberties with my sums along the way, we can see that a 9% risk of a CV event aged 70 converts into approximately a one-year reduction in life expectancy. Terms and conditions apply.

You might well be thinking, goodness me, this all gets very complicated, very quickly. The answer is that, yes, it does. It is why actuaries – very clever, and very rich accountants – get paid such a lot of damned money for working out how much life insurance should cost, and suchlike. With a large slice of profit stuck on top. Including, of course, enormous additional actuarial fees.

Indeed, my back of an envelope figure would probably make any actuary keel over with a heart attack. Bet they didn't calculate for that... suckers. However, I was not aiming for perfection here because that would make this the world's most boring book, instead of just being the world's second most boring book. Sitting alongside – '*Fun stats for actuaries.*'

I simply wanted to give you a sense of the impact of how risk converts to life expectancy. A figure that's never going to be fully accurate, or set in concrete, because people change their risks all the time. Often in ways that are impossible to predict on an individual basis. In addition, of course, you cannot averagely die, nor can you be 2.7% dead. I can only do averages here.

Setting aside all such problems, the fact is that life expectancy remains by far the most important and useful figure. Percentage risks are close to meaningless, especially if you don't know what the underlying risk was in the first place. In fact, I shall make this statement stronger. If you have no idea about the underlying risk of an event occurring, a percentage increase in risk is totally meaningless.

It is the same type of nonsense as claiming that drug X can reduce the risk of dying of a heart attack by, say, 40%. I hate to point it out, but the risk of dying is always... one. As in one, 100% going to happen. There is nothing you can do about that. All you can do is extend the amount of time it takes before you shuffle off this mortal coil.

The other significant benefit of converting everything into life expectancy is that it allows different interventions to be compared.

For example, if you exercise regularly, you can expect to increase life expectancy by five years: exercise vs no exercise.[186]

Knowing that figure it becomes simple to match it to my woman's cardiovascular risk, in a way that means something. Five years versus one year. Before working out my 70-year-old woman's life expectancy, you had two numbers bellowing across a void of incomprehension. Five years vs 9%. Say what?

Moving to another example, it has been estimated that smoking reduces life expectancy by 10 years. If a smoker were to stop smoking before the age of 40, this can reduce their risk of dying (due to smoking) by about 90%. Thus, you get an extra 9 years, or 3,285 days.[187]

Using such figures, it becomes straightforward to compare the benefits, or harms, of smoking and exercise. If you never smoke, you gain 10 years. If you stop smoking aged 40, you gain 9 years, if you exercise you gain 5. If you never smoke, *and* exercise you get 15.

You may now be wondering, what happens to my 70-year-old woman if she exercises? Sorry, Qrisk3 is not bothered in the slightest about exercise. Which is a pretty damned significant omission. Exercise doesn't matter? I think this might give you some insight into another of the problems with all the risk calculators. They count only those things which can be easily counted.

"Everything that can be counted does not necessarily count; everything that counts cannot necessarily be counted."

Albert Einstein

Anyway, now that we are looking at things through the lens of life expectancy, it becomes relatively straightforward to compare and contrast other factors. For example, exercise and obesity.

From a number of discussions that I've had over the years I get the sense that most people believe a lack of exercise, and obesity, have a pretty similar impact. Indeed, the general consensus seems to be that obesity is probably worse for you. Is this true?

To find out, we can return to Qrisk3 to study the effect of a raised body mass index (BMI) on cardiovascular risk. Yes, I am continuing to lean on Qrisk3 here. Mainly because it uses the mainstream figures, so I cannot be accused of making things up to suit myself. Also, they have done the complex calculations, so I don't need to do them all again. Frankly, I don't think I could. Because my rudimentary maths knowledge would rapidly fall apart at the seams.

In the case of obesity, I inputted new data for a 60-year-old man. To keep things as simple as possible I included no other significant risk factors – as with my 70-year-old woman. This is a man as healthy as healthy can be. I based him on myself, obviously. Perhaps not as handsome as I. Nor as witty.

I named him Bob and made him of average height – five feet nine inches (175 cm). Which is my height, on a good day, with a following wind. I set his weight at 75 kg, which *was* me on a good day, about 30 years ago. This represents a body mass index (BMI) of 25. Which is at the upper end of 'normal.'

Qrisk3 informed me that Bob's 10-year risk of a cardiovascular event was precisely 6.1%. So, I raised Bob's weight all the way up to 150 kilograms, giving Bob a BMI of 50, which is super-morbidly obese. Which is why I called him Bob, as this is about all he could manage in a swimming pool.

After turning his obesity dial all the way up to eleven, his risk went up by 0.3%. Reaching the giddy heights of 6.4%.

In case you are wondering, I did try to do this calculation aged 70. Which would make the comparison as close as possible to my woman. However, when I doubled the BMI in a 70-year-old man, the cardiovascular risk remained stubbornly unaltered.

What did this mean with regard to Bob's life expectancy? Well, without going through all the figures again, which is probably a great relief to all concerned, I can tell you that by becoming morbidly obese, Bob's life expectancy was reduced by around 12 days.

Moving away from Bob, who was much relieved that he was not going to drop dead from heart attack – so he ate a pack of celebratory donuts – I thought it would be interesting to create a little graph (Figure 26), comparing the impact of three risk factors on life expectancy. Obesity, lack of exercise and smoking.

Yes, I am playing a couple of games here. I have compared a lifetime of smoking, to 20 or 30 years of being obese. In addition, I ascribed no age to the lack of exercise.

I am simply trying to emphasize a point here. Which is that, when it comes to the risk of death, some things are vastly... and when I say vastly, I mean vastly, more important than others. This only becomes clear once you compare one thing with the other, using the same outcome measurement. In this case, life expectancy.

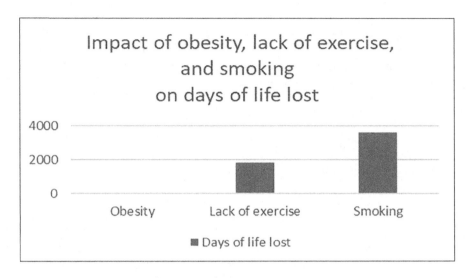

Figure 26

In fact, the extraordinarily modest impact of obesity on life expectancy is a topic I covered in some detail in my book *Doctoring Data*. When I analysed the evidence, I found the body mass index (BMI) associated with the longest life expectancy lay between 25 to 30. This is currently considered 'overweight.'

It was not until the body mass index got above 35 that it had any discernible impact on how long you lived. Even then the effect was pretty minuscule. In truth, a very low body mass index turned out to be far more dangerous than being obese. But no-one warns you against losing weight... Stop dieting, you might die! You may want to try looking up the life expectancy of those with anorexia nervosa some time.

Of course, body mass index does tangle up with central obesity, and raised blood pressure and diabetes... and Uncle Tom Cobley and all. However, in isolation, forget about it. It has almost zero effect on life expectancy. Indeed, a moderately raised body mass index means you will live longer. To quote from one Canadian study.

"Our results are similar to those from other recent studies, confirming that underweight and obesity class II+ are clear risk factors for mortality, and

217

*showing that when compared to the acceptable BMI category, **overweight appears to be protective against mortality**. Obesity class I was not associated with an increased risk of mortality."* [188]

I turned the figures from this paper into a simple graph that can be seen below (Figure 27). Highest risk of death, when the BMI was below 18.5. Lowest between 25–30. The risk of death with a BMI of 30–35 (Level 1 obesity) was lower than with a healthy BMI 18.5 to 25.

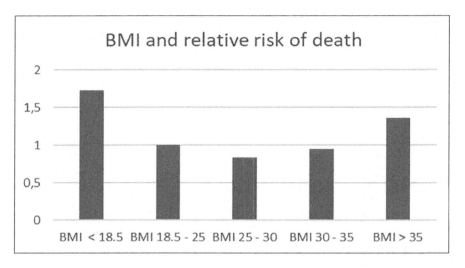

Figure 27

I know from bitter experience that this fact is the single thing that creates apoplexy in most people. Being overweight means that you live longer! How very dare you! You are a charlatan and a fool – a few even ruder names have been used.

A number of people simply refuse to believe it, and I don't know what to do about that. Facts that create painful cognitive dissonance are usually attacked with great venom, followed by dismissal. First of the fact, then of me... anyway, getting back to the main point.

The main point is that I want to try to give you some sense of the harms, or benefits of various things, using the most important outcome measure that there is. Namely, life expectancy. I don't think I have ever seen anyone else do this, or even attempt to do this? Possibly because it is just so damned tricky.

In addition, as you may have noticed, I have begun to discuss overall mortality, not just cardiovascular mortality. Smoking, for example, can kill you in several different ways: lung damage (chronic obstructive lung disease), lung cancer, and cardiovascular disease. To name but three.

However, I don't think there is any great point is separating out the benefits, or harms, from each other. It doesn't really matter which type of damage from smoking ends up killing you. Dead is dead.

When the discussion moves to diabetes, this can also kill you through several different mechanisms: cardiovascular disease, kidney failure, increased risk of infections, and suchlike. Once again, there is nothing much to be gained in teasing out the impact of one vs. the other In short, from now on, it is mainly going to be about overall mortality.

So, there we go. Having cleared up life expectancy, I am now going to move onto the factors, or actions, or whatever term is best here, that can do damage, or provide the most benefit. I am going to break this down into three sections. Endothelial damage, blood clotting, and 'miscellaneous.'

Endothelial damage is by far the most important of the three, and so it makes up by far the longest, section. The miscellaneous section is a quick review of actions that don't quite fit with anything else e.g., increasing magnesium intake, or taking thiamine as a supplement. These things do not (necessarily) have any significant impact on endothelial damage, or blood clotting, but they can prevent you dying from cardiovascular disease in other ways. So, they remain important.

CHAPTER 10

Endothelial damage – endothelial protection

As discussed, there are many hundreds of things that can damage the endothelium. I am certainly not going to go through them all here. For example, sickle cell disease, rheumatoid arthritis, Kawasaki's disease, COVID19, sepsis, Avastin/Bevacizumab, and suchlike.

Instead, I am going to look at the most important factors that can damage the endothelium, in the greatest number of people.

At this point I am going to add homocysteine into the discussion – something that I only mentioned in passing earlier. The reason for doing this, is that it has an additional health impact which makes it almost impossible to leave out. I think you're going to agree with me on this.

Which takes us to the most important factors that can lead to endothelial damage, in the greatest number of people are:

1. Raised blood sugar levels/type 2 diabetes

2. HPA-axis dysfunction/mental illness/use of steroids (cortisol)

3. Smoking

4. Air pollution

5. Raised blood pressure

6. Periodontal disease

7. Drugs/cocaine

8. Use of prescription drugs e.g., drugs to reduce acid in the stomach

9. Homocysteine

Although I have shaved down this list, even in its much-truncated form I am not going to discuss them all, at least not separately. For example, HPA-axis dysfunction whether or not caused by mental illness and/or use of steroids is all covered within 'diabetes'. As for smoking, the action required can be summed up by a single word... stop. Gum disease/periodontal disease... see your dentist. Drugs/cocaine... stop.

Which means that I am only going to look in greater detail here at:

1. Diabetes

2. Air pollution

3. Raised blood pressure

4. Use of prescription drugs to reduce stomach acid

5. Homocysteine

After this, I am going to outline a few things you can do to protect the endothelium.

1. Raised blood sugar levels/type 2 diabetes.

Number of people with the problem ~ **10 million**
Maximum reduction in lifespan **20 years**

(I am not talking about type I diabetes, caused by a lack of insulin).

This is almost certainly the single most important cardiovascular risk factor, impacting on the greatest number of people. In the UK there are around 10 million people with type 2 diabetes, and/or prediabetes. Around 60 million in the US. Looked at in isolation it can knock at least 10 years off your life expectancy.[189]

In truth though, it is much worse than this. With diabetes there are significant add-on problems such as: kidney failure, raised blood pressure, increased blood clotting factors and suchlike. If you bring them all to the party, you can probably double the years of life lost to 20.

Because of this massive burden, I am going to spend more time looking at diabetes than anything else. I am also using the term 'diabetes' to cover all manifestations of raised blood sugar. (Even though the direct translation of *diabetes* is – passing a lot of urine).

222

There are three main reasons why you may have diabetes, and they can all tangle up with each other:

- Taking corticosteroids/steroids (having a high blood cortisol level)
- Stress/strain mental illness (HPA-axis dysfunction)
- Obesity/central obesity

Although they represent different underlying pathways, when it comes down to it, they all end up in much the same place. Which is that insulin can no longer keep the blood sugar level under control.

This leads to a high insulin level, and a high blood sugar level at the same time. A state that is commonly referred to as 'insulin resistance'. I don't like it as a term (another potential book I fear), but it will do as a convenient shorthand.

Before delving deeper, I feel the need to pause for a moment to pop in a couple of disclaimers. First, I want to make it crystal clear that I am not going to suggest anyone stops taking steroids if they are on them for a medical reason.

As for stress/strain HPA-axis dysfunction. If this is due to depression, or bipolar disorder, or PTSD, then the management of these conditions is beyond the scope of this book. Please try to get proper medical attention and support. Having said this, the same actions that work for everyone else will also work here. If, to a lesser extent, because you will still have an underlying driver of 'insulin resistance' that you can do little about.

Having got that out of the way, here goes. What can you do to reduce insulin resistance, lower your blood sugar levels – and thus protect your endothelium?

Well, whatever the underlying cause, there are essentially two ways to get the blood sugar level down and keep it down.

- Burn up the stores of sugar in your body
- Avoid refilling the stores

First, some background on how the body deals with 'sugar.'

How sugar is stored in the body

The average person can store about 1,500 calories of sugar in their body. Around 1,000 in the muscles, and 500 in the liver. More if you're massive, less if you're titchy. Whatever size you are, once your sugar stores are full, they are full.

Just to tie off a small loose end, you also have around 5 grams (25 calories worth) of sugar floating about in your bloodstream at any given time. About twice as much if you have diabetes, obviously.

When I say sugar I mean, to all intents and purposes, glucose. This is by far the most important form of sugar that we consume, store, and utilise for energy. It is entirely possible to eat other sugar(s). The main one is fructose, which is found in fruit and corn oil syrup, and suchlike. However, apart from some very specialised cells, the body does not use fructose, or any other type of sugar, for energy.

In turn this means that all other sugars are either rapidly turned into glucose, or else they are converted into fat/fatty acids. A small amount of this conversion takes place in the digestive system, but the vast majority occurs in the liver. As a general rule, most clever biochemical things happen in the liver.

When it comes to storage, glucose is not actually stored as 'glucose'. Instead, thousands of individual glucose molecules are stuck together, end to end, to create a massive multi-glucose 'polymer', called glycogen. This can be very rapidly broken down again for use. This happens if, for example, the sugar level in the blood starts to fall. Or the muscles need rapid access to energy.

Now that you know these few essential facts, let's have a think about what it means. For the purposes of this discussion, the critical issue is the following. If you reach glycogen storage capacity in the liver and the muscles, then that's that. There is absolutely nowhere else for it to go.

So, when your glycogen stores are full, and you continue to eat sugar, the liver has only one choice, which is convert the excess glucose into fatty acids. It does this using the process called de novo lipogenesis (fats made from new), which I described earlier in the book. The process needs a pretty high insulin level to drive it. So, the insulin level goes up.

At this point you are now, officially, in a state of insulin resistance. Your muscles are full of glycogen – so they can store no more. Your liver is full of glycogen – so it can store no more. Insulin levels have risen to force the system of *de novo* lipogenesis into action.

I don't know if I should define this as insulin resistance, or simply call it being 'full of glucose'. If you are fit and healthy, and slim, and you stop eating, this insulin resistant state rapidly reverses. If, however, you are becoming obese, and you never stop eating for any length of time (to the point where calorie consumption constantly remains higher than energy use), this state will become permanent. You will be, in effect, diabetic.

Stepping back for a moment, I feel the need to clear up something important. The vast majority of glucose that we eat comes in the form of carbohydrates. Few of us eat pure sugar.

Even what we call 'sugar', the white stuff you sprinkle on cornflakes, and suchlike, is actually a combination of one glucose molecule attached to one fructose molecule – otherwise known as sucrose. Which means that 'sugar' is actually a carbohydrate, not a sugar, although we call it sugar. As usual, the terminology is a bloody nightmare. Sugar is not sugar... it is sugar.

When you eat sugar/sucrose, or any other carbohydrate, it is broken down into glucose and fructose or, say, galactose, before being absorbed. Commonly consumed sugars, as shown in Figure 28, are single molecules of:

- Glucose

- Fructose

- Galactose

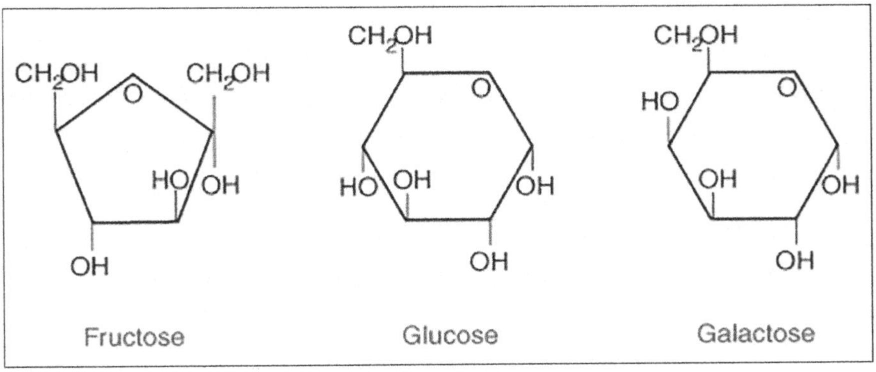

Figure 28

You may have already known this, but I've spoken to many patients with diabetes who cannot understand why their 'sugar' level spikes when they eat bread, or potatoes, or pasta, or fruit or suchlike. *'But I don't eat any sugar doc?'*

I usually refrain from telling them what I really think at this point. I simply point out that, as far as your body is concerned, all these things are just 'sugar'. Even a tree is just a massive sugar lump. It is constructed, primarily, from trillions of molecules of glucose, all bound tightly together. The reason why we can't eat wood is because the glucose molecules are stuck together too tightly for our puny human enzymes to break them apart. Woodworms, we ain't.

Just as a quick golly gee whizz fact. Crab shells and lobster shells are constructed from chitin. Chitin too, is made from glucose molecules, even more tightly bound together than in wood. Yes, crabs are surrounded by sugar armour. Obviously, we cannot digest chitin, we have to crack it with pincers.

The type of plants/carbohydrates we can actually eat are things such as potatoes, rice, wheat, fruits, and other various 'vegetables', swedes, and broccoli, peas, and beans and suchlike.

Even though the glucose molecules in these plants are less tightly bound than in trees, we still need to cook most of them in order to break apart the strongest bonds. Or else they will pass straight through, like fibre. Yes, fibre, super healthy because it goes shooting from one end to the other without touching the sides. You might as well eat a baseball bat.

After cooking, our enzymes can then finish off the 'breakdown' job of turning the carbs into 'sugars.'

In summary, in whatever form we choose to eat them, once they arrive in our digestive tract, all carbohydrates are broken down into simple sugars – mainly glucose – they are then transported directly to the liver.

Key point: Carbohydrates = glucose

It is within the liver that the fate of glucose is then decided. There are three options:

- Release into the bloodstream
- Store as glycogen
- Convert to fat

And that, gentle reader, is probably all that you need to know. From this simple framework, you can work out what drives diabetes, and how to reverse it. You probably don't think so. But you can.

If you can't work it out, here is the answer that I prepared earlier. You can avoid developing diabetes, or reverse diabetes, by emptying out your glucose/glycogen stores. There are two ways to do this.

- Burn up the stores

- Don't eat carbohydrates, as you will fill the stores straight back up again

And that's it.

The best way to burn up glucose is with short bursts of intensive exercise. Indeed, when it comes to diabetes, not all exercise is the same. The type of exercise that works best is 'short burst.' [190]

As little as 10 minutes of high intensity exercise, 3 or 4 times a week, can be enough. The reason why short sharp exercise works best, is because it's mainly *an*aerobic (does not use up oxygen) and relies entirely on using glucose, rather than fat, for fuel.

The added advantage of anaerobic (high intensity, no oxygen, exercise) is that it is horribly inefficient. With aerobic metabolism, one gram of fat produces around nine calories of energy, and one gram of glucose provides about four or five calories of energy.

However, if you burn one gram of glucose using the anaerobic system, it will only produce about a half a calorie. Which makes it possible to empty your glucose stores very fast (Some is recycled, as lactate, which is converted back to glucose in the liver, but a lot is just… gone)

Here is a story from Diabetes.co.uk.

"A pensioner with type 2 diabetes claims to have effectively cured himself of the disease by exercising intensely for less than half an hour a week. John Hall, 67, from Coventry, has been battling type 2 diabetes for the past seven years after being diagnosed with the metabolic condition the day after his 60th birthday.

"John decided to take a different approach to exercise and started participating in a programme called Progressive Accelerating Cardiopulmonary Exercise, or Pace for short, at his local community centre. The exercise programme combines warm-ups and a series of high intensity aerobic activity, including running and jumping, into just two or three 12-minute sessions a week.

"After only four months of attending the short, intense, exercise classes, John says he has seen a huge drop in blood glucose, blood pressure and cholesterol levels, which before were nearly twice as high as what they should be.

"When I went back to the doctors two weeks ago, they were absolutely astounded. They said 'what on earth have you been doing?'" After managing to reverse the progression of his type 2 diabetes, John said he no longer considers himself as a diabetic and feels free to enjoy life." [191]

Moving on, there's little point in emptying your glycogen stores with short burst exercise, if you then simply proceed to stuff yourself with carbohydrates. Because the muscles and the liver will just fill up once again. At which point you slither down the snake, back to square one on the diabetes board.

Which means that the other action you need to take, if you want to keep insulin resistance at bay, or to reverse it, is to cut down on carbohydrates. In this way, the stores can only slowly be refilled.

In their 'unfilled' state, muscles are free to mop up any excess glucose that is floating about in the bloodstream. The liver is also free to convert glucose into glycogen and store it. There is no need for *de novo* lipogenesis, so the insulin level drops. And, because insulin drives fat storage, and prevents fat being released for use as energy, you can also now access fat, and start to burn it up.

Is there any evidence that reducing carbohydrate consumption works, as described? There is plenty, but I am going to focus on the work of a colleague, and friend, who has been working in this area for several years, Dr David Unwin.

At one point he was discounted as a dangerous maverick for his views on a low carb diet. At the time of writing he has become the Royal College of General Practitioners expert clinical advisor on diabetes. In 2016 he won the NHS innovator of the year award and was made General Practice National champion of Collaborative Care and Support Planning in Obesity and Diabetes.

In short, his ideas are now becoming far more widely accepted by the medical mainstream. His advice has moved from being considered highly controversial, quack medicine, towards grudging acceptance. In the UK at least. I wrote a blog about his research, and I include a section of it here. It starts with his own worlds.

"A few years ago, I was interested to find out how a patient had improved her diabetic control. She confessed she had ignored my advice and learnt a much better way to look after herself, from the internet. I suppressed my

wounded pride and looked at the Low Carb Forum on Diabetes.co.uk There were thousands of type two diabetics on there, ignoring their doctors – and getting great results (now that is just not allowed)."

Yes, Dr Unwin did not criticize, or ignore, instead he was intrigued. Could this possibly be true. Could a high fat, low carbohydrate diet be beneficial? It went against everything he had been told about healthy eating, and weight loss, and type 2 diabetes. Fat has twice the calories, per gram, as carbohydrates... and suchlike. Eating fat, he believed, makes you fat, and then you develop diabetes, and heart disease.

Dr Unwin did more research, then he made the decision to work with patients, mainly those with diabetes, to see if a low carbohydrate diet could be beneficial. Lo and behold, it was... very beneficial. In fact, he found that it was like a miracle cure.

In 2014 he published a paper on his research on a small number of patients. *"Low carbohydrate diet to achieve weight loss and improve HbA1c in type 2 diabetes and prediabetes: experience from one general practice."*

"It was observed that a low carbohydrate diet achieved substantial weight loss in all patients and brought about normalisation of blood glucose control in 16 out of 18 patients. At the same time, plasma lipid profiles improved, and BP fell allowing discontinuation of antihypertensive therapy in some individuals...

*"**Conclusions**. Based on our work so far, we can understand the reasons for the internet enthusiasm for a low carbohydrate diet; the majority of patients lose weight rapidly and fairly easily; predictably the HbA1c levels are not far behind. Cholesterol levels, liver enzymes and BP levels all improved. This approach is simple to implement and much appreciated by people with diabetes."*

Next, he published results of a much larger study, on nearly 200 patients over 6-year period. It is called. *"Insights from a general practice service evaluation supporting a lower carbohydrate diet in patients with type 2 diabetes mellitus and prediabetes"* published in *BMJ nutrition.*

Here are the main findings, which I nicked directly from his press release:

- 46% drug-free T2 diabetes remission

- Significant improvements in weight, blood pressure and lipid profiles

- 93% remission of prediabetes

- £50,885 annual saving on the Norwood GP practice NHS diabetes drug budget

- If every GP practice in England spent the same on drugs for diabetes per patient as Norwood the NHS could save £277,000,000

- Older patients can do as well as younger ones with a low carb approach

- The participants who started with the worst blood sugars saw the greatest improvements in diabetic control

- Four individuals came off insulin altogether

- Total weight loss for the 199 participants was 1.6 metric tons.

This paper was attacked, of course. There are massive financial interests involved in this area. For example, as Dr Unwin pointed out, if every GP practice in the UK used the low carb approach, the NHS could save £277,000,000 (~$350 million) in drug costs. Scaled up to the US, with much higher drugs costs, we could be looking at around $2Bn/year. Around the world, who knows, just vast sums of money.

So, you can imagine the joy that this paper will be met with in pharmaceutical company boardrooms around the world. The words 'lead' and 'balloon', spring to mind. Equally the massive low-fat high carb food manufacturers will be throwing their hands up in horror – '*my bonus, my bonus... nooooo.*' You can take your low carb yoghurts and....'

Yes, high fat low carbohydrate diets work in reversing diabetes. Let me repeat that statement, they work. Nothing else gets close. In fact, the dietary advice over the last 40 or 50 years – to eat carbohydrates and not fat – has been one of the main driving forces behind the explosion in obesity and diabetes in the Western World.

The experts are currently fighting a desperate and vicious rearguard action to protect their reputations and funding. Attacking Dr Unwin, and anyone else who dares point out that they have been talking nonsense for half a century. I think, I hope, they are losing – will lose. In a few years' time the high carb approach will simply be a warning footnote in history.

What you may also notice from Dr Unwin's research is that there was a substantial reduction in blood pressure on the low carb approach. So much so that, in many cases, people managed to stop their antihypertensive treatment altogether. That is, in addition to stopping their diabetes drugs.

The reason for this additional benefit is that a high insulin level raises blood pressure. Which means that, if you can get the insulin levels down, the blood pressure will usually fall. This is not actually a new finding. The effect of insulin on blood pressure has been known for decades. Here is a paper from as far back as 1991 called "*Insulin resistance in hypertension – a relationship with consequences?*"

"Resistance to the action of insulin on glucose metabolism, with the ensuing compensatory hyperinsulinemia [raised insulin levels], *is closely linked to essential hypertension. Acutely, insulin has been shown to stimulate sympathetic nervous system activity and … to promote sodium retention and to cause vascular wall changes, including increased cholesterol biosynthesis and smooth muscle proliferation.*

"If these mechanisms operate on a chronic basis, the continuous exposure to elevated plasma insulin levels may play a pathogenetic role in the development of high blood pressure, and also of a predisposition toward atherosclerosis in patients with hypertension." [192]

As you can gather from this, insulin is not the entirely benign substance that it is generally made out to be. Certainly not when the level is too high. It causes the kidneys to retain sodium (salt). It also stimulates the sympathetic nervous system, both of which drive up blood pressure.

Perhaps most critically at this point in the discussion, is the fact that a high insulin level stimulates fat storage, thus obesity. Therefore, getting the level down will almost certainly lead to weight loss. So, yes, carbohydrates are delicious and wonderful, and I would never suggest that people stop eating them altogether. However, for many people, excess consumption can result in metabolic and physiological catastrophe.

Anyway, that's pretty much it. Two very simple solutions for preventing and reversing diabetes. High intensity exercise, and a reduction in carbohydrate consumption. Doing both is best. By doing so, you clear out glucose stores, and also stop them getting filled up again. Insulin resistance… gone.

The other important thing to do, and I say this with a heavy heart, is to reduce alcohol consumption. Alcohol, as you probably know is created by the process of fermentation, whereby bacteria transform sugars into alcohol. Which means that alcohol, and sugars, are pretty closely related substances.

Indeed, if given the choice, the body will use alcohol for energy, before it turns reluctantly to glucose. Only once the glucose stores are staring to drain away will the body turn to fat for energy. Alcohol → glucose → fat. (If things are getting very hairy, the body will start breaking down proteins, and convert parts of them into glucose. This normally starts to happen about 22 miles into a marathon... a.k.a. 'the wall').

Therefore, if you drink too much alcohol, it becomes exceedingly difficult to burn up your glucose stores. If you drink in the evening, then head for bed, your body will be powered by booze all night. You will not have 'fasted' at all by the time you break your fast. No glucose will have been used up and you will remain insulin resistant. You will certainly get nowhere near your fat stores. Losing weight becomes exceedingly difficult.

The impact of alcohol on obesity is one of the reasons why Sumo wrestlers drink a lot of beer. Around six pints per meal. They do so, because they know it helps to promote the weight gain they need, to avoid being picked up and thrown out of the dohyo by another very large gentleman whose heart is full of murderous intent.

However, despite being heavy drinkers, and hugely overweight, it is very unusual for Sumo wrestlers to develop diabetes. Fattest population in the world, virtually no diabetes. How so? Because they train very hard, for long periods of time – every single day. In turn they burn up their glucose stores, every single day.[193]

Once they stop exercising, however... kaboom.

In the opposite direction, and of particular interest in this discussion, there is a group of people who are very, very, thin. They have no adipose tissue at all. This is because have a very rare genetic condition known as congenital generalised lipodystrophy (CGL). It is also called Berardinelli-Seip syndrome. They are the leanest people on the planet. Lucky them?

In fact, I have used them many times as a pop-question with a number of doctors. Having described Berardinelli-Seip syndrome I then ask the follow-up question; how many do you think have type 2 diabetes? Almost everyone answers that, obviously, none of them can possibly have diabetes, because they are super slim with not an ounce of fat.

Of course, the correct answer is that every single one of them has diabetes. It is always extremely severe, with stratospherically high blood sugar levels, super-high insulin levels, fatty livers, VLDL levels through the roof, pancreatitis... The absolute works. Thinnest people in the world – yet they all have terrible problems with diabetes.

Why?

Well, if you think about it, you already have the answer. They have severe diabetes, because they have absolutely nowhere to store excess glucose. Once they have their 1,500 calories of glycogen stored, they are now officially... full up. Ping!

Of course, as with everyone else, their livers can convert the excess glucose into fat, but where can they then put it? Into the non-existent fat cells? No, that's not going to work is it? In effect, those with Berardinelli-Seip are trapped in the ultimate 'back-pressure' situation.

They are full of glucose. In order to try to clear it from the liver, the insulin level climbs higher and higher to flog *de novo* lipogenesis. In turn, the VLDL level in the blood goes sky high – VLDL transports fat out of the liver to fat cells. This puts massive back pressure on fat generation. With nowhere else to go glucose will then inevitably leak out from the liver, so the blood sugar level climbs higher and higher. The end result is unavoidable.

Of course, if they do manage to eat precisely what they require to meet their energy needs, each day. Or, if they manage to use up all the energy they consume, every day, there will be no problem.

This could be achieved with great discipline. Unfortunately, they have another issue to deal with. Which is that, with no fat cells, no leptin is produced. With no leptin, which is the most powerful appetite suppressant known to man, they are starving hungry all the time. This is because their body its screaming at them that they *are* starving. Which makes it very difficult for them to keep energy consumption under control. (I believe labradors do not produce leptin either, which is why they will always be hungry, and want to eat all the time – and get fat).

In the end Berardinelli-Siep results in metabolic catastrophe.

"Metabolic derangements are mostly responsible for the serious comorbidities associated with lipodystrophy; some of which are chronic

complications of poorly controlled diabetes, acute pancreatitis, hepatic cirrhosis, proteinuria and renal failure, and premature cardiovascular disease." [194]

Fascinatingly, here we have a group of super-thin diabetics, who develop diabetes for exactly the same reason as the super-fat diabetics. Which is that they have run out of place to store excess energy. Whilst they are certainly not lucky in any way shape or form, they do provide a perfect model to explain what does cause diabetes.

You might argue they must have other abnormalities creating problems. It cannot just be because they are super-thin. Although I don't actually agree with this, I did consider it. Therefore, I thought it would be interesting to try to find someone who had been metabolically 'normal', who then developed Berardinelli-Seip, and then went on to have full-blown diabetes – as a direct result.

Which leads us to the case of a woman with malignant melanoma, who was treated with the anti-cancer drug nivolumab. Yes, you've never heard of it, and almost certainly never will again. Put that to the back of your mind. The important thing here is that this drug triggered an auto-immune reaction which then attacked and killed her fat cells. Which meant that she developed late onset Berardinelli-Seip syndrome.

Suddenly, she became extremely slim, with a BMI of 16. She was also starving hungry, due to having no leptin. She rapidly developed super-high insulin and glucose levels – six times normal – and her VLDL level went through the roof. At the same time her liver filled up with fat. Yes, what she represents is a case of severe diabetes as a direct result of rapid *loss* of body fat. [195]

In a world where obesity is believed to be *the* cause of type 2 diabetes, her story makes no sense. In a world where the cause of type 2 diabetes is that the liver, and muscles, are full of glucose – and there is nowhere else to put it – this makes perfect sense.

So, in short, yes, it is all that simple. It is why the answers are also simple. High intensity exercise and a low carbohydrate diet – and cut down on the booze. Accept no alternatives.

Reducing cortisol levels

As explained earlier, the other major cause of insulin resistance is a high cortisol level. This is because cortisol acts as a direct antagonist to insulin at most sites in the body. A raised cortisol can be due to psychological 'strain' or taking steroids which are, basically, cortisol. So, both causes are pretty much the same cause, really.

In either case it becomes even more important to reduce glucose intake and clear out glucose stores, to avoid making the situation worse. Which means that exercise, and a low carbohydrate diet, are doubly important here.

In addition to this, you must do everything you can to reduce HPA-axis dysfunction. Relaxation, meditation, mindfulness, yoga. I say this because there is good evidence that they can all be highly beneficial.

"Biofeedback and relaxation were associated with significant decreases in average blood glucose, A1C, and muscle tension compared with the control group. At 3-month follow-up, the treatment group continued to demonstrate lower blood glucose." [196]

I was also fascinated by a German study, where the researchers looked at the benefits of yoga following a heart attack, in men. It was found that their systolic blood pressure could be lowered by up to 21 mmHg using yoga alone.[197] Which is a damn sight better than almost any single blood pressure lowering medication. I believe they had to tell them it wasn't actually Yoga because German men are a bit like that. *'Yoga, Gott in Himmel. Nein danke.'*

In truth, I don't think it really matters which relaxation technique you use, so long as you enjoy it. It is a very personal thing. Use the technique you feel most comfortable with, whichever works for you... get on with it.

I like controlled breathing exercise best, because I am lazy. Breathe in for five seconds, breathe out for five seconds. Concentrate only on how you are breathing and clear your mind of everything else. Not tricky in my case, as there is very little to clear. Ten minutes a day is all you need. It can help to re-set the HPA-axis.

For those who are interested in the deeper science, you can read the Nature paper *"Voluntary upregulation of heart rate variability through biofeedback is improved by mental contemplative training."* [198]

"To summarise, we have shown that a mental training intervention increases the ability to voluntarily increase HF-HRV [high frequency heart rate variability, which is a key measure of HPA-axis dysfunction]. This has implications for the use of such interventions in healthy and impaired populations. Mental training may prove particularly fruitful for people who exhibit altered or reduced vagal

flexibility, as found in children at risk of psychopathology and people suffering from depression or social phobia. Such programs may also be helpful for people suffering from psychotic symptoms, who have been found to benefit from increased high frequency heart rate variability control in a biofeedback study."

In addition to this, it is a good idea to identify sources of negative stress in your life. Be it work, relationships, next-door neighbours, Facebook, Twitter, husband, wife. If they are upsetting you, try to avoid, mitigate, change, stop reading, or divorce.

In addition, try to steer clear of anger, and other negative emotions. One fascinating study from the US looked at the language used on Twitter, and then related this to heart disease mortality. It was called *"Psychological Language on Twitter Predicts County-Level Heart Disease Mortality"*.

What they found was that the words and phrases used on Twitter were an amazingly accurate predictor of cardiovascular mortality. Better than any of the cardiovascular disease calculators.[199]

The main finding was that if you live an area where people post far more nasty, angry, things on Twitter, you were more likely to die from heart attacks. Below, in Figure 29, is a map of the North-eastern United States comparing deaths from heart disease vs. Twitter predicted heart disease (Called AHD here – atherosclerotic heart disease).

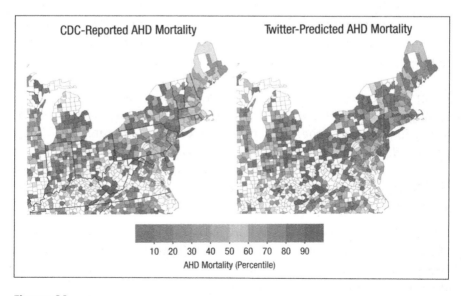

Figure 29

236

I further enjoyed some of their conclusions:

"Although less is known at the individual level about the protective effects of positive psychological variables than about the risk associated with negative variables, our findings align with a growing body of research supporting the cardiovascular health benefits of psychological well-being. Engagement, which has long been considered an important component of successful aging, emerged as the strongest protective factor in our study. Use of positive-emotion words was also protective, which is in line with numerous findings that positive emotions convey protection from illness and disease."

The entire area of HPA-axis dysfunction, stress, cortisol central obesity and diabetes could form the basis of several books. However, for now, I shall sum it up with a quote from Woody in Toy Story. *'Play nice.'*

2: Air pollution/small particulate matter

Number of people with the problem ~ **10 million**

Maximum reduction in lifespan **4 years**

Air pollution, small particulate air pollution, is much less of a problem than it used to be. In the 1950s the 'smog' from coal fires and car exhausts was truly dreadful. The great London smog of 1952 was estimated to have killed 10,000-12,000 people over a period of only 5 days. It led to the clean air acts of 1956 and '62.

In addition to the widespread atmospheric air pollution, many people worked in terribly polluted environments. Coal mines, iron smelters, locomotive works. In Crewe, near to where I now live, there was a massive locomotive factory which is now defunct. To insulate the engines, they used a great deal of asbestos.

Within the factory, the workers used asbestos sheets to build smart little sheds to sit in, and have a nice cup of tea, and a smoke. They also made kick-about footballs, from binding together the spare asbestos strands that were lying about all over the place. This did not end well. One patient, reduced to breathing through an oxygen concentrator, told me all about it as I listened with horrid fascination.

Which means that in many workplaces there were millions of men, almost entirely men, suffering from pneumoconiosis and asbestosis, and silicosis, and hatters breathing in mercury vapour. To explain this one. To make hats you use felt. To make felt, you use mercury at high temperatures. The mercury vapour is then breathed into the lungs, before finding its way into the brain. Hence the character of the Mad Hatter from Alice in Wonderland. Which was based on real life Mad Hatters. Otherwise known as 'people who make hats, who then suffer from brain mercury poisoning'.

There was also far more smoking. My childhood memory of going to the cinema was that, about halfway through the film, a cloud of smoke was hanging just above your head, and you could see the light beam of the projector flickering through it. Restaurants and bars were also heavy with cigarette smoke. Clothes stank of smoke, even if you didn't smoke.

In one hospital in Scotland where I worked there was an actual smoking room for the medical staff. If I remember correctly, it was in the accident and emergency department. The walls of the room were a dull, sickly, brown, and you could literally scrape sticky brown goo off with your fingernail. Lovely. Was this, I wonder, the inspiration for champagne beige?

Then, of course, there was lead pollution, with hundreds of thousands of tons of lead pumped out of car exhausts each year. Frankly, I'm amazed humanity survived the corrosive lung and endothelium destroying toxic pollution that everyone breathed in day after day in the recent past.

Nowadays, whilst things have certainly improved, air pollution still exists. Mainly in the form of diesel exhaust particulate matter. This is obviously far worse in cities, mainly close to major roads where heavy goods vehicles ply their trade. It has been estimated that people who live in such highly polluted environments, may lose four years of life expectancy.[200]

How can this be avoided? Moving to the countryside is not really possible for many people. Which means that the only realistic option is to wear a mask outside, as they do in much of the Far East. I must say that I hesitate to recommend doing this, because I hate the idea of walking about masked up.

However, until they get rid of most diesel-powered vehicles, and we all happily go electric, if you live in the centre of, say, London, and you walk about the streets next to busy roads, it may be the best idea.

Having said this, you do need a proper mask that filters out small particulate matter. There is no point in sticking an old sock over your face and hoping for the best. As a wise man once said. Using a cloth mask to keep out nanoparticles, is like trying to pick up sand using a tennis racquet.

3: Raised blood pressure (Eighteen months)

Number of people with the problem ~ **10 million**
Reduction in lifespan, average **18 months**

Many millions of people have a high blood pressure which batters away at their endothelial cells, day after day. This makes it highly significant, on a population-wide level. However, the impact on life expectancy may not be as great as you might have been led to believe.

Using Qrisk3 as the font of all human knowledge. If you have a systolic blood pressure of 160 mmHg, rather than 120 mmHg, this will reduce your life expectancy by around a year and a half. Assuming the high blood pressure starts at the age of 40.

To arrive at this figure, I created another super healthy 60-year-old man whom I shall call 'Ace'. I whacked Ace's blood pressure up from 120 mmHg to 160 mmHg. His 10-year risk rose from 6.1%, to 9%.

This resulted in around a six-month reduction in life expectancy. If you move Ace back in time, and start his raised blood pressure aged 40, he lost about a year and a half. I think this might be a slight underestimate. It's a tricky one, as these figures always are.

A year and a half is certainly significant, if rather dwarfed by such things as smoking, a lack of exercise and diabetes. So, what can you do about it? The first thing I need to say is – disclaimer alert – if your blood pressure is very high, and you cannot get it down in any other way, it will need to be treated with drugs. Terms and condition apply. It may also be caused by an underlying medical condition that requires treatment.

And, whilst I do not wish to be accused of meddling with anyone's mainstream treatment, I am going to recommend that if you need drugs, you should start with the class known as angiotensin converting enzyme inhibitors (ACE-inhibitors). These all end in -*pril*. As in rami*pril*, or enala*pril*, or perindo*pril*.

Luckily, in this case, the mainstream view is pretty much the same as mine – *finally* they are learning. Which is that ACE-inhibitors should be used first line. They don't lower the blood pressure by any more than other drugs. However, they have an additional, and important benefit, which is that they are extremely good at stimulating nitric oxide synthesis, with all the additional benefits that this provides.

*"Levels of circulating nitrite/nitrate, the end-metabolites of **nitric oxide**, were also significantly affected by ACE inhibition** ... Our findings provide further evidence in favor of differential effects associated with ACE inhibitor therapy and suggest that **the clinical benefits associated with these drugs may not solely reflect a class effect** extending their benefit beyond blood pressure-lowering effect."* [201]

The ACE-inhibitor with the greatest benefit on nitric oxide is perindopril. So, I recommend using this one, if possible. Warning, all ACE-inhibitors can cause a nasty dry cough. If this happens, and you can't cope with it, switch to an angiotensin receptor blocker (ARB) instead. Which will still have some impact on nitric oxide. The drugs in this class all end in *sartan*. As in cande*sartan*, or irbe*sartan* or val*sartan*.

Moving on from drugs. At the risk of sounding like Mr Motivator, exercise is good. It increases nitric oxide synthesis, and it lowers the blood pressure in many other ways.

A low carbohydrate diet is also highly beneficial. One of the main reasons for this, touched on earlier, is that it lowers insulin levels. Whilst insulin is clearly important stuff, when the level gets too high, it can be extremely damaging.

This is primarily because it is a potent activator of a thing called the renin-angiotensin-aldosterone-system (RAAS). A system designed for two main purposes. Purpose one, to keep hold of sodium. Purpose two, to keep your blood pressure up.

How does it work? Moving away from insulin, and keeping things as simple as possible, if your blood pressure falls, or your sodium levels fall, the kidneys take immediate note of this fact, and release a hormone called renin, which is the R in RAAS. This then drives the production, further down the line, of another hormone called angiotensin II – which is the first A in RAAS.

Angiotensin II then charges about the body doing all sorts of different things. It narrows the arteries; it stops water and sodium

240

being released from the kidneys – thus retaining sodium. It triggers the sympathetic nervous system into action, increasing heart rate etc. etc. All these things are designed to keep your blood pressure up. Because, if your blood pressure falls too much, then so will you. Resulting in such things as broken hips. A particular problem in the elderly.

(ACE-inhibitors work by preventing angiotensin I from being converted to the active form... angiotensin II. It is the reason why this class of drugs are called angiotensin-converting-enzyme *inhibitors* (ACE-inhibitors) Essentially, by blocking angiotensin II production, they lower the blood pressure).

This is all well and good, it's a cracking little system. Unfortunately, angiotensin II is the sworn enemy of both nitric oxide, and endothelial cells. In fact, it can directly kill them. As discussed in the paper *"Angiotensin II Induces Apoptosis* of Human Endothelial Cells (Protective Effect of Nitric Oxide)."* [202]

As you can now see, from a cardiovascular health perspective, activating RAAS for any length of time is an exceptionally bad idea. Indeed, for cardiovascular health, you really need to keep the RAAS monster snoring gently in its cave.

You can do this in many ways, such as, not getting angry, deep breathing, being nice, and suchlike. Because, as you already know, stress and strain increase cortisol release. This, in turn, also activates the RAAS. Yes, everything in this world truly is connected to everything else.

So, what else disturbs the slumbers of the RAAS 'endothelium destroying' monster?

Ironically, one of most important things is salt/sodium restriction. I say ironically, because salt restriction is universally promoted as a way to reduce blood pressure, and thus protect against cardiovascular disease.

This idea first appeared on the scene decades ago, when it was discovered that cutting down on salt can lower the blood pressure. In truth, the effect is vanishingly small. Indeed, on an individual level it is virtually unmeasurable. For most people the effect is around two to three mmHg, absolute max. [203]

In the real world, if you take the blood pressure on your own arm a couple of times, within a short space of time, you will find there is a

---

* Apoptosis means... death.

far greater difference than two to three millimetres of mercury. I know, because I regularly do it with patients, just to make sure their readings are reliable. The figures vary by far more than three millimetres of mercury between every single reading. Every time, guaranteed.

Given that salt restriction causes such minuscule differences in blood pressure, any benefit was never really going to be that great. Using Qrisk3, a three millimetre rise in blood pressure leads to a 0.2% increase in risk. This translates to about 15 days in life expectancy. Well within the statistical boundaries of 'bugger all.'

In addition, even this microscopic potential benefit must be balanced against the fact that if you reduce your salt intake, the kidneys will fight to keep hold of it. Because the kidneys consider sodium to be to a critical substance, even if the medical profession treats it with barely disguised disdain.

Which means that the kidneys react to low sodium levels by releasing renin. This then fires the rest of the RAAS into action:

*"... **patients with a sodium intake reduction** of 40 to 100 mmol/24 hours presented **significant increases in plasma renin and aldosterone** by a factor of 1.8 to 2.5 and two-fold, respectively."* [204]

Aldosterone, the other key hormone within the renin-angiotensin-aldosterone-system (the other A in RAAS), can also lead to havoc in the cardiovascular system. It causes, and I quote, *"increased arterial 'stiffness', endothelial cell shrinkage, and a significant drop in nitric oxide synthesis"*. All bad.[205]

All of which means that, if you restrict salt intake, there is a considerable risk that you will do far more harm than good. Indeed, many animal studies have demonstrated that salt restriction directly promotes atherosclerosis. By the way, you are not allowed to do studies like the one described below on humans. For which we should be eternally grateful.

*"In the mouse model of atherosclerosis, any reduction in dietary salt intake (from high to normal or normal to low) is proatherogenic (promotes atherosclerosis) because of activation of the RAAS. In contrast, **increasing salt in the diet suppresses RAAS dependent atherogenesis.**"* [206]

But what of humans? Here are the results from the on-going, and massive, National Health and Nutrition Examination Survey that takes place in the US on a rolling basis.

"The inverse association of sodium to CVD mortality seen here raises *questions regarding the likelihood of a survival advantage accompanying a lower sodium diet. These findings highlight the need for **further study of the relation of dietary sodium to mortality outcomes.**"* [207]

'Inverse association' means that the more you restrict sodium intake, the greater the risk of cardiovascular mortality. Yes, you did just read that. To be frank, the difference here is not that great, and probably not worth getting too worried about. I estimate an average reduction in lifespan of about a month.

However, if you really work hard enough to significantly cut salt intake, long term, things could get a lot worse. Fortunately, despite all the guidelines, and constant haranguing, few people manage to restrict salt intake to the point where the RAAS monster becomes truly angry. Just as well.

The wrong salt

Now, having just digested that, it is time for you to forget all about salt, and start worrying about salt. I shall just give you a moment to digest that statement... The reality is that you should not, and never should have been worried about (NaCl) salt. The focus should be on potassium (salt), not sodium (salt). Yes, there are many more salts in the world than are dreamt of in your philosophy, Horatio. What we call 'salt' is just one of many. Ah yes, the exquisite joy of scientific terminology once more.

Salt is not salt; it is a salt.

You may not be aware of it, but your entire body works because of the balance between sodium and potassium. Cells pump sodium out, and pump potassium in, to create what is known as an action potential across the cell membrane, which drives a vast number of your critical cellular processes.

When this system kicks into reverse (depolarises) it creates the electrical impulses that travel along nerves, allowing you to move, think and... basically exist. It also drives muscle contraction and... anyway, it all gets mind-bogglingly complicated.

So, I will focus on only one issue here. Which is that you must have the correct balance between sodium and potassium in your body. This absolutely does *not* mean that you should consume less sodium (see under the dangers of RAAS activation). It means that you should consume more potassium.

"Our Stone Age ancestors consumed about 16 times more potassium than sodium. Modern tribes of hunter-gatherers have similarly high ratios. That's a far cry from the average American diet, which has about twice as much sodium as potassium."

What happens if you don't eat enough potassium?[208]

*"Normal body levels of potassium are important for muscle function. Potassium relaxes the walls of the blood vessels, lowering blood pressure and protecting against muscle cramping. **A number of studies have shown an association between low potassium intake and increased blood pressure and higher risk of stroke.** On the flip side, **people who already have high blood pressure can significantly lower their systolic blood pressure by increasing their potassium intake.**"[209]*

Thus, in answer to the question. How can you lower blood pressure without reducing NaCl intake, and thus prodding the RAAS monster into life. The answer is simple. Consume more potassium.

In truth, the passage above does not really highlight how critical potassium can be for your health and wellbeing. Let me return to one of my touchstone clinical trials, the Scottish heart health study. Here, it was found that a higher potassium intake reduced the risk of death *to a greater degree* than diabetes increased it. There was a nearly threefold reduction in risk.[210]

As the authors of the study remarked, there was:

"... an unexpectedly powerful protective relation of dietary potassium to all-cause mortality."

This represents the greatest benefit from potassium that I have ever seen, in any study. We are looking at several years of increased life expectancy here. At least five, possibly ten. I tend to favour the lower figure, although I am not sure why. Whichever figure is true, it demonstrated very clearly that in a population with a high rate of cardiovascular disease, potassium consumption is absolutely critical.

Remember, when this study was done, Scotland had the highest rate of cardiovascular disease in the world, and possibly the lowest consumption of fresh fruit and vegetables.

When I grew up in Scotland you had neeps and tatties (turnip/ swede and potatoes), and that was about it. Maybe a frozen pea or two. As for an aubergine... the average Scot would have run in terror from that strange scary, purple thing. Leafy greens, that's what happens to the golf course in autumn.

Moving on from the Scots genetic aversion to vegetables, the lesson from this is to forget about salt... it's salt that matters... Potassium salt. Consume more of it and you can stop worrying about sodium, forever. How much do you need? At least four grams a day. Increased consumption of fruit and vegetables is a good way to achieve this.

Here are the fruits and veggies highest in potassium, starting with fruit.

- Bananas, oranges, cantaloupe, honeydew melons, apricots, grapefruit (some dried fruits, such as prunes, raisins, and dates)

- Spinach

- Broccoli

- Potatoes

- Sweet potatoes

- Mushrooms

- Peas

- Cucumbers

- Aubergine/zucchini

- Pumpkins

- Leafy greens

If you feel like it, you can also use lo-salt, instead of salt-salt. This is KCl, not NaCl. Which means that it is not actually 'lo' in salt at all. It is only 'lo' in sodium. KCl is still, chemically, a 'salt'.

And you do need chloride in the body as well – although no-one *ever* discusses this – because a low chloride level is associated with increased mortality. Who knew? Well, in truth, anyone who ever looked. Here is the title of one paper on the subject *"Serum Chloride Is an Independent Predictor of Mortality in Hypertensive Patients."* [211]

Just about the only way that the vast majority of people get sufficient chloride is by consuming NaCl (salt). When you eat sodium chloride do people think the chloride ion simply disappears into a black hole and does nothing in the body... ho hum. NaCl... sodium and chloride. One of each. I have read a great deal around this area, including a paper entitled *'Chloride, the queen of electrolytes.'* The point is made in this paper that, unlike sodium, with hundreds of thousands of studies dedicated to it, you can find out almost nothing about chloride. Despite the fact it is essential for cellular function.

Now, I think it is time for a quick blood pressure summary. If you want to reduce blood pressure, without drugs. Here are your four best approaches:

- Exercise

- Low carb diet

- Increase potassium intake, do *not* reduce NaCl intake (you need your sodium *and* your chloride)

- Reduce stress/strain

If you need drugs, I recommend:

- ACE-inhibitor/angiotensin receptor blocker (ARB)

- Aldosterone inhibitor (old fashioned, but good)

4. Use of prescription drugs to reduce stomach acid.

Number of people with the problem ~ **6 million**

Reduction in lifespan, maximum **2 years**

I wasn't certain whether to include this topic, because it doesn't concern most people. However, around six million people do take drugs to reduce stomach acid. Which means that it is not a niche issue. These drugs help with acid reflux, stomach ulcers and suchlike.

They are also used to protect the stomach when people are taking anti-inflammatories for arthritis. Drugs such as naproxen and ibuprofen, diclofenac, and suchlike.

These are often called non-steroidal anti-inflammatory drugs (NSAIDS). They can all damage the stomach lining, as can aspirin, leading to gastric ulcers. Almost everyone over the age of 60, who takes an anti-inflammatory drug, will be given an additional drug to protect the stomach. (Steroids also damage the stomach lining; in case you were wondering).

The most commonly used class of anti-acid drugs are called proton pump inhibitors (PPIs). The 'proton pump' makes the acid in the stomach. If you 'inhibit' the pump, less acid is produced. There are other drugs which are used to do this in a slightly different way e.g., ranitidine, cimetidine. These are not the problem. This section is all about the proton pump inhibitors. A class of drugs that end in ... *prazole*. Such as ome*prazole*, lanso*prazole*, panto*prazole.*

It is true that they reduce acid production very effectively, and significantly cut down the risk of stomach ulcers and suchlike. The issue of concern here is that they also reduce nitric oxide synthesis in endothelial cells.

*"According to a majority of experimental and clinical observations, PPIs appear to have adverse cardiovascular effects. These effects may be mediated in part through **an impairment in vascular homeostasis characterized by NO deficiency** and should be considered when PPIs are prescribed, especially, in patients at increased cardiovascular risk."*[212]

What is the size of the cardiovascular problem?

"In a further data-mining exercise examining records from 2.9 million patients, PPIs were associated with a 1.16-fold risk of myocardial infarction, and a 2-fold increased risk of cardiovascular mortality."[213]

A doubling of cardiovascular mortality. So, if my 70-year-old woman were to take a proton pump inhibitor, her risk of cardiovascular death would double from 2.7 to 5.4%. Which would reduce her life expectancy by a further year (at least). If she took them from the age 60, she would have a greater than 2-year reduction in life expectancy.

Which is significantly more damaging than a high blood pressure. Yes, it is true that proton pump inhibitors are not supposed to be taken long-term, but I don't think I have seen a patient taken off one by their doctor – ever. With six million people taking them in the UK, and around 35 million in the US, this represents a major health issue.

If you really need to reduce the acid in your stomach – long term – maybe think about taking ranitidine or cimetidine, or suchlike. There, direct medical advice. I am now certain to be stuck off the medical register.

5: Homocysteine

Number of people with the problem: **around 2 million (I think)**

Reduction in life expectancy: **Max 10 years**

So, on to homocysteine. It is a protein that can be found in the bloodstream. Although, it must be said, in pretty minuscule quantities. However, if the level rises, it is exceedingly toxic to endothelial cells.

There are children who have the condition known as *hyper*homocysteinemia and they have very serious issues. One of which is rapid onset cardiovascular disease. This is the condition that Kilmer McCully was studying, before getting unceremoniously booted out of Harvard for daring to, even indirectly, criticise the cholesterol hypothesis.

I am not discussing *hyper*homocysteinemia here. I am looking at a more moderately raised homocysteine, which affects many more people.

"Elevated homocysteine (Hc) levels have a well-established and clear causal relationship to epithelial damage leading to coronary artery disease. ***Furthermore, it is strongly associated with other metabolic syndrome variables, such as hypertension, which is correlated with type 2 diabetes mellitus (T2DM).****"* [214]

As you can see, there are additional links here between homocysteine and cardiovascular disease, via raised blood pressure and diabetes. This brings homocysteine even more tightly into the cardiovascular fold. However, moving sideways, there is something else about homocysteine that you need to know about. Which is that it greatly increases the risk of Alzheimer's.

"High levels of a substance in the blood called homocysteine tops the list of potentially new risk factors for heart disease, stroke, ***and now dementia****. A new study suggests that high homocysteine levels are linked with mental declines associated with Alzheimer's disease in elderly people."* [215]

Just to complicate things further, diabetes also increases homocysteine levels and, for extra added complexity, a raised homocysteine increases the level of insulin resistance. [216]

Diabetes is also a significant risk factor for dementia:

"The exact connection between Alzheimer's disease (AD) and type 2 diabetes is still in debate. However, poorly controlled blood sugar may increase the risk of developing Alzheimer's. This relationship is so strong that some have called Alzheimer's 'diabetes of the brain' or 'type 3 diabetes (T3D)'."[217]

Here, once again, we have a kind of swirling mass of risk factors for diabetes, cardiovascular disease and Alzheimer's. Tricky to separate them. Simple answer, get them all down if possible.

Outside of diabetes, is there anything else that can raise homocysteine? Age, as usual plays a part. Homocysteine levels tends to rise as you get older. Other causes are smoking and (possibly) excess coffee drinking. There is also chronic kidney disease – which wraps back around into diabetes – so it is the old dance of interacting factors once more.

Anyway, stripping this down to basics. One thing is very clear. You really do not want to have a high homocysteine level. The next obvious question is – what can you do about it? There is a rather obvious clue in the passage that follows:

*"Elevated levels of homocysteine is an indication of inadequate folate and vitamin B-12 in the diet, writes lead author Giovanni Ravaglia, a researcher with University Hospital S. Orsola-Malpighi in Bologna, Italy. His paper appears in the March American Journal of Clinical Nutrition... **High homocysteine levels can be treated very easily with vitamins, including folate, niacin, and B-12.**"*[218]

There is another clue below:

*"In observational studies, lower homocysteine levels are associated with lower rates of coronary heart disease and stroke. **Folic acid and vitamins B6 and B12 lower homocysteine levels.**"*[219]

Just to clear up one small confusing point. Folate is a B vitamin, vitamin B_9. However, it is often just called folate – don't ask me why. You generally take it as a supplement called 'folic acid'. Because, because, why give a thing one name, when you can give it three – and switch about between them in a random fashion. Nothing about the naming systems in medicine makes any sense to me anymore. I just go along with them, and deal with things the best I can.

249

Moving on and focussing on Alzheimer's at this point. If low levels of B vitamins can cause Alzheimer's, can supplementation provide benefits?

"In an initial, randomized controlled study on elderly subjects with increased dementia risk, we showed that high-dose B-vitamin treatment (folic acid 0.8 mg, vitamin B6 20 mg, vitamin B12 0.5 mg) **slowed shrinkage of the whole brain volume over 2 years.***"* [220]

In a follow-up study, this group of researchers found that, in those with higher homocysteine, who already had signs of dementia, B-vitamins reduced brain destruction and slowed, even halted, the progression of Alzheimer's. In their own words, from the paper *"Preventing Alzheimer's disease-related gray matter atrophy by B-vitamin treatment"*:

"...we showed that high-dose B-vitamin treatment (folic acid 0.8 mg, vitamin B6 20 mg, vitamin B12 0.5 mg) slowed shrinkage of the whole brain volume over 2 years. Here, we go further by demonstrating that **B-vitamin treatment reduces, by as much as seven-fold, the cerebral atrophy in those gray matter (GM) regions specifically vulnerable to the AD (Alzheimer's Disease) process,** *including the medial temporal lobe.* **In the placebo group, higher homocysteine levels at baseline are associated with faster GM atrophy, but this deleterious effect is largely prevented by B-vitamin treatment. We additionally show that the beneficial effect of B vitamins is confined to participants with high homocysteine.***"* [221]

In short, if you have a high homocysteine level, and you want to avoid – or significantly slow down – the progression of Alzheimer's, take B-vitamins. This truly is a no-brainer. When I say high, what I am talking about here is levels above about 12 to 15 micromoles per litre (12-15 µmol/l). This is considered 'moderately' raised. Anything above 30 is called high, where you definitely, absolutely should do something.

Dose of B vitamins to take daily:

- folic acid (vitamin B_9) 0.8 mg

- vitamin B_6 20 mg

- vitamin B_{12} 0.5 mg

What is the worst thing that can possibly happen here? That you wasted money on some vitamins that don't do a great deal of good. To me this is like playing the lottery. Costs a couple of pounds a week. You may win nothing, but the jackpot is enormous. You may well avoid dementia, and you will reduce the risk of cardiovascular disease at the same time.

As a quick footnote, I should mention that this is a highly contentious area. As is anything to do with vitamins. The mainstream pharmaceutical-medical industry is pretty much hell-bent on attacking vitamins from all direction. They claim that vitamins have no benefits and don't work for anything, ever. '*I said ever!*' In addition, if you dare to take vitamins they say there is a risk of significant harm.

I think it is best to simply ignore them on this issue. They are protecting profits. We do not want people taking cheap harmless vitamins, when they could be taking massively expensive drugs instead. For that would never do.

I have covered one of the main attacks on B-vitamins below. Specifically, with regard to studies on dementia. Exactly the same issues apply to attacks on cardiovascular studies.

Attacks on using B-vitamins in dementia.

There have been a number of studies looking at the use of B-vitamins in preventing dementia. They were brought together in a 'meta-analysis.'[222] A meta-analysis is a posh term denoting an attempt to combine all the relevant trials that have been done in a therapeutic area, in order to construct a 'meta' study, or meta-analysis.

These wide-ranging analyses can be very useful, in areas where there have been a large number of different studies done, with variable results. However, 'meta-analyses' often mash together studies with very different populations, using different doses of drugs, or vitamins, even completely different drugs or vitamins, for different lengths of time.

Just to add to the potential messiness, the studies may look at completely unrelated outcomes. Some will study mood, others, mental decline, others, quality of life. It can get very messy. Meta-analyses are often treated as though they are the very pinnacle of medical research. Tablets of stone handed down by Gods. In reality, they need to be treated with a large pinch of salt (KCl).

Due to the many complexities involved, I am not going through this meta-analysis in great detail. I will restrict myself to a few key criticisms. Just for starters the authors claim to have reviewed the impact of vitamin B supplementation on 'cognitive aging' on 22,000 participants. The title was:

"Effects of homocysteine lowering with B vitamins on cognitive aging: meta-analysis of 11 trials with cognitive data on 22,000 individuals."

In fact, the total number they looked at was 20,431 – which is a lot nearer to 20,000 than 22,000. But, hey ho, what's 1,500 people between friends? However, in my book, deliberate figure inflation is an important indication of researchers trying to 'big up' their findings.

Moving on, and this is significantly more mission critical, in only 7,199 did anyone bother to measure cognitive function at the start of the trial and then again, at the end. Which, straight off, means that the vast bulk of this meta-analysis is utterly meaningless.

How can you possibly know what happened to anyone's cognitive state if you only measured it once? Did it improve, did it worsen – not the faintest. There were other major problems. A few of which were noted by others:

*"First and foremost, this meta-analysis **excluded** trials on mild cognitive impairment (MCI) and Alzheimer's disease. As a possible consequence, most of the trials included in this meta-analysis either did not see any significant cognitive change (between the start and the end of the trial) in the placebo group or **did not look at such change**."*[223]

Yes indeed, they excluded people with existing cognitive impairment, or Alzheimer's, which are the very groups that you want to study.

"...people included in these trials included in the meta-analysis were healthy and did not show any cognitive decline, whether they received B-vitamin treatment or not. So, B-vitamins could hardly prevent or slow down something not happening in the first place."

Just to make this point a little clearer. In the minority of studies, where they bothered to measure cognitive function at the start, and also at the end, they found that very, very few people developed any degree of cognitive impairment in either group. Not in the treatment group, or the placebo groups. As virtually nothing happened to anyone, nothing could have been proved one way or another.

Attempting to study the progress of dementia, in people who do not have dementia, and who may never get dementia, nor have signs of cognitive decline... is like doing a blood pressure lowering study on people who do not have a raised blood pressure.

Then, on finding that no-one had a cardiovascular event in either arm of the trial, you proceed to claim that blood pressure lowering does not work. Because there was no difference between those given the drug, and those taking the placebo. Do you think this makes any sense? Answers on a postcard, that should be sent to the Willie Wonka chocolate factory. Care of A. N. Idiot. Despite such critical, fatal, flaws, this analysis was greeted as though it was utterly definitive. B-vitamins have no effect, end of. This is what the head of Alzheimer's research UK had to say.

"Although one trial in 2010 showed that for people with high homocysteine, B vitamins had some beneficial effect on the rate of brain shrinkage, this comprehensive review of several trials shows that B vitamins have not been able to slow mental decline as we age, nor are they likely to prevent Alzheimer's. While the outcome of this new and far-reaching analysis is not what we hoped for, it does underline the need for larger studies to improve certainty around the effects of any treatment."[224]

New and far-reaching analysis. Comprehensive review... ho hum. If I were given the job of marking this meta-analysis, I would hand it back in a rather grumpy fashion. *'I asked you to look at the benefit of lowering homocysteine, using B-vitamins, in people with cognitive problems, or early-stage Alzheimer's. Yet, you have not even bothered to look at these groups. In fact, you deliberately excluded them.*

In addition, you did not exclude trials where the researchers failed to measure mental decline. Added to this, in most of these trials, no-one even had a high homocysteine level to start with, so they cannot – by definition – have had low levels of B-vitamins. So, how could vitamin B supplementation possible have been of any benefit... I am most disappointed. Please try again, and this time READ the brief.'

As it turns out, this analysis was done by exactly the same people who rule the world of cholesterol lowering, known as the cholesterol treatment triallists collaboration (CTT) in Oxford. This paper came under the banner of the 'B-vitamin treatment triallists collaboration'. Who knew such a group existed? One thing that can be said for certain is that these people really do not like vitamins. They may interfere with enormously profitable pharmaceutical world dominance.

CHAPTER 11

Endothelial damage – life gained, life lost

Anyway, there you have it. A look at the most important things that damage the endothelium – with a short detour into Alzheimer's. As I said at the start, I have not attempted to cover all possible ways that you can do damage. I restricted myself to the most important factors, impacting the greatest number of people.

You may also remember that I began this section with a list of nine factors, which I then faffed about with a bit, and will now faff about with a bit more. For example, I did not have exercise on my list to start with, but I include it now.

I am also changing HPA-axis dysfunction into significant mental illness. Because the impact of these conditions on life expectancy has been estimated:

An analysis by the University of Oxford calculated the following reductions in life expectancy:

Bipolar disorder   = 9 to 20 years

Schizophrenia   = 10 to 20 years

Recurrent depression = 7 to 11 years[225]

The same group also looked at drug use, and found that drug and alcohol abuse can be the most damaging thing of all:

Drug and alcohol abuse = 24 years

Which means that, even though my list has altered during the process of discussion, there are still nine critical things that make up my 'Top of the Pops'. I have included the maximum years of life lost they can cause.

1. Drug and alcohol abuse = 24 years
2. Raised blood sugar levels/type 2 diabetes. = 20 years
3. Significant mental illness = 20 years
4. Smoking = 10 years
5. Lack of exercise = 5 years
6. Air pollution = 4 years
7. Use of PPIs = 2 years
8. Raised blood pressure = 18 months
9. Periodontal disease = 18 months

Despite the somewhat fluid nature of my list, and all the inherent difficulties of creating it, I believe that attempting to define the reduction in life expectancy in this way, represents the most useful way of looking at harm.

Just to give a couple of examples of what it means in real life. If we assume, for the sake of argument, that everyone is designed to live to 100 – on average. That is, if nothing goes horribly wrong on the way, like a car crash, or cancer, or suchlike, then we can establish how the various factors listed about can cut down this maximum figure.

For example. Take someone who smokes (10 years) and has longstanding diabetes (20 years) and raised blood pressure (18 months). You can establish that this is likely to knock 31.5 years off their life expectancy. Which means that they will only make it to 68.5 years – or thereabouts. Which, from what I have seen in medical practice, sounds about right.

What this list also makes clear is that, perhaps very worst thing to suffer from, is severe mental illness. Not only do those with such conditions have major HPA-axis dysfunction and, often, frank diabetes, they almost always have additional health issues such as drug use, smoking, suicide attempts, terrible teeth...

"The average life expectancy of Norwegians with schizophrenic disorders is 62 years. If you also have a drug problem, it goes down to 47 years. 'It's difficult to understand why this isn't prioritized by the health services,' says a veteran psychiatric researcher."[226]

Fifty-three years of life straight down the plughole. More than a half of a potential lifespan. This is about as low as life expectancy gets. At least for any population within a wealthy Western country. In Russia, after the fall of the Berlin wall and break-up of the Soviet Union, life expectancy fell to 57, for men. Again, pretty damned awful.

On the positive side, if you tick nothing on that list, you may well make it to 100 and those hundred years should be mostly healthy. Of course, if you're born with super powerful, extra-long-lived genes, you will make it past your centenary. If, that, is, you really want to. I am not certain that I do.

CHAPTER 12

Positive things you can do to keep your endothelium healthy

I suppose one criticism of my nine-item list is that it primarily covers everything *not* to do. Which could be seen as a little negative, censorious even. Surely there must be things that can keep us all, super-healthy. We can all make it to 200 if we try.... Sorry, probably not. Maybe a 110? Well, good luck with that. Let me know how you get on. On second thoughts, you will have to tell my great grandchildren.

Having said this, there are a number of actions that have been shown to optimise endothelial cell health. I have split them into two groups:

1. Protect and sustain the glycocalyx.

2. Increase nitric oxide synthesis.

1. Protect and sustain the glycocalyx

The glycocalyx is the first line of defence against endothelial damage. As we saw in Figure 10, it mainly consists of strands, or filaments, of glycoproteins (a mixture of glucose and proteins). It provides a strong anticoagulant layer and stops platelets and white blood cells sticking to the endothelium – and suchlike.

So, is there anything you can do to grow your endothelial garden and keep it blooming? Well, although a high glucose level is damaging, a high protein level protects it. Mainly by providing the raw material that allow it to be kept strong and healthy. Feed and grow.

The most abundant protein in the blood is called albumin, which is manufactured in the liver. Cells around the body absorb albumin, and make the various proteins they need from it, and suchlike. The amino acids found in albumin are also used to make the glycocalyx. In fact, albumin is bound within the glycocalyx layer, for exactly this reason:

"Plasma proteins such as albumin are physiologically bound within the glycocalyx, thus contributing to stability of the layer." [227]

"Albumin is physiologically bound within the glycocalyx, protecting against shedding and contributing to the maintenance of vascular integrity and normal capillary permeability. Owing to these properties, albumin has the potential to improve outcomes in clinical scenarios characterized by damaged glycocalyx." [228]

Recent studies have demonstrated that for every 10g/L drop in albumin, the risk of CVD doubles. The normal range of albumin is generally considered to be 35-55 g/L.[229] Which is actually a hell of a lot, when you consider that with homocysteine, for example, we are talking about micrograms – a million times less.

When you get down to it, the glycocalyx needs proteins to make it, repair it and replenish it. Therefore, it would seem a good idea to take supplements containing the same type of proteins that are found in the glycocalyx. Which means supplements such as chondroitin sulphate, glucosamine and hyaluronan.

Many people already use these to help with arthritis. They can (severe pharmaceutical company woo-woo warning) improve the health of the cartilage – which also contains a high concentration of glycoproteins. Not only can they help with arthritis, there is strong evidence that they can also reduce the risk of CVD.

"Habitual glucosamine use was associated with a 15% lower risk of total CVD events and a 9%-22% lower risk of individual CVD events (CVD death, coronary heart disease, and stroke)." [230]

"Osteoarthritic patients treated with high doses of chondroitin sulfate (CS) have a lower incidence of coronary heart disease." [231]

Japanese researchers also found that chondroitin sulphate acts as a potent anticoagulant reducing the risk of blood clots forming on the arterial walls.[232] Almost certainly because a healthy glycocalyx stops blood clots forming.

So yes, it does appear that you can keep the glycocalyx much healthier by taking protein supplements. The main ones are:

- Chondroitin sulphate

- Glucosamine

- Hyaluronan

All three can reduce the risk of CVD. Not massively, but significantly. If you do have a thinned glycocalyx (and this can be measured) I would make damned sure that I did take them. No question. How much can this increase in life expectancy? I am guessing at a year. However, there are no good figures here. Which means that I am somewhat making it up.

By the way, this advice is not currently controversial. This is simply because there is hardly anyone in the medical profession that has even heard of the glycocalyx, let alone have any idea what you can do to keep it in good shape. As soon as they become aware of it, this advice will become CONTROVERSIAL.

'Supplements are of NO damned use whatsoever. This nonsense makes me so angry.... Aaarrrrggghhhh!' Thud. Sound of key opinion leader choking on his vintage after-dinner, paid for by the pharmaceutical industry, port.

2. Increased nitric oxide synthesis

There are many, many, things that can improve nitric oxide synthesis. Many of them I have covered before under such factors as exercise, relaxation techniques, diabetes, ACE-inhibitors, and suchlike. At this point I am talking more about specific things that have been shown to increase nitric oxide synthesis. Regardless of whatever else is going on.

Here is a list of my 'favourite things' (we'll explain any you might not be familiar with in the following pages). I hate to say it, but, as usual, a couple of these are highly controversial. I will leave you to guess which ones.

1. Increased sun exposure

2. L-arginine

3. L-citrulline

4. Co-enzyme Q10

5. Sildenafil

6. Breathe through your nose

7. Certain vegetables

8. Dark chocolate

9. Red wine

10. Meat/animal organs e.g. liver

My especially favourite things on this list are numbers one, eight and nine. Lying in the sun, eating chocolate, and drinking wine. Otherwise known as watching an exercise class bursting various blood vessels whilst I lounge about on a sunbed by the pool. *'Keep going, you're all doing very well... red wine anyone?'*

Looking at other items on the list. I am less keen on vegetables. I have nothing particularly against vegetables. It's just that some of them are a bit on the tedious and tasteless in many cases. Kale... what is all that about. You buy a packet the size of a large pillow, and it ends up as a small green spot that needs to be scraped off the bottom of the saucepan. Spinach is not much better.

One thing I do like about this list is that it probably seems a bit ridiculous. Breathing through your nose! What is he on about? I must admit I thought this was ridiculous too Then I studied the science, and you know what... it's true. As you can possibly tell, I am a great fan of bonkers scientific claims that turn out to be true.

'You wrap Sellotape round a pencil, and you get a layer of graphene? Ho, ho, you earthlings are so funny.'

'Thank you, I shall claim my Nobel prize now.'

1. Increased sun exposure

Of all the things I recommend, getting out into the sun is the easiest. It is also the most enjoyable, with possibly the greatest benefits. Just being outside is beneficial. For example:

"Walking outdoors was associated with improved mood but walking indoors was not."[233]

Even if you don't do the exercise bit, being outside significantly improves your mood. It also makes your brain work better, otherwise known as cognitive function.

"Among depressed participants, a dose-response relationship was found

262

between sunlight exposure and cognitive function, with lower levels of sunlight associated with impaired cognitive status." [234]

In fact, I heartily advise all depressed patients to get outside and walk as much as possible. It can have astonishingly beneficial effects. Gardening is also good, as is simply lounging about on a comfy chair, gin and tonic in hand… Sorry, must control alcohol consumption.

Another direct benefit of sun exposure is that it increases vitamin D levels. Vitamin D is synthesised in the skin, under the influence of sunlight. Vitamin D is made from the same molecule the body uses to make most hormones (vitamin D is really a hormone, not a vitamin). That molecule is, of course, cholesterol. The chemical of doom… without which you would rapidly die.

There can be no doubt about the benefits of achieving optimal vitamin D levels. Moving away from cardiovascular disease for a moment, here is a study from Japan, looking at cancer.

*"In this large prospective study, higher vitamin D concentration was associated with lower risk of total cancer. These findings support the hypothesis that **vitamin D has protective effects against cancers at many sites**."* [235]

Oh look, sunshine improves mood, cognitive function, and cancer. Moving back to cardiovascular disease

*"…studies have reported that vitamin D deficiency is associated with increased risk of CVD, including hypertension, heart failure, and ischemic heart disease. Initial prospective studies have also demonstrated that **vitamin D deficiency increases the risk of developing incident hypertension or sudden cardiac death in individuals with pre-existing CVD**."* [236]

Mood, cognitive function, cancer, and cardiovascular disease. How long can this list get?

At this point I need to add that the benefits of sunlight are not all down to vitamin D. There is something even more important going on here. Which is that sun exposure helps the body to synthesize nitric oxide. [237]

We already know that nitric oxide lowers blood pressure and prevents blood clots. Less well known is that it also improves insulin sensitivity. So, it lowers blood sugar levels, and insulin levels. Nitric oxide has even been demonstrated to reverse type 2 diabetes. [238]

Mood, cognitive function, cancer, CVD, high blood pressure and diabetes.

Yes, you are the sunshine of my life. Why do you think it feels so good when you go and lie in the sun? Because IT IS GOOD FOR YOU. With all these benefits it ought to give you several more years of healthy life, and it appears that it does.

A study was done in Sweden, mentioned earlier, looking at women with *"active sunlight exposure habits."* Which is a poncy medical way of saying... sunbathes a lot. They compared these evil sunbathing harlots to another group of women who avoided the sun. What did the researchers find?

*"Non-smokers who avoided sun exposure had a life expectancy similar to smokers in the highest sun exposure group, indicating that **avoidance of sun exposure is a risk factor for death of a similar magnitude as smoking**. Compared to the highest sun exposure group, **life expectancy of avoiders of sun exposure was reduced by 0.6-2.1 years**."* [239]

This was a 20-year study, so a lifetime of sun exposure could give you 3 to 8 years of added life expectancy. Possibly 10, if you compare avoiding sunlight to smoking, as these researchers did.

To those who cry, but what of melanoma? I respond, *'what of melanoma?'* Whilst no-one wants to get it, it remains a very uncommon cancer, killing about a tenth the number who die of either say, breast, or prostate cancer. Added to this, the evidence that sun exposure actually causes malignant melanoma is weak, at best.

Here from an article written in the British *Journal of Dermatology* (no less), which was entitled *"Melanoma epidemic: a midsummer night's dream."*

It stated a number of pretty startling things:

- The rise in reported malignant melanoma is due to 'diagnostic drift' whereby benign lesions are reported as stage one melanoma

- The distribution of melanomas does not correspond to areas of sun exposure. You would expect them on the face, the arms, the legs, more than anywhere else. Not true

- There needs to be a re-evaluation of the role of UV radiation and recommendations for protection from it

- There needs to be a new direction for research into the cause [240]

Yes, this was actually written by dermatologists. Members of the

264

very speciality who constantly harangue us to never, ever, go out into the sun. At least not without slathering every inch of your body with clothing, or high-powered suntan lotion.

These guys came to a different conclusion. Which is that sun exposure almost certainly does not cause malignant melanomas. It appears that this universally held belief is simply another medical meme. There are many other papers supporting this position – if you choose to look.

I think that, key amongst their findings was that:

*"The distribution of melanomas does **not** correspond to areas of sun exposure."*

Which, alone, should demolish the idea of causality. If factor X is thought to cause Y, then more of thing X should cause more Y. In the case of sun exposure, it doesn't. End of.

Even if I have failed miserably to convince you that sunshine will not kill you with malignant melanomas, life is also about balancing risks. You're never going to reach zero – ever. Which means that even if sun exposure does cause an increase in malignant melanoma, you are not looking at a common cancer.

It kills fewer than 1 in 30,000 people annually. Or about 2,000 every year in the UK. Even if you doubled that risk, it is still extremely unlikely that you will die from it.

On the other hand, if we look at, say, prostate cancer, this kills 1 in 5,000 a year – or 6 times as many as malignant melanoma. Reduce the risk by 20%, and you will prevent more deaths than are killed by malignant melanoma, in total. What of all cancers?

A study in the *Journal of the American Medical Association* found up to a **38%** reduction in metastatic, and all forms of fatal cancer in those given vitamin D supplementation.[241]

So, we may... and when I say may, I mean almost certainly not, prevent a few hundred deaths from malignant melanoma by telling people to avoid the sun. On the other hand, by reducing sun exposure we could be wiping out many thousands by increasing the risk of CVD, cancer, depression and type 2 diabetes.

In addition to all this, sunshine simply makes us feel good. It also costs precisely nothing. Just be careful that the pharmaceutical industry doesn't try to patent it and charge you for each photon.

2. L-arginine, 3. L-citrulline, 4. Co-enzyme Q10

I have brought these three supplements under one umbrella. They don't work in the same way, but they all increase nitric oxide production.

In the case of L-arginine and L-citrulline the reason why they increase nitric oxide levels is because they are directly involved in its creation. Indeed, the enzyme nitric oxide synthase (NOS) uses l-arginine to create nitric oxide.

As a by-product you end up with l-citrulline. The body can convert L-citrulline back into L-arginine and the cycle continues. Which means that on optimal intake of L-arginine, and L-citrulline leads to optimal nitric oxide synthesis.

Nitric oxide production is not really an issue when you are young and fit and have all the nitric oxide and l-arginine that you need. However, as you get older, over about 60, and especially if you have raised blood pressure and/or diabetes, I would advise taking both. I would certainly do so if you are vegetarian or vegan, as the best source of l-arginine is meat/animal produce which you ain't eating.

Co-enzyme Q10 also raises nitric oxide synthesis a bit. It does so by using a completely different mechanism, which I am not getting into here. The main reason for mentioning co-enzyme Q10 is because it is critical for those many millions chewing gloomily on statins. This is because statins block the synthesis of co-enzyme Q10, and the level can drop by over 50%.

This creates significant problems beyond nitric oxide production. Co-enzyme Q10 is critical in the production of a substance called adenosine tri-phosphate (ATP). ATP is, effectively, the substance that every cell in your body uses as fuel. Virtually every biochemical and physiological process in your body is powered by ATP.[242]

Which means that, if you take a statin, you should also take co-enzyme Q10 at the same time. To quote the *Journal of the American College of Cardiology* – no less.

*"**Statins block** production of farnesyl pyrophosphate, an intermediate in **the synthesis of ubiquinone or coenzyme Q10 (CoQ10)**. This fact, plus the role of CoQ10 in mitochondrial energy production, has prompted the hypothesis that **statin-induced CoQ10 deficiency** is involved in the pathogenesis of statin myopathy*."[243]*

---

* Muscle pain and weakness

266

I sometimes wonder how much co-enzyme Q10, taken orally, actually makes it to the mitochondria – where the ATP is made. Some, not much, a lot... probably some. However, if you are taking statins, which many millions do, I would strongly advise taking co-enzyme Q10 as a supplement.

I think I should just mention that, in one of life's great ironies, statins also increase nitric oxide production, specifically in endothelial cells. In my opinion this is how they reduce the risk of cardiovascular disease – by the exceedingly small amount that they do. It has nothing to do with cholesterol lowering.

Just type 'statins nitric oxide synthesis' into Google, and you will find great waterfalls of information cascading down upon you. Such as this. Short and sweet:

"...statins improve nitric oxide production and vasodilatation."[244]

5. Sildenafil

Sildenafil (Viagra) is one of the most potent stimulants of nitric oxide there is. It was originally developed to treat angina. It does this by opening coronary arteries narrowed by atherosclerosis. In truth, I don't think anyone really had much idea about how it actually worked at first, at least with regard to the impact on nitric oxide.

It certainly came as a surprise to Pfizer when they found that Viagra was rather more effective at opening up the arteries somewhat lower-down in the male anatomy. A chance discovery that was revealed by the fact that the male volunteers in the early-stage clinical trials did not hand spare tablets back. Something previously unheard of.

It is also used for mountain sickness. It dilates the pulmonary blood vessels, lowers the pulmonary blood pressure, and therefore stops fluid leaking out and filling up the lungs. It is also used to treat those with pulmonary hypertension at ground level. In addition, it prevents elderly male nursing home residents from falling out of bed.

So, does it reduce the risk of cardiovascular disease? Well, there's never been an interventional trial, by which I mean, give Viagra to 10,000, and a placebo to another 10,000 to see what happens. There would be no money to be made doing this.

However, researchers in Manchester did do a long-term observational study where they looked carefully at the use of sildenafil in men, with diabetes, who had also suffered a heart attack.

There were significant reductions in risk. The two most important were:

- The risk of a heart attack dropped by 38%

- Overall mortality fell by 15.4% (40.1% vs 25.7%)[245]

These men were certainly in a very high-risk group. A previous heart attack *and* diabetes. Which is why the mortality rates were so high. Four in 10 died in the control group, in under 10 years.

Even with such a high rate of death, a 15.4% reduction in the risk of dying, over 7.5 years, equates to around 10 years additional life expectancy. For any actuaries in the audience, yes, this one becomes a bloody complex sum. But I am going with 10 years.

Let us now compare and contrast this with the largest 'high risk' statin trial. Which was the Heart Protection Study (HPS). This lasted five years, and the reduction in overall mortality was 1.8%.[246] Which makes Viagra five point seven times more effective than a statin, at reducing the risk of death. Let's call it six, for luck.

I will let you decide which of these two medications you feel provides a longer and significantly higher quality of life. I will give you a clue. It begins with an s (or a V), and it isn't a statin. Would it also work for women – I don't see why not.

6. Breathe through your nose

Stop, are you breathing through your mouth, or your nose? Bet you had no idea until I asked. Now you are suddenly aware of it. Sorry about that. Now stand in a corner and don't think about a tiger for 30 minutes.

When I started looking at this area, I found it fascinating that nitric oxide is manufactured in the nasal passages before being released into the surrounding air. Then, when you breathe it in, it produces all sorts of beneficial effects, including increased oxygen uptake. Because it opens up the blood vessels in the lungs.

"Intriguingly, NO gas from the nose and sinuses is inhaled with every breath and reaches the lungs in a more diluted form to enhance pulmonary oxygen uptake via local vasodilation."[247]

Essentially, if you breathe through your nose, nitric oxide gets into your lungs and your blood vessels. This dilates the airways and the blood vessels in the lungs, and elsewhere. Nitric oxide also acts as a potent viral and bacterial killer. So, it protects the lungs from infection (see under COVID19) and almost certainly helps to prevent nanoparticles entering your bloodstream.

Here is what Cleveland HeartLab®, have to say about taking long, deep breaths through your nose. "*It helps release nitric oxide; a chemical that has been shown to:*

- Expand blood vessels

- Increase blood flow

- Lower blood pressure

- Reduce stress and produce an all-over calming effect

- Prevent the build-up of artery-clogging plaque" [248]

Yes, it's that simple.

7. Vegetables/8. Dark Chocolate/9. Red wine 10. Meat etc

There are many things you can eat, or drink that increase nitric oxide synthesis. Such things as red wine and dark chocolate – discussed earlier. Here are a few of the vegetables and fruits and suchlike that can also do it:

- Beets

- Garlic

- Leafy greens

- Citrus fruits

- Nuts and seeds

- Watermelon

In addition, meat, of any sort is good. Because meat contains L-arginine (as discussed earlier).

And that, I think is enough in the way of lists. I have read way too many books on health and healthy eating over the years. They get sent to me for review, from time to time. They often seem to end up as a series of endless lists of things to do or eat. Which just depresses me. I know am never going to do all that. Never, ever. No matter how pure my intentions may be to start with.

So, rather than creating endless lists, here is a more general rule to follow. Eat food that looks like food. Real food, natural food. Food without a list of ingredients 10 feet long on the side. Fish, meat, vegetables, fruit, cream, eggs. You should be able to get everything that you require from 'natural' food. All the vitamins, minerals, potassium, and things that boost your nitric oxide.

In addition, try to buy food that is produced locally, if possible. Food that hasn't been irradiated, and stuffed with chemicals, to stop it rotting on the long journey across mighty seas.

I believe that one important reason why many people do need supplements, is because many of the essential nutrients in our foodstuffs have been pulverised out of existence in a massive factory somewhere. Yes, the manufacturers then jam a load of them back in again. However, I feel that it's probably best not to strip them out in the first place.

I agree that it is more expensive to eat fresh natural food. It also takes more time to prepare and cook. A Pot Noodle takes about a minute. Crunchy Nut Cornflakes, which I have to admit are pretty difficult to resist, simply need to be emptied into a bowl with milk poured on top. A MacDonald's is also super-convenient.

I am not suggesting that you become a Trappist monk, or a terrible food bore who eats only authentic sour-dough bread from Ulan Bator, or various poncy rubbish like quinoa with the finest hand crafted, toasted pumpkin seeds. I eat MacDonald's, from time to time. I enjoy them when I do, even with the added sharp twinge of guilt. *'Forgive me father, for I have MacDonalded.'*

I also enjoy a Crunchy Nut Cornflake. Even more than one, from time to time. I do draw the line at Pot Noodles because, well, just because. However, I do attempt to eat cooked meals that include fresh ingredients, most of the time. Friday night is, however, take-away curry night. Yum, yum.

Even with eating mostly natural food, I still take vitamin D in the winter months, and I always stir up a gram of soluble vitamin C – when I can remember. Sharp, is not the word for it. In addition, I take hyaluronan/chondroitin when I spot it on Amazon. Mainly because I have a knackered cartilage in my knee.

Indeed, I actually do most of the nitric oxide boosting thing on my list, at least some of the time. I most certainly drink red wine and go out in the sun. Again, no great hardship here. I must admit that my dark chocolate can sometimes seem less then fully dark. Ninety per cent cocoa... a tad on the sharp side for me. Lindt chocolate balls however... Keep thee behind me Satan. I mean, something that delicious just has to be good for you.

What of the B-vitamins for Alzheimer's? I think it is about time that I started taking them too. As Woody Allen once said. My brain is my second favourite organ. I intend to look after it.

CHAPTER 13

Blood clotting

Now it is time to move on to blood clotting. The other key part of the thrombogenic process. However, I do want to make it clear up front that it is not necessary to have problems with blood clotting to kick atherosclerosis into gear. Repeated damage to the endothelium is enough – all by itself.

However, if your blood is more likely to clot. Or, when it does clot, the clots are bigger and more difficult to shift, it means that any damage to the endothelium will be magnified. The cardiovascular disease process is accelerated. Which makes it a good idea to avoid things that make your blood significantly clottier (*hyper*coagulable).

Just to start with a quick look at one of the major clotting factors that floats about in your bloodstream, which is fibrinogen. Here from the paper *"Update on fibrinogen as a cardiovascular risk factor."*

*"Mounting data support a causal connection between high-normal fibrinogen levels and atherosclerotic cardiovascular disease. **There is clearly a thrombogenic component to atherosclerosis and the onset of clinical manifestations**... Fibrinogen should be added to the list of major cardiovascular risk factors. Trials of intervention to lower fibrinogen in high-risk coronary candidates are needed."[249]*

Depressingly, despite the polite request in the paper above, there were no trials, and fibrinogen was not added to the list of major cardiovascular risk factors. Why not? Because it interfered with the cholesterol hypothesis of course. This paper is now nearly 30 years old.

The Scottish Heart Health study also found that a raised fibrinogen level was a hugely important risk factor. Here are two charts, looking at the most important factors driving overall mortality in men, and women (Figure 30). The full lists are much longer, I have just covered the top few here.

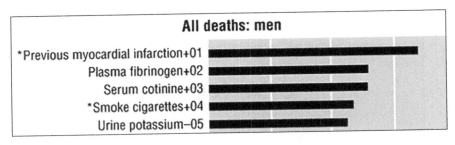

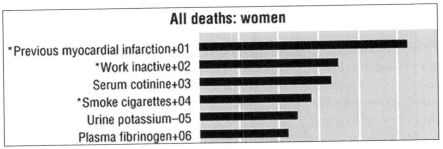

Figure 30

As a quick explanation. A plus sign, as in *'Previous myocardial infarction +01'*, means an increased risk. A minus sign, as in, *'Urine potassium -05'* means a decreased risk. I should also add that serum 'cotinine' is a blood tests that measures how many cigarettes you smoke – so it is really the same risk factor as smoking. Heavy smokers will simply have higher cotinine levels.

The main point I am trying to illustrate here is that fibrinogen is an extremely powerful risk factor for both men and women. In the top five. In men, a raised fibrinogen was more deadly than smoking. Worse even than diabetes – which was actually next on the list.

The impact of blood clotting is highlighted even more clearly if we look at a condition called von Willebrand's disease. Yes, there is a clotting factor that resides in your endothelium called *'von Willebrand factor'*. Named after a certain Mr von Willebrand I would imagine. (Can you be *Mr* and a *von* at the same time... probably not). He was actually Finnish.

This factor binds to platelets and factor VIII, amongst other things, and builds bigger, stickier thrombi. I did say blood clotting was complicated, and anyone who can get their head around the entire system has my undying admiration. Anyway, moving on:

274

- Some people have too much von Willebrand – and they are more clotty

- Some people have too little von Willebrand – and they are less clotty

A study on those with too little von Willebrand factor found that they had a greatly reduced risk of developing cardiovascular disease: 15% vs. 26%. Close to a 50% reduction.[250]

On the other hand, a study on those with too much von Willebrand factor found that those with too much, had a three-fold increase in the risk of coronary heart disease.[251]

Ergo, if you have a high level of von Willebrand factor, you are six times more likely to suffer from cardiovascular disease than if you have a low level. Which should give you a very clear picture about the increased risks associated with hypercoagulability.

So, should everyone just take an anticoagulant and be done with it? Well, probably not. For most of us, our blood is exactly as clotty as it needs to be. If you make it less clotty, you will reduce the risk of cardiovascular disease, but you will increase the risk of serious bleeding problems at the same time.

For example, there are people who take potent anticoagulants on a regular basis. Usually because they have a condition called atrial fibrillation. This is where the atria (upper chambers of the heart) do not beat regularly. They 'twitch' and contract in a highly irregular fashion. Or, to put it another way, they 'fibrillate'. Atrial fibrillation is not that uncommon, there are well over a million people in the UK who have it. Over the age of 65, nearly one in 10 people have it.

Because the atria are 'fibrillating' the blood does not get pushed through the chambers of the atria efficiently. It can get stuck in whirls and eddies, and small clots can easily form on the walls of the atria. This is pretty much the same mechanism that occurs in a deep venous thrombosis (DVT).

If these clots, which may be no bigger than a grain of rice, break off and get flung out of the heart, they can often travel into the brain, where they block a blood vessel, causing a stroke. This is why atrial fibrillation appears on Qrisk3 – as a risk factor for stroke – nothing to do with atherosclerosis.

To stop this happening, people with atrial fibrillation often take warfarin. Nowadays there are also newer, far more expensive anticoagulants to take. They all prevent clots forming and reduce the risk of stroke by interfering with the system that turns fibrinogen into fibrin. These same anticoagulants are also taken if people suffer a deep vein thrombosis or are at a high risk of one developing. Or have had a couple in the past.

All good, but there is a downside. Which is that there is an increased risk of bleeding. If someone who's taking anticoagulants bashes their head, they could more easily bleed into the brain, which can be fatal. If they have a small stomach ulcer, it can bleed and bleed – and kill them and suchlike. Which means you have to be pretty certain that the risk of a clot is significantly greater than the risk of a bleed. Which is true in atrial fibrillation, but not so for most other people.

Even low dose aspirin can cause major problems. It can trigger bleeding in the stomach and bowels. This is why aspirin (which hampers platelets sticking together) goes in and out of favour for cardiovascular disease prevention. Yes, it reduces the risk of cardiovascular disease, somewhat, but it also increases the risk of bleeding somewhat. On the whole, for most people, forget about it.

As a general rule, unless you are at greatly increased cardiovascular/ clotting risk I would not take anticoagulants. One exception to this may be fish oils (omega 3). These can reduce blood clotting, via a whole series of different mechanisms.[252] The effect is not enormous. However, there does not appear to be any increased bleeding risk attached. Which makes them almost completely safe.

Although I did once write an article pointing out that the Inuit – before their culture MacDonaldised – who ate a lot of fish, and oily fish at that, also had a lot of nosebleeds. On the plus side they had virtually no cardiovascular disease. They sure now do.

There is another situation where almost everyone will be prescribed anticoagulants. Which is during, and after, a heart attack. During a heart attack people were, and often still are, prescribed clotbusters such as tissue plasminogen activator. This is to break apart the clot that is blocking an artery.

Tissue plasminogen activator is also given when someone has a stroke. (Not, however, if the stroke is due to a bleed, rather than a clot – for obvious reasons). Today, with strokes, it is increasingly common to simply reach in and pull the clot out. Which, as you can imagine, is not as simple to do as I perhaps made it sound.

After someone has survived a heart attack, they will almost always be prescribed an 'anti-platelet' – which stops platelets sticking together. It doesn't destroy them, as the term anti-platelet may imply. The anti-platelet of choice used to be aspirin. Nowadays it is usually clopidogrel. In the trade we call this, very expensive aspirin.

As a quick aside, I do find it somewhat ironic that the mainstream management of strokes and heart attacks is almost entirely 'blood clot management.' Break them up, pull them out, squash them flat with a stent, prescribe various drugs to stop them forming again.

Blood clots, blood clots, blood clots all the way. Yet, still, the mainstream still refuses to believe that blood clots have anything to do with causing atherosclerosis in the first place. Um, isn't the evidence right there in front of your eyes? Oh well.

Having said all of this I am still not suggesting that people should take anticoagulants – unless they have a specific reason to do so. Although there are a couple of conditions which I will get to, where I do recommend their use. Before that I want to cover a few things that increase blood clotting and therefore should, in general, be avoided.

1. Physical stress (hot and cold)

2. Dehydration

3. Not moving

4. Acute mental stress

5. Non-steroidal anti-inflammatory drugs (NSAIDS)

1. Physical stress (Hot and cold)

Many years ago, I looked at the health of deep coal miners in the Soviet Union, as you do. I found that average age of death in this population was significantly lower than 50. Almost all of them died of heart attacks. In addition, most of them had several previous 'silent' heart attacks – noted on post-mortem examination. The articles were all in Russian, so they have a certain grammatical style. Interesting which is, very.

What is clear is that these men worked extremely hard and were regularly exposed to massive temperature changes. Sub-zero above ground, baking hot below. Which resulted in them being the most heart-attacky population in the world. At least I am pretty sure they topped this particular list.

Yes, they had all sorts of other things going on as well. Smoking, heavy drinking, coal dust, social stresses. However, even then...

*"It is shown that miners engaged in deep coal mines develop myocardial infarction (MI) at a young age, **the mean age being 42.8 years**. The foregoing clinical picture was characterized by an atypical, painless course... The leading factors that promote MI development are **intense hard physical work combined with a heating microclimate. This is evidenced by the high rate of its occurrence during work and the first 1 to 4 hours after work (74.2 percent).**"*[253]

Soviet miners highlight the fact that if you move rapidly from hot to cold, or vice-versa, you put your circulation under enormous strain. Blood vessels open and close in the periphery, the blood itself becomes hypercoagulable.

Changing tack from the Soviet Union to North America, we can see the same effect of taking heavy exercise, with the additional stress of working hard at extreme temperatures. I am talking here about clearing the drive of snow in winter, followed by a heart attack. Indeed, middle-aged men are strongly advised not to shovel snow from their driveways, especially in Canada.[254]

The drive does look lovely when you finish. The inscription on the gravestone does not look quite so lovely. The simple fact is that extreme physical stress is most definitely a trigger for clots to form. Add in temperature changes, and things get even worse. So, just be careful out there, and don't overdo it on cold mornings. Warm up, warm down. Take an aspirin. Or buy a snowblower – much more fun. As an added benefit, you can cover the next-door neighbour's drive with snow.

2. Dehydration

Dehydration can also trigger blood clots. It is one of the major reasons why long-haul flights are a trigger for deep vein thrombosis – and other thromboses as well. The increased risk with flying is not simply because you are sitting the same position for several hours. The air pressure is lower, more water escapes from the lungs. Many people drink alcohol when flying, and dehydration becomes an even more major issue.

So, if you are flying, don't simply wear pressure stockings. You also need to drink plenty, and not too much booze. Doing this, you will not just prevent clots in your legs, you will prevent them elsewhere.

3. Not moving

At one time patients were commanded to remain immobile in bed for six weeks following a heart attack. They couldn't even get up for a pee, or a poo. This long-term immobility triggered blood clots all over the place. Mainly deep vein thromboses in the legs. These clots often broke off, then travelled to the lungs and got stuck, blocking blood flow in the lungs and killing millions and millions over the decades.

The lesson from this is that you really need to move around. Indeed, you must move around, and not simply on long haul flights. I am not just talking about preventing heart attacks and strokes here. Pulmonary emboli are very much included in my list here.

Because, you know, if a blood clot is going to kill you, it matters not how exactly it does. Stroke, heart attack, pulmonary embolism. Blood clot, blood clot... blood clot. Dead, dead... and dead, in that order. In addition, as you now know, a blood clot arriving in the lungs is quite likely to turn into an atherosclerotic plaque. If it doesn't kill you first.

4. Acute mental stress

This one is very simple. Acute psychological stress triggers your HPA-axis into a state of high alert. One thing this does is to promote a hyper-coagulant state. This makes sense from a survival point of view. If your primitive brain senses that it is under attack, and it doesn't really differentiate between an angry bear and an angry boss, it prepares your blood to be ready to clot at a moment's notice.

"A truly physiologic prothrombotic stress response to acute mental stress is part of the fight-or-flight response, but can be exaggerated and prolonged in vulnerable individuals, thereby leading to excess/pathologic hypercoagulability. Plausible psychobiological processes have been identified to partially explain how acute stress affects hemostasis (blood clotting). As a prothrombotic state plays a key role in atherothrombotic CVD and VTE (Venous ThromboEmbolism), excess/pathologic stress-hypercoagulability provides one mechanism that might underlie thrombotic manifestations triggered by emotional upset and psychological trauma such as ACS [Acute Coronary Symptoms]."[255]

Yes indeed, if you get very upset or angry, this can trigger a big old blood clot that may well end up killing you. A fact that has been known for centuries. In the good old days, when someone suddenly dropped dead it was often referred to as death from 'apoplexy'. If you look up the definitions of the word apoplexy, it includes the following:

Apoplexy = stroke

Apoplexy = heart attack

Apoplexy = extreme anger

The fact that this one word connects anger to strokes and heart attacks is not a coincidence. Well over 200 years ago John Hunter, a famous surgeon and pathologist of his time, and who also suffered from angina, knew very well that strong emotions were a very dangerous thing for him:

"A sufferer from angina, Hunter found that his attacks were often brought on by anger. He declared, 'My life is at the mercy of the scoundrel who chooses to put me in a passion.' This proved prophetic: at a meeting of the board of St. George's Hospital, London, of which he was a member, he became involved in a heated argument with other board members, walked out of the meeting and dropped dead in the next room." [256]

As I mentioned earlier in the book 'Play nice.' Do not allow yourself to become enraged at the drop of a hat. Although as Aristotle acknowledged there are two very different types of anger. Type one – getting upset/enraged/apoplectic: type two – righteous anger.

"Anybody can become angry – that is easy, but to be angry with the right person and to the right degree and at the right time and for the right purpose, and in the right way – that is not within everybody's power and is not easy."

Or, to put it another way, don't let other people trigger your HPA-axis willy-nilly, but it is not a bad thing to be angry when it is required – and under control. And if you can manage to do that... chapeau.

5. Non-steroidal anti-inflammatory drugs (NSAIDS)

These drugs have been around for a long while now. They are not all the same. Aspirin, for example, is an anti-inflammatory drug. However, it is not usually defined as a non-steroidal anti-inflammatory – even though that is precisely what it is. It is not a steroid, and it reduces inflammation. What else would you call it? A banana?

He searched for logic here, he searched for logic there... he gave up with medical terminology.

Anyway, non-steroidal drugs are very commonly used for pain and arthritis. Many people take them over the counter in such forms as ibuprofen, or voltarol, or naproxen. So, it is difficult to know exactly how many people take them. Millions for certain, but I am not sure how many millions. I think almost everyone has taken one of these drugs, at one time or another. Either as tablets or rubbed on as gel. Even a patch. Yes, we now truly live in an age of wonders.

The main ones are:

- Ibuprofen – also called neurofen

- Naproxen – also called naproxen (in the UK)

- Diclofenac – also called voltarol

There is also celoxicab, mefanemic acid, etoricoxib and indomethacin. There are a few others too, less commonly used. They are all pretty damned good at what they do. My knee can vouch for that. However (aspirin aside, because it has a separate anti-coagulant effects) they all increase the risk of blood clots. They can also damage the endothelium by blocking a substance called cyclo-oxygenase 2 (COX-2).

"In fact, COX-2 inhibition can damage the endothelium, leading to a prothrombotic state which increases the CV risk. Recent observational studies and a meta-analysis have shown that even the administration of some nonselective NSAIDs such as aceclofenac, diclofenac and high doses of ibuprofen can increase the risk of CV events, especially when prescribed for long periods of time."[257]

The clotting problem with non-steroidal is often made worse by the fact they are prescribed along with proton pump inhibitors such as omeprazole. So, I am not really talking about short term use here, only longer term.

Highlighting the potential scale of the problems with non-steroidals, a few years ago there was a big medical scandal when a new one was launched. It was specifically designed to reduce inflammation in the body, without damaging the lining of the stomach. Which meant that there would be, in theory at least, no ulcers.

This was made possible because the drug, Vioxx, was designed to inhibit COX-2, not COX-1 (COX-1 is the type of COX mainly found in the stomach, which protects the stomach lining). It was therefore known as a selective COX-2 inhibitor. In theory, this was a good idea, but you may have already spotted the problem.

Yes, if it powerfully inhibited COX-2, then it was almost certainly going to increase cardiovascular risk. This was a problem that would almost certainly have emerged early on in the clinical trials. However, Merck, the pharmaceutical company involved in developing this drug, decided it would be a splendid idea to camouflage the data on cardiovascular disease deaths.

In fact, their actions come direct from the playbook of how to manipulate science in order to make money – and thus kill thousands of people. Here from the article *"Merck Manipulated the Science about the Drug Vioxx."*

"To increase the likelihood of FDA (Food and Drug Administration) approval for its anti-inflammatory and arthritis drug Vioxx, the pharmaceutical giant Merck used flawed methodologies biased toward predetermined results to exaggerate the drug's positive effects. Internal documents made public in litigation revealed that a Merck marketing team had developed a strategy called ADVANTAGE (Assessment of Differences between Vioxx And Naproxen To Ascertain Gastrointestinal tolerability and Effectiveness) to skew the results of clinical trials in the drug's favor.

"As part of the strategy, scientists manipulated the trial design by comparing the drug to naproxen, a pain reliever sold under brand names such as Aleve, rather than to a placebo.

"The scientists highlighted the results that naproxen decreased the risk of heart attack by 80 percent, and downplayed results showing that Vioxx increased the risk of heart attack by 400 percent. This misleading presentation of the evidence made it look like naproxen was protecting patients from heart attacks, and that Vioxx only looked risky by comparison. In fact, Vioxx has since been found to significantly increase cardiovascular risk, leading Merck to withdraw the product from the market in 2004.

"Tragically, Merck's manipulation of its data – and the FDA's resulting approval of Vioxx in 1999 – led to thousands of avoidable premature deaths and 100,000 heart attacks." [258]

Perfect day. Merck pretended that naproxen significantly reduced the risk of heart attacks, so they could claim that the *increase* in heart attacks seen with Vioxx only occurred because it wasn't as good as naproxen at reducing the risk.

The reality is that naproxen increases cardiovascular risk, and Vioxx increased the risk of heart attacks far more. By at least *400%* more. Merck ended up being fined very nearly a billion dollars for this particular piece of lying scumbaggery, but you know what I feel about the size of this punishment?

I think that several heads should have been placed on stakes outside Merck HQ. These people quite deliberately falsified, then hid data. Actions that ended up killing thousands of people. A billion dollar fine represents about a 5% annual tax payment to these guys. I would imagine it hardly made a dent in their annual bonus. Well, you know what they say. Kill one man and they put you in jail. Kill a thousand and they make you king.

Anyway, non-steroidal drugs. Be careful. They make you clottier. And if you take a proton pump inhibitor, and a non-steroidal, at the same time – you may want to have a think about that. If it were me, I certainly would.

Now to move onto a couple of specific pro-coagulant conditions that need to be mentioned.

1. Raised lipoprotein(a) Lp(a)

2. Hughes' syndrome/antiphospholipid syndrome

1. Raised lipoprotein(a) Lp(a)

A raised Lp(a) is far from uncommon. Here from the study *"Lipoprotein(a): An independent, genetic, and causal factor for cardiovascular disease and acute myocardial infarction."*

"High Lp(a) level ≥50 mg/dl is found in 10%–30% of the population with an estimated 1.43 billion people affected globally." [259]

At least you won't be lonely if you have a high Lp(a) level. There are well over a billion of you on the planet. It can increase the risk of CVD death by two to three-fold. Both of these facts are non-controversial, so why does no-one screen for it? The answer is because pharmaceutical companies have no treatments for it, yet.

Leaving that aside, is there anything you can do about it. Up to now, three things have been consistently shown to lower Lp(a). If not by much:

- Niacin (vitamin B3)

- Coenzyme Q10

- Vitamin C

A more recent observation is that a low carbohydrate diet may be effective in reducing Lp(a) levels.[260] In truth, although this study was published in *BMJ nutrition*, this was actually a study on one person. Although larger investigations have also demonstrated the same thing.[261]

Unfortunately, there is, as yet, no clear evidence of reduction in CVD if you lower Lp(a), mainly because it has proved very difficult to do. However, to quote the American Heart Association. *"We are on the cusp of having elevated plasma concentrations of lipoprotein (a) as a therapeutic target for cardiovascular disease (CVD)."* [262]

Translation – pharmaceutical companies have finally turned their attention to Lp(a) and have found medications with which to lower it. Very, very, expensive medications that change cell signalling, and suchlike, by re-programming cellular DNA. The posh term for this is antisense therapy. Whenever a medication does something complex, and fancy, this means MONEY!

The words used by healthcare organisations having to pay for this will be *'How bloody much?'* Followed by *'You must be joking.'* Alas, my friends, the pharmaceutical industry does not joke. They can be more accurately described as being akin to a rhinoceros. They possess a very thick hide, and they charge madly in all directions.

So, what can you do if you have a high Lp(a)? I would advise that you take some vitamin B_3 (niacin) That is, if you can tolerate it, it can cause unpleasant flushing. I would also advice a gram of vitamin C a day, and 30 mg or so of co-enzyme Q10. In addition, I would cut down on the carbohydrates. I would be especially keen on doing this, if I developed type 2 diabetes.

I would also strongly advise aspirin to reduce clot formation. It has been found that aspirin can reduce the CVD risk by over 50% in those with high Lp(a). So low dose aspirin, 75 mg daily is definitely a good idea.[263]

Best ways to lower Lp(a), or reduce the risk of having a high Lp(a)

- Do NOT smoke

- Check for other clotting factors e.g., factor V Leiden

- Do not take drugs that increase blood clotting risk, if possible, e.g., ibuprofen, naproxen, or suchlike... or cocaine

- Take 75 mg aspirin a day

- Take B3/niacin, as much as you can tolerate

- Take co-enzyme Q10 ~ 30 mg a day

- Take one gram of vitamin C per day

- Reduce carbohydrate intake

Of course, you have to find a doctor who is willing to measure your Lp(a) level in the first place. And good luck with that. Just watch them furtively looking up Lp(a) on Google first.

2. Hughes' syndrome/antiphospholipid syndrome

Moving onto the last clotty syndrome, which is Hughes' syndrome. This is not common, affecting maybe 1 in a 1,000 people, perhaps 1 in 500. I did wonder whether or not to bring it up, because it is certainly not an issue for the vast majority.

However, even though it is relatively uncommon, it is thought to cause over 50% of strokes in people under the age of 50. Yes, one half.[264]

Around 1 in 10 strokes occur before the age of 50, which means that antiphospholipid syndrome accounts for 5% of all strokes. Which makes it a massively important health problem.

Especially so as the early strokes that occur with Hughes' syndrome often lead on to 'multi-infarct dementia'. This is dementia due to a build-up of small stroke after small stroke (infarcts), gradually destroying the brain. Which is a devastating disability. Compare and contrast the echoing silence here, with the massive efforts to detect familial hypercholesterolaemia.

Other studies have shown that it may drive a quarter of a million thrombotic (blood clotting) events each year in the US, so about 50,000 in the UK. Of course, not all are fatal, but a significant number are. In addition, a large number of these clots will end up as pulmonary emboli – which can certainly be fatal.

Bringing the issues together:

"It is estimated to account for 6% of all pregnancy morbidity, 13.5% of stroke, 11% of myocardial infarction and 9.5% of all deep vein thromboses."[265]

Thus, when it comes to many forms of cardiovascular disease, Hughes' syndrome punches way above its weight. Perhaps only one in 500 people have it, yet it causes over 10% of all severe cardiovascular events. Many of these happen at a tragically young age. So, should you screen for it? After all, it is rarely detected before anything goes seriously wrong.

I would say, probably not, unless there is a strong family history of strokes and heart attacks, at a young age. Or, if a female relative has lost a series of pregnancies. (the increased blood clotting problem can cause major blood supply issues for the foetus, leading to miscarriages).

At which point, probably, yes, try to convince your family doctor to look for it – and good luck with that. You test for antiphospholipid antibodies, and here is the official advice from the National Health Service.

"A diagnosis of APS can usually be confirmed if you have had:

- *1 or more confirmed blood clots*

- *1 or more unexplained late miscarriages at or after week 10 of your pregnancy*

- *1 or more premature births at or before week 34 of your pregnancy*

- *3 or more unexplained early miscarriages before week 10 of your pregnancy"* [266]

As you can see, this advice is more for women, than men. But, yes, men suffer from Hughes' syndrome too, in around the same numbers. However, if you don't become pregnant, it is less likely to show up – before something else drastic happens. The first symptom of Hughes' syndrome may well be... suddenly dropped dead.

Moving back to testing, if a close relative has antiphospholipid syndrome diagnosed, then I would certainly get yourself checked. At which point, take the advice on treatment that you are offered by the specialists. Some form of anticoagulant is best. Starting with that old favourite... aspirin.

And that is that for blood clotting.

CHAPTER 14

Miscellaneous factors

If we are looking at heart health, which we are, I think we need to wrap up by looking at other things that can damage your heart, or weaken your heart, or cause it to suddenly stop beating. Factors that may only be indirectly related to atherosclerosis. Or, indeed, have nothing to do with atherosclerosis at all. But they are still important.

For example, atrial fibrillation which I have already discussed. This is only tentatively connected to atherosclerotic plaques – if at all. However, it can still kill you from a stroke, which is one of the two biggest killers when it comes to cardiovascular events. So, it is worth checking your pulse, and if it is not regular, get your doctor to check it again. Atrial fibrillation can be silent, because it does not cause significant symptoms in most people who have it.

So, what other things should you look out for... or do?

I am going to restrict this to five:

1. Magnesium

2. Vitamin C

3. Thiamine

4. Chelation therapy

5. Enhanced External Counter Pulsation therapy EECP

1. Magnesium

Most people are probably blissfully aware that they need magnesium in the diet, and if you do not have enough how would you know? As with Hughes' syndrome, the first recognisable symptoms may be... suddenly dropping dead.

Israel provides an example of what happens when magnesium goes missing from the environment, with no-one noticing. For many years, most of the water in Israel has been provided by desalination. This process does not just get rid of salt (NaCl). It also gets rid of all the other salts, and minerals.

In normal circumstances, people get the majority of their magnesium from drinking water. Because of this, there was clearly the potential for a deficiency problem building in Israel, as their water contained nothing but H_2O.

Did anyone notice? As in, did anyone say, 'golly I feel low in magnesium today'. Nope. Did anyone die. Yup, they did. As outlined in the paper "Association between exposure to desalinated sea water and ischemic heart disease, diabetes mellitus and colorectal cancer; A population-based study in Israel."[267]

There were possibly as many as 4,000 deaths a year:

"An estimated 4,000 Israelis die in an average year due to an inadequate amount of magnesium in their bodies – and the amount they get from natural potable water sources is increasingly declining due to the growing desalination of sea water. The figure is 10-fold the death toll from road accidents."[268]

The population of Israel is just over nine million. The equivalent death rate in the UK would be 30,000 and deaths a year, or 180,000 in the US. A silent killer indeed.

Yes, magnesium is critical stuff. It is extremely important for health, especially heart health. For one thing, it is required for the correct functioning of the electrical system in your heart. Because of this, it increases the risk of atrial fibrillation. Here from the paper "Low serum magnesium and the development of atrial fibrillation in the community: the Framingham Heart Study."

"...individuals in the lowest quartile of serum magnesium were ~50% more likely to develop AF ... compared with those in the upper quartiles."[269]

Unfortunately, despite its importance, we don't feel magnesium depleted. We do not crave magnesium rich foods – as if we would have any idea what they are. The symptoms of severe deficiency are also non-specific.

It's not just Israel. Here from the paper: "Subclinical magnesium deficiency: a principal driver of cardiovascular disease and a public health crisis."

"*Furthermore, because of chronic diseases, medications, decreases in food crop magnesium contents, and the availability of refined and processed foods, the vast majority of people in modern societies are at risk for magnesium deficiency.*"[270]

Have you ever heard of *any* of this? Did you even know you had magnesium in your body – or that it did anything important? I suspect not.

"*...magnesium deficiency can lead to serious morbidity and mortality and has been implicated in multiple cardiovascular diseases such as hypertension, cardiomyopathy, cardiac arrhythmia, atherosclerosis, dyslipidaemia and diabetes. Unfortunately, the western diet is often low in magnesium due to the refining and processing of foods, and hypomagnesaemia is often underdiagnosed in hospitalised patients.*"[271]

My advice, take a supplement. Especially if you live in an area with 'soft' water – which means not many minerals. Doubly especially if you have atrial fibrillation. It might just go away. How much do you need to take? Around 400 mg a day is fine.

2. Vitamin C

I have talked about vitamin C before. Mainly with regard to Lp(a). The cardiovascular importance of vitamin C is that is required for the synthesis of collagen – the most important support molecule in your body. Think of collagen as like the steel bars in concrete. If collagen is not made, various bits of your body start to crack and break down. One of the first bits to break down are the walls of your blood vessels.

So, if you lack vitamin C (scurvy) one of the first clinical signs is bleeding gums, because the blood vessels here crack open – where you can see the blood. Then you bleed everywhere else, then you die. Lp(a), on the other hand, is designed to block the cracks in blood vessels and stop the bleeding. Lp(a) is found in animals that cannot make their own vitamin C. Great apes, fruit bats, guinea pigs... human beings.

Cutting a very long story short. If you have a high Lp(a) you really don't want any cracks in your blood vessels, because Lp(a) will come along and help to construct a very strong and resilient blood clot that will be very difficult to remove.

So, even if vitamin C does not lower Lp(a) levels that much, it is still important to take it if you have a high Lp(a) level, because you certainly do not want cracks to form. It is probably a good idea for everyone else to take some as well.

Linus Pauling was the great vitamin C promoter. He felt that high dose vitamin C could prevent cardiovascular disease completely, by stopping any damage to arterial walls. Whilst I entirely agree that vitamin C deficiency (however you define it) is a cause of atherosclerosis. It is definitely not *the* cause. I think he went over the top in what he claimed.

He also suggested taking 10 grams a day. I tried this and couldn't get off the toilet for a week (slight exaggeration). A full spray paint job. If you ever suffer from constipation, take 10 grams of vitamin C. I will guarantee the problem goes away – very fast. I take one gram a day. I think this is probably enough.

However, if you are suffering from an infection – of almost any sort – I would increase this to the maximum you can tolerate. Because vitamin C boosts immune function, protects the endothelium. Additionally, the body burns through a lot of vitamin C when fighting off infections, so you need as much as you can get:

"Vitamin C deficiency results in impaired immunity and higher susceptibility to infections. In turn, infections significantly impact on vitamin C levels due to enhanced inflammation and metabolic requirements. Furthermore, supplementation with vitamin C appears to be able to both prevent and treat respiratory and systemic infections."[272]

As I wrote earlier in the book, infective agents are seriously damaging to the endothelium, and you need vitamin C to help protect it.

3. Thiamine

Thiamine is also called vitamin B_1. It is actually prescribed quite a lot by doctors. Who'd a thunk? A vitamin that the medical profession doesn't dismiss as useless. It is mainly given to people who drink too much alcohol, who often end up deficient in Thiamine. This is mainly because alcohol prevents thiamine absorption.

All sorts of problem then ensue. One of the well-known ones is Korsakoff's syndrome: confused mental state, loss of memory, difficulty walking and suchlike – which wraps us back around in using B vitamins for Alzheimer's again.

Yes B-vitamins are very good for the brain, and also the effective functioning of the brain. In fact, vitamin B_{12} deficiency results in the destruction of nerve cells all around the body, not just the brain. As a quick aside nitrous oxide (not nitric oxide) inhalation strips Vitamin B12 from the body very fast. So young people using nitrous oxide, for kicks, will end up perilously low in vitamin B12. This can result in irreversible nerve damage.

Another significant downside of thiamine deficiency is heart failure. This is because thiamine is essential for energy production in all cells, which is especially important in the highly energetic heart muscle cells.

Heart failure means that the heart is no longer capable of pumping blood through the body, so fluid starts to build up in the ankles and the lungs and suchlike. This can commonly happen after a heart attack – where a part of the heart is no longer able to function. It affects about a million people in the UK, mainly the elderly. In around a third of cases, thiamine deficiency can be found.

So, whilst this is not an issue for most, heart failure remains a highly important 'heart' condition, and it can be improved with thiamine supplementation – which is why I include it here.

"Thiamine deficiency appears to be not uncommon in patients with HF (heart failure), and supplementation with thiamine has been shown to improve cardiac function, urine output, weight loss, and signs and symptoms of HF." [273]

4. Chelation therapy – for raised levels of lead (or other heavy metals) – or for those with diabetes?

We now move the furthest distance possible in woo-woo territory with chelation therapy. Chelation therapy uses a substance, or substances, which can be taken orally, or by injection. They then bind with lead (and other heavy metals), and the resultant compound is excreted by the kidneys. Chelation therapy is a well-established and non-controversial way of removing lead from the body. Normally when the levels are very high/toxic.[274]

What is significantly more controversial is the use of chelation therapy in people with lower blood levels. Or maybe even in people where there is not a high level at all.

"Medical practitioners have treated atherosclerotic disease with chelation therapy for over fifty years. Lack of strong of evidence led conventional practitioners to abandon its use in the 1960s and 1970s. This relegated chelation therapy to complementary and alternative medicine practitioners, who reported

291

*good anecdotal results. Concurrently, **the epidemiologic evidence linking xenobiotic* metals with cardiovascular disease and mortality gradually accumulated, suggesting a plausible role for chelation therapy**. On the basis of the continued use of chelation therapy without an evidence base, the National Institutes of Health released a Request for Applications for a definitive trial of chelation therapy."* [275]

Under some pressure, the National Institutes of Health in the US did fund a study. It was called: *"Trial to Assess Chelation Therapy (TACT)"*. In a breach of normal scientific politeness (a term covers over much anger and spite), it was attacked viciously, right from the very start. Here from Medscape in 2008.

*"The trial employs nearly **100 unfit co-investigators**... The trial's outcome will be unreliable and almost certainly equivocal, thus defeating its stated purpose. **We conclude that the TACT is unethical, dangerous, pointless, and wasteful. It should be abandoned**."* [276]

Well, those were lovely and kind comments are they not. As I was once told *'If you can't think of anything nice to say, say nothing.'* Advice which I have almost totally ignored ever since.

In the world of medical research, trials are often attacked *after* they are published. Very few are subjected to poisonous vitriol whilst they are still recruiting patients. Poisonous vitriol such as this might lead some people to suspect that various individuals, or large companies, did not want to see a positive result with chelation therapy. *'We need patented drugs my precious, druuuuuugs, my precious.'*

At one point this trial had to be temporarily suspended, due to angry claims that it was unethical. However, it did restart, and battled on, fighting against a very stiff headwind.

The end result? Well, despite the fact that many people were desperate to prove that chelation doesn't work. It did.

*"With a result that is likely to surprise and baffle much of the mainstream medical community, **a large NIH-sponsored trial has turned up the first substantial evidence in support of chelation therapy for patients with coronary disease**. Known as TACT (Trial to Assess Chelation Therapy), the highly*

---

* Cracking word xenobiotic, I love it. Very sci-fi. Sadly, and rather prosaically, it just means something found in the body that shouldn't really be there e.g., a heavy metal.

controversial trial was presented today at the AHA by Gervasio Lamas. The trial was sponsored by two NIH institutes, the National Center for Complementary and Alternative Medicine and the National Heart Lung and Blood Institute."[277]

It worked spectacularly well in people with diabetes, where there was an extremely significant benefit. A 41% (relative risk) reduction in relative risk of CV events. The probability of this result being a chance finding was 0.00002 (two in one million).

A clinical trial is considered to have 'succeeded' if the probability of the result being a chance finding is less than 0.05 (5 in 100). Chelation also worked better in those given high dose vitamins at the same time. Woo-woo medicine to the power ten.[278]

Yes, chelation therapy worked, it should also be pointed out that it worked in people who did not necessarily have high levels of heavy metals in their blood in the first place. You could say that this trial was almost deliberately set up to fail, but even whilst being attacked from all sides – it worked.

A second TACT trial is now ongoing, specifically to look at people with diabetes. I hope they are going to use a combination B-vitamin/ chelation trial. Let us wait to see what it shows. In the meantime. High levels of heavy metals = consider chelation therapy.

Personally, if I had diabetes, I would also seriously consider chelation therapy. I would definitely do so if I had a high level of lead (or any other heavy metal). A high level of lead means anything greater than 0.24 µmol/l (5 µg/dl).

5. Enhanced External Counter Pulsation therapy (EECP)

This is the form of 'treatment' that impacts the least number of people discussed, which makes it footnote, of a sort. If you do not have severe cardiovascular disease, with heart failure, and angina, you need know nothing about Enhance External Counter Pulsation therapy.

However, it is still available on the NHS, just clinging on by its fingertips. It is widely used in some other countries. In the UK, hardly anyone knows anything about it. No GP I have spoken to in the UK has ever heard of it. Despite this almost complete silence, for those with severely blocked coronary arteries and severe angina, it is important to know that it exists.

Enhanced External Counter Pulsation therapy uses inflatable cuffs wrapped around the legs to squeeze the blood vessels in your legs, in time with your heartbeat. This pushes more blood back into the heart. This triggers the formation of new, small, blood vessels that can bypass the narrowings and blockages in your coronary arteries. These new blood vessels are called collateral circulation.

It sounds completely woo-woo, and I believe that it originated in China. However, despite its origins and seeming bonkersness, the simple fact is that it works. If you have problems with angina, which have proven untreatable in any other way. Go pester your GP to get this treatment organised.[279]

CHAPTER 15

Keeping cardiovascular disease at bay

And so gentle reader, we come to a close. I haven't discussed everything here. But I have covered the things that I believe to be most important. I do not expect everyone to do everything I have recommended. I certainly don't. At least not every day. Frankly, I am far too lazy.

I thought I would finish off by reminding you of a study done in the UK, where the researchers looked at many different factors that had been gathered by GPs on their patients – 378,256 patients in total, analysed over 10 years. It was, if you like, a super-expanded Qrisk3, with almost 50 different factors analysed.[280]

The study was called *"Can machine-learning improve cardiovascular risk prediction using routine clinical data?"* Here is what they found to be the top 10 risk factors for CVD, in order, with number one being highest risk, and number 10 lowest risk:

1. Chronic obstructive pulmonary disease
2. Oral corticosteroid prescribed
3. Age
4. Severe mental illness
5. Ethnicity South Asian
6. Immunosuppressant prescribed
7. Socio-economic-status quintile 3
8. Socio-economic status quintile 4
9. Chronic kidney disease
10. Socio-economic status quintile 2

If you remove age, which you can do nothing about, we are left with only a few different factors in the top ten. With chronic obstructive pulmonary disease at number one. Well, well, who'd a thunk? Not me, until I saw this study.

Then we have steroids and other immunosuppressants (steroids are immunosuppressants) and severe mental illness. With these three we are looking at, essentially, the same mechanisms of action. Which centres on cortisol/HPA-axis dysfunction with insulin resistance. All of which also wrap back around into chronic kidney disease.

The other four are all socio-economic factors.

Where is diabetes? It is wrapped into most of the other factors.

Where was LDL? Well, it came 46th... out of 48. Essentially, it was of no significance at all. None. I wrote to the authors of this paper to find out why they failed to mention this complete and utter lack of impact of LDL. The reply was a masterclass in obfuscation. I cannot blame them. See under Kilmer McCully. So long as you don't directly mention LDL, you can get away with demonstrating that it has nothing to do with cardiovascular disease. It slips under the radar.

I think that the main thing that this list highlights is that there are not too many things that most people need to greatly worry about. Do not breathe in really nasty toxic stuff. Keep your cortisol levels down and keep your HPA-axis healthy by remaining calm and by nurturing your friends and family. Do the type of exercise you most enjoy, get out in the sunshine... just get outside. Eat, local, natural food.

As for supplements. Here are the ones I believe to be most important:

- Vitamin D – in the winter

- Vitamin C

- Potassium

- Magnesium

- L-arginine/citrulline

If you already have diagnosed heart disease

- Chondroitin sulphate

- Thiamine

- Co-enzyme Q-10

- Consider Viagra...

- Consider aspirin, low dose, especially if you have a clotting disorder

- Avoid non-steroidal drugs, long term, if possible

- Avoid proton pump inhibitors, long-term, if possible

If you have diabetes

- Low carb diet

- Short burst exercise

- Reduce alcohol

- Consider chelation therapy

And always, smile, count your blessings and do things that make you feel good about yourself. Volunteer, join a club, meet people. Nurture yourself.

And... if you do have serious medical problems, do not avoid mainstream medicine. I do not wish to give the impression that mainstream medicine has no solutions, nothing of benefit in this area. If you have a heart attack – get thee to the hospital. If your blood pressure, or blood sugar are flying out of control – get thee to a doctor. The model of cardiovascular disease they are using is, I believe, wrong. However, many of the solutions still work.

CHAPTER 16

The end

I hope I have given you a clearer idea about cardiovascular disease. What causes it, and how to keep it at bay. In my view it has been a crying shame that the ideas of Rokitansky, Duguid, Ross and Smith – to name but four – never managed to gain any traction. The cholesterol hypothesis came, it saw, it conquered. Sweeping all other ideas into the dust, where they currently remain.

When I first came across their thinking it immediately made sense to me. I became determined to fill in the gaps and try to bring everything into a coherent picture. All of the scattered pieces of the jigsaw laid down in their rightful place.

In the end it became my obsession to fit smoking, to rheumatoid arthritis, to high blood pressure, to lack of exercise to diabetes, to mental illness, to chronic kidney disease to... on and on the factors stretched. I was getting nowhere. In the end it was Paul Rosch who pointed me in the right direction. Do not focus on individual causes. Focus on process, then see if the factors fit into the process. If they don't, your process is wrong.

I think, I certainly hope, that everything does fit within the 'thrombogenic process.' I have found nothing that does not – so far. I am sure that at some point in the future it will be found to be flawed and will require updating, reviewing, and suchlike. Science is always a journey, never a destination. All we can try to do it move understanding a few steps further forward. A few more bricks in the cathedral walls. *'See that Cathedral of Science... one of those small bricks halfway up the outer wall, that you can't really see. I put that there.'*

Then you die a happy man, or woman, aged 103 – from a sudden heart attack. Best way to go, in my opinion.

References

1 Mandy Oaklander. Cholesterol Is Not a 'Nutrient of Concern,' Report Says. Time Magazine. February 11, 2015. http://time.com/3705734/cholesterol-dietary-guidelines/

2 CBS News. Exchange between Dr Robert Olson and Senator George McGovern from The United States Senate Select Committee on Nutrition and Human Needs. Washington, July 26, 1977.

3 Harcombe *et al.* Evidence from randomised controlled trials did not support the introduction of dietary fat guidelines in 1977 and 1983: a systematic review and meta-analysis. BMJ Open Heart. 2015. https://openheart.bmj.com/content/2/1/e000196

4 Keys A, Anderson JT. The relationship of the diet to the development of atherosclerosis in man. In: National Research Council DoMS, ed. Symposium on atherosclerosis. Washington: National Academy of Sciences – National Research Council. 1954.

5 https://www.zoeharcombe.com/2018/06/swiss-re-bmj-nutrition-conference/

6 Ramsden *et al.* Re-evaluation of the traditional diet-heart hypothesis: analysis of recovered data from Minnesota Coronary Experiment (1968-73). BMJ. 2016. https://www.bmj.com/content/353/bmj.i1246

7 Sharon Begley. Records Found in Dusty Basement Undermine Decades of Dietary Advice. Scientific American. April 19, 2017. https://www.scientificamerican.com/article/records-found-in-dusty-basement-undermine-decades-of-dietary-advice/

8 Harcombe & Baker. Plant Sterols lower cholesterol but increase risk for coronary heart disease. The Journal of Biological Sciences. 2014. https://thescipub.com/abstract/10.3844/ojbsci.2014.167.169

9 Ramsden *et al.* The Sydney Diet Heart Study: a randomised controlled trial of linoleic acid for secondary prevention of coronary heart disease and death. The FASEB Journal. 2013. https://faseb.onlinelibrary.wiley.com/doi/abs/10.1096/fasebj.27.1_supplement.127.4

10 Jacobs D *et al.* Report of the conference on Low Blood cholesterol: Mortality associations. Circulation Vol 86, No 3. September 1992

11 Petursson *et al.* Is the use of cholesterol in mortality risk algorithms in clinical guidelines valid? Ten years prospective data from the Norwegian HUNT 2 study. J Eval Clin Pract. 2012. https://www.ncbi.nlm.nih.gov/pmc/articles/PMC3303886/

12 http://www.fathead-movie.com/index.php/2010/03/22/dr-uffe-ravnskov-fat-and-cholesterol-are-good-for-you/

13 Michelle Stacey. The Fall and Rise Of Kilmer McCully. The New York Times Magazine. August 10, 1997. https://www.nytimes.com/1997/08/10/magazine/the-fall-and-rise-of-kilmer-mccully.html

14 Ian Leslie. The Sugar Conspiracy. The Guardian. April 7, 2016. https://www.theguardian.com/society/2016/apr/07/the-sugar-conspiracy-robert-lustig-john-yudkin

15 Kearns *et al*. Sugar Industry and Coronary Heart Disease Research. JAMA Intern Med. 2016. https://jamanetwork.com/journals/jamainternalmedicine/article-abstract/2548255

16 Alliance for Human Research Protection. Why was Dr John Yudkin ridiculed & marginalized? September 30, 2016. https://ahrp.org/why-was-dr-john-yudkin-ridiculed-marginalized/ "Sugar Bakers Paid to Shift Blame to Fat" *The New York Times*, Sept. 13, 2016

17 Banta *et al*. The Global Influence of the Seventh-Day Adventist Church on Diet. Religions. 2018. https://www.mdpi.com/2077-1444/9/9/251/htm

18 Howard Markel. The Secret Ingredient in Kellogg's Corn Flakes Is Seventh-Day Adventism. Smithsonian Magazine. July 28, 2017. https://www.smithsonianmag.com/history/secret-ingredient-kelloggs-corn-flakes-seventh-day-adventism-180964247/

19 Ravnskov *et al*. Lack of an association or an inverse association between low-density-lipoprotein cholesterol and mortality in the elderly: a systematic review. BMJ Open. 2015. https://bmjopen.bmj.com/content/6/6/e010401

20 Ravnskov *et al*. LDL-C does not cause cardiovascular disease: a comprehensive review of the current literature. Expert Review of Clinical Pharmacology. 2018. https://www.tandfonline.com/doi/full/10.1080/17512433.2018.1519391

21 http://healthbulletin.org.au/articles/review-of-cardiovascular-health-among-aboriginal-and-torres-strait-islander-people/

22 https://qrisk.org/three/

23 Hopkins & Williams. A survey of 246 suggested coronary risk factors. Atherosclerosis. 1981. https://www.atherosclerosis-journal.com/article/0021-9150(81)90122-2/pdf

24 Poulter. Coronary heart disease is a multifactorial disease. American Journal of Hypertension. 1999. https://academic.oup.com/ajh/article/12/S6/92S/106550

25 Zaman *et al*. The role of plaque rupture and thrombosis in coronary artery disease. Atherosclerosis. 2000. https://www.sciencedirect.com/science/article/pii/S0021915099004797

26 https://en.wikipedia.org/wiki/Tight_junction

27 Greene & Campbell. Tight junction modulation of the blood brain barrier: CNS delivery of small molecules. Tissue Barriers. 2016. https://www.ncbi.nlm.nih.gov/pmc/articles/PMC4836485/

28 Fedson & Rordam. Treating Ebola patients: a 'bottom up' approach using generic statins and angiotensin receptor blockers. International Journal of Infectious Diseases. Volume 36. 2015. https://www.sciencedirect.com/science/article/pii/S120197121500106X

29 Gertz *et al*. Composition of atherosclerotic plaques in the four major epicardial coronary arteries in patients greater than or equal to 90 years of age. Am J Cardiol. 1991. https://www.ncbi.nlm.nih.gov/pubmed/2035446

30 Stary *et al*. A Definition of Advanced Types of Atherosclerotic Lesions and a Histological Classification of Atherosclerosis. A Report From the Committee on Vascular Lesions of the Council on Arteriosclerosis, American Heart Association. 1995. https://www.ahajournals.org/doi/full/10.1161/01.CIR.92.5.1355

31 Beckerman. Cholesterol and Artery Plaque Buildup. WebMD. August 22, 2020. https://www.webmd.com/cholesterol-management/cholesterol-and-artery-plaque-buildup#1

32 Origin of atherosclerosis in childhood and adolescence. The American Journal of Clinical Nutrition, Volume 72, Issue 5, November 2000. https://academic.oup.com/ajcn/article/72/5/1307s/4730131

33 Velican & Velican. Progression of coronary atherosclerosis from adolescents to mature adults. Atherosclerosis. 1983. https://www.sciencedirect.com/science/article/abs/pii/0021915083901508

34 Ventura. Rudolph Virchow and Cellular Pathology. Profiles in Cardiology. Edited by Hurst & Fye. Clin. Cardiol. 2000. https://onlinelibrary.wiley.com/doi/pdf/10.1002/clc.4960230717

35 Pub(C)hem. Compound summary. Cholesterol. https://pubchem.ncbi.nlm.nih.gov/compound/cholesterol#section=Top

36 Pasterkamp & Virmani. The erythrocyte: a new player in atheromatous core formation. Heart. 2002. https://www.ncbi.nlm.nih.gov/pmc/articles/PMC1767211/

37 Zhong et al. Total cholesterol content of erythrocyte membranes is associated with the severity of coronary artery disease and the therapeutic effect of rosuvastatin. Ups J Med Sci. 2012. https://www.ncbi.nlm.nih.gov/pmc/articles/PMC3497225/

38 Weisel. Role of Red Cells in Thrombosis and Hemostasis. Blood. 2015. https://ashpublications.org/blood/article/126/23/SCI-39/136388/Role-of-Red-Cells-in-Thrombosis-and-Hemostasis

39 Beckerman. Cholesterol and Artery Plaque Buildup. WebMD. August 22, 2020. https://www.webmd.com/cholesterol-management/cholesterol-and-artery-plaque-buildup#1

40 Rath et al. Detection and Quantification of Lipoprotein(a) in the Arterial Wall of 107 Coronary Bypass Patients. Arteriosclerosis VOL 9, No 5. September/October 1989. https://www.ahajournals.org/doi/pdf/10.1161/01.ATV.9.5.579

41 Pepin et al. Quantification of apo[a] and apoB in human atherosclerotic lesions. Journal of Lipid Research Volume 32, 1991. http://www.jlr.org/content/32/2/317.full.pdf

42 Nordestgaard & Langsted. Lipoprotein (a) as a cause of cardiovascular disease: insights from epidemiology, genetics, and biology. Journal of Lipid Research. 2016. http://www.jlr.org/content/57/11/1953.long

43 Anahad O'Connor. A heart risk factor even doctors know little about. The New York Times. January 9, 2018. https://www.nytimes.com/2018/01/09/well/heart-risk-doctors-lipoprotein.html

44 Romagnuolo et al. Inhibition of plasminogen activation by apo(a): role of carboxyl-terminal lysines and identification of inhibitory domains in apo(a). Journal of Lipid Research. 2014. https://www.ncbi.nlm.nih.gov/pmc/articles/PMC3966697/

45 Undas et al. Lipoprotein(a) as a modifier of fibrin clot permeability and susceptibility to lysis. Journal of Thrombosis and Haemostasis. 2006. https://onlinelibrary.wiley.com/doi/full/10.1111/j.1538-7836.2006.01903.x

46 Zwaal et al. Lipid–protein interactions in blood coagulation. Biochimica et Biophysica Acta (BBA) – Reviews on Biomembranes. 1998. https://www.sciencedirect.com/science/article/abs/pii/S0304415798000185

47 Boffa & Koschinsky. Lipoprotein(a): truly a direct prothrombotic factor in cardiovascular disease? Journal of Lipid Research. 2016. http://www.jlr.org/content/57/5/745.full

48 Pathobiology of the Human Atherosclerotic Plaque. pp ISBN-14: 978-1-4612-7968-6. Seymour Glabog, Williman P Newmman III, Sheldon A. Schaffer pp 360.

49 Smith & Thompson. Fibrin as a factor in atherogenesis. Thrombosis Research. 1993. https://www.sciencedirect.com/sdfe/pdf/download/eid/1-s2.0-0049384894900493/first-page-pdf

50 Smith. Fibrinogen and atherosclerosis. Review Wien Klin Wochenschr. 1993. https://www.ncbi.nlm.nih.gov/pubmed/8379153

51 Gawaz *et al.* Platelets modulate atherogenesis and progression of atherosclerotic plaques via interaction with progenitor and dendritic cells. Journal of Thrombosis and Haemostasis. 2007. https://onlinelibrary.wiley.com/doi/pdf/10.1111/j.1538-7836.2008.02867.x

52 Stary *et al.* A Definition of Advanced Types of Atherosclerotic Lesions and a Histological Classification of Atherosclerosis. Circulation. 1995. https://www.ahajournals.org/doi/full/10.1161/01.CIR.92.5.1355

53 Zaman *et al.* The role of plaque rupture and thrombosis in coronary artery disease. Atherosclerosis. 2000. https://www.sciencedirect.com/science/article/pii/S0021915099004797

54 Mann & Davies. Mechanisms of progression in native coronary artery disease: role of healed plaque disruption. Heart. 1999. https://www.ncbi.nlm.nih.gov/pmc/articles/PMC1729162/

55 Smith & Thompson. Fibrin as a factor in atherogenesis. Thrombosis Research. 1993. https://www.sciencedirect.com/sdfe/pdf/download/eid/1-s2.0-0049384894900493/first-page-pdf

56 Nissen. Statin Denial: An Internet-Driven Cult With Deadly Consequences. Editorial Ann Intern Med. 2017. https://annals.org/aim/article-abstract/2645554/statin-denial-internet-driven-cult-deadly-consequences

57 https://www.dailymail.co.uk/health/article-6764117/Devastating-investigation-reveals-impact-deadly-statin-denier-propaganda.html

58 Significance of the endothelial glycocalyx. Deranged Physiology. Required Reading. Infectious diseases antibiotics and sepsis. 2015. https://derangedphysiology.com/main/required-reading/infectious-diseases-antibiotics-and-sepsis/Chapter%201.3.1/significance-endothelial-glycocalyx

59 Significance of the endothelial glycocalyx. Deranged Physiology. Required Reading. Infectious diseases antibiotics and sepsis. 2015. https://derangedphysiology.com/main/required-reading/infectious-diseases-antibiotics-and-sepsis/Chapter%20131/significance-endothelial-glycocalyx

60 Astrup et *al.* Thromboplastic and Fibrnolytic Activity of the Human Aorta. Circulation Research, Volume VII. November 1959.

61 National Institute for Care and Health Excellence. Do not do recommendation details. MI: Secondary prevention (CG48). May 2007. https://www.nice.org.uk/donotdo/for-patients-who-have-had-an-myocardial-infarction-mi-highintensity-warfarin-inr-3-should-not-be-considered-as-an-alternative-to-aspirin-in-firstline-treatment

62 Woolf et *al.* Experimental mural thrombi in the pig aorta. The early natural history. Br J Exp Pathol. 1968. https://www.ncbi.nlm.nih.gov/pmc/articles/PMC2093824/?page=3

63 Altabas. Diabetes, Endothelial Dysfunction, and Vascular Repair: What Should a Diabetologist Keep His Eye on? International Journal of Endocrinology. 2015. https://new.hindawi.com/journals/ije/2015/848272/

64 Luttun & Verfaillie. Will the real EPC please stand up? Blood. 2007. https://ashpublications.org/blood/article/109/5/1795/23187/Will-the-real-EPC-please-stand-up

65 Lin *et al.* Endothelial Progenitor Cell Dysfunction in Cardiovascular Diseases: Role of Reactive Oxygen Species and Inflammation. BioMed Research International. 2013. https://new.hindawi.com/journals/bmri/2013/845037/

66 António *et al.* Reduced levels of circulating endothelial progenitor cells in acute myocardial infarction patients with diabetes or pre-diabetes: accompanying the glycemic continuum. Cardiovasc Diabetol. 2014. https://www.ncbi.nlm.nih.gov/pmc/articles/PMC4082424/

67 Chen *et al.* Value and level of circulating endothelial progenitor cells, angiogenesis factors and mononuclear cell apoptosis in patients with chronic kidney disease. Clin Exp Nephrol. 2013. https://www.ncbi.nlm.nih.gov/pubmed/22814956

68 Ding *et al.* Impairment of circulating endothelial progenitor cells (EPCs) in patients with glucocorticoid-induced avascular necrosis of the femoral head and changes of EPCs after glucocorticoid treatment in vitro. Journal of Orthopaedic Surgery and Research. 2019. https://josr-online.biomedcentral.com/articles/10.1186/s13018-019-1279-6

69 Liu & Huang. Cardiovascular roles of nitric oxide: A review of insights from nitric oxide synthase gene disrupted mice. Cardiovascular Research. 2008. https://academic.oup.com/cardiovascres/article/77/1/19/463897

70 Burnett. Novel nitric oxide signaling mechanisms regulate the erectile response. International Journal of Impotence Research volume. 2004. https://www.nature.com/articles/3901209

71 VIAGRA®Clinical Pharmacology (sildenafil citrate). Pfizer. https://www.pfizermedicalinformation.com/en-us/viagra/clinical-pharmacology

72 Weller. Sunlight Has Cardiovascular Benefits Independently of Vitamin D. Blood Purif. 2016. https://www.karger.com/Article/FullText/441266

73 Lindqvist *et al.* Avoidance of sun exposure as a risk factor for major causes of death: a competing risk analysis of the Melanoma in Southern Sweden cohort. Journal of Internal Medicine. 2016. https://onlinelibrary.wiley.com/doi/full/10.1111/joim.12496

74 Chang *et al.* Age Decreases Endothelial Progenitor Cell Recruitment Through Decreases in Hypoxia-Inducible Factor 1α Stabilization During Ischemia. Circulation. 2007. https://www.ahajournals.org/doi/full/10.1161/CIRCULATIONAHA.107.715847

75 Toprakçı, *et al.* Age-associated changes in nitric oxide metabolites nitrite and nitrate. International Journal of Clinical and Laboratory Research. 2000. https://link.springer.com/article/10.1007/BF02874163

76 Hopkins & Williams. A survey of 246 suggested coronary risk factors. Atherosclerosis. 1981. https://www.atherosclerosis-journal.com/article/0021-9150(81)90122-2/pdf

77 Marmot. Closing the health gap. Scandinavian Journal of Public Health. 2017. https://journals.sagepub.com/doi/full/10.1177/1403494817717433

78 The Marmot Review. Fair Society, Healthy Lives. Strategic Review of Health Inequalities in England post 2010. http://www.instituteofhealthequity.org/file-manager/Presentationsandrecordings/all-marmot-review-slides.pdf

79 Mobarrez *et al.* The Effects of Smoking on Levels of Endothelial Progenitor Cells and Microparticles in the Blood of Healthy Volunteers. PLoS ONE. 2014. https://www.ncbi.nlm.nih.gov/pmc/articles/PMC3938677/

80 Messner & Bernhard. Smoking and cardiovascular disease: mechanisms of endothelial dysfunction and early atherogenesis. Arterioscler Thromb Vasc Biol. 2014. https://www.ncbi.nlm.nih.gov/pubmed/24554606

81 Solomon *et al.* Induction of platelet aggregation after a direct physical interaction with diesel exhaust particles. J Thromb Haemost. 2013. https://www.ncbi.nlm.nih.gov/pubmed/23206187

82 Wildfire smoke associated with more ER visits for heart, stroke ailments among seniors. American Heart Association. April 11, 2018. https://www.sciencedaily.com/releases/2018/04/180411090420.htm

83 Landen *et al.* Mining Publication: Coal Dust Exposure and Mortality From Ischemic Heart Disease Among a Cohort of U.S. Coal Miners. The National Institute for Occupational Safety and Health (NIOSH). October 2011. https://www.cdc.gov/niosh/mining/works/coversheet667.html

84 Setiawana *et al.* Subchronic inhalation of particulate matter 10 coal dust induces atherosclerosis in the aorta of diabetic and nondiabetic rats. Biomarkers and Genomic Medicine. 2014. https://www.sciencedirect.com/science/article/pii/S2214024714000112

85 Weng *et al.* Can machine-learning improve cardiovascular risk prediction using routine clinical data? PLoS ONE 2017. https://journals.plos.org/plosone/article?id=10.1371/journal.pone.0174944

86 Wani *et al.* Lead toxicity: a review. Interdiscip Toxicol. 2015. https://www.ncbi.nlm.nih.gov/pmc/articles/PMC4961898/

87 Lanphear *et al.* Low-level lead exposure and mortality in US adults: a population-based cohort study. The Lancet. 2018. https://www.thelancet.com/journals/lanpub/article/PIIS2468-2667(18)30025-2/fulltext

88 Weisskopf *et al.* A prospective study of bone lead concentration and death from all causes, cardiovascular diseases, and cancer in the Department of Veterans Affairs Normative Aging Study. Circulation. 2009. https://www.ncbi.nlm.nih.gov/pubmed/19738141

89 Solenkova *et al.* Metal pollutants and cardiovascular disease: mechanisms and consequences of exposure. Am Heart J. 2014. https://www.ncbi.nlm.nih.gov/pubmed/25458643

90 Shin *et al.* Lead-induced procoagulant activation of erythrocytes through phosphatidylserine exposure may lead to thrombotic diseases. Chem Res Toxicol. 2007. https://www.ncbi.nlm.nih.gov/pubmed/17226925

91 Bøtker & Møller. ON NO – The Continuing Story of Nitric Oxide, Diabetes, and Cardiovascular Disease. Diabetes. 2013. https://diabetes.diabetesjournals.org/content/62/8/2645

92 Sena *et al.* Endothelial dysfunction — A major mediator of diabetic vascular disease. Biochimica et Biophysica Acta (BBA) – Molecular Basis of Disease. 2013. https://www.sciencedirect.com/science/article/pii/S0925443913002718

93 Carr. Diabetes mellitus: a hypercoagulable state. J Diabetes Complications. Jan-Feb 2001. https://pubmed.ncbi.nlm.nih.gov/11259926/

94 Ark *et al.* Type 2 diabetes mellitus is associated with an imbalance in circulating endothelial and smooth muscle progenitor cell numbers. Diabetologia. 2012. https://link.springer.com/article/10.1007/s00125-012-2590-5

95 Nieuwdorp *et al.* Loss of Endothelial Glycocalyx During Acute Hyperglycemia Coincides With Endothelial Dysfunction and Coagulation Activation In Vivo. Diabetes. 2006. https://diabetes.diabetesjournals.org/content/55/2/480

96 Stehouwer. Microvascular Dysfunction and Hyperglycemia: A Vicious Cycle With Widespread Consequences. Diabetes. 2018. https://diabetes.diabetesjournals.org/content/67/9/1729

97 Ohishi. Hypertension with diabetes mellitus: physiology and pathology. Hypertens Res. 2018. https://www.ncbi.nlm.nih.gov/pubmed/29556093

98 Kuusisto *et al.* Atherosclerosis-like lesions of the aortic valve are common in adults of all ages: a necropsy study. BMJ Heart. 2005. https://heart.bmj.com/content/91/5/576

99 Judith Marcin. How is essential hypertension diagnosed? Healthline. September 17, 2018. https://www.healthline.com/health/essential-hypertension#diagnosis

100 Public Health England. Health matters: combating high blood pressure. Guidance. January 24, 2017. https://www.gov.uk/government/publications/health-matters-combating-high-blood-pressure/health-matters-combating-high-blood-pressure

101 Perrot *et al.* Pulmonary hypertension after pulmonary emboli: an underrecognized condition. CMAJ. 2006. https://www.ncbi.nlm.nih.gov/pmc/articles/PMC1471826/

102 Reddy *et al.* Nitric oxide status in patients with chronic kidney disease. Indian J Nephrol. 2015. https://www.ncbi.nlm.nih.gov/pmc/articles/PMC4588324/

103 Krenning *et al.* Endothelial progenitor cell dysfunction in patients with progressive chronic kidney disease. American Journal of Renal Physiology. 2009. https://journals.physiology.org/doi/full/10.1152/ajprenal.90755.2008

104 Cedars Sinai. Rheumatoid Vasculitis. Health Library. https://www.cedars-sinai.org/health-library/diseases-and-conditions/r/rheumatoid-vasculitis.html

105 Esdaile *et al.* Traditional Framingham risk factors fail to fully account for accelerated atherosclerosis in systemic lupus erythematosus. Arthritis Rheum. 2001. https://www.ncbi.nlm.nih.gov/pubmed/11665973

106 Edwards *et al.* Endothelial Progenitor Cells: New Targets for Therapeutics for Inflammatory Conditions With High Cardiovascular Risk. Front. Med. 2018. https://www.frontiersin.org/articles/10.3389/fmed.2018.00200/full

107 Emmi *et al.* Thrombosis in vasculitis: from pathogenesis to treatment. Thromb J. 2015. https://www.ncbi.nlm.nih.gov/pmc/articles/PMC4399148/

108 Dhar & Sokol. Thrombophilia in Systemic Lupus Erythematosus: A Review of Multiple Mechanisms and Resultant Clinical Outcomes. Open access peer-reviewed chapter. September 19, 2013. https://www.intechopen.com/books/pregnancy-thrombophilia-the-unsuspected-risk/thrombophilia-in-systemic-lupus-erythematosus-a-review-of-multiple-mechanisms-and-resultant-clinical

109 Stojan & Petri. Atherosclerosis in Systemic Lupus Erythematosus. J Cardiovasc Pharmacol. 2013. https://www.ncbi.nlm.nih.gov/pmc/articles/PMC4406345/

110 American College of Rheumatology. Antiphospholipid Syndrome. Fast Facts. March 2019. https://www.rheumatology.org/I-Am-A/Patient-Caregiver/Diseases-Conditions/Antiphospholipid-Syndrome

111 Kathryn Watson. All About Antiphospholipid Syndrome (Hughes Syndrome). Healthline. August 31, 2018. https://www.healthline.com/health/hughes-syndrome

112 Kim & Park. Acute and Chronic Effects of Cocaine on Cardiovascular Health. Int J Mol Sci. 2019. https://www.ncbi.nlm.nih.gov/pmc/articles/PMC6387265/

113 Bachi *et al.* Vascular disease in cocaine addiction. Atherosclerosis. 2017. https://www.ncbi.nlm.nih.gov/pmc/articles/PMC5757372/

114 Talarico *et al.* Cocaine and coronary artery diseases: a systematic review of the literature. J Cardiovasc Med (Hagerstown). 2017. https://www.ncbi.nlm.nih.gov/pubmed/28306693

115 Holzer *et al.* Cerebral vasculitis mimicking migraine with aura in a patient with Crohn's disease. Acta Neurol Belg. 2009. https://www.ncbi.nlm.nih.gov/pubmed/19402574

116 Dr Stojan. How Lupus affects the body. John Hopkins Lupus Center. https://www.hopkinslupus.org/lupus-info/lupus-affects-body/lupus-nervous-system/

117 Mohammad Hassan A Noureldine *et al.* Antiphospholipid syndrome (APS) revisited: Would migraine headaches be included in future classification criteria? Immunol Res. 2017. https://www.ncbi.nlm.nih.gov/pubmed/27423434

118 Conference coverage. Why the Eye Should Be a Focus When Treating Migraine. Neurology Reviews. 2016. https://www.mdedge.com/neurology/article/114974/headache-migraine/why-eye-should-be-focus-when-treating-migraine

119 Adelborg *et al.* Migraine and risk of cardiovascular diseases: Danish population based matched cohort study. BMJ. 2018. https://www.bmj.com/content/360/bmj.k96

120 Platt *et al.* Mortality In Sickle Cell Disease – Life Expectancy and Risk Factors for Early Death. NEMJ. 1994. https://www.nejm.org/doi/full/10.1056/NEJM199406093302303

121 Elsharawy & Moghazy. Peripheral Arterial Lesions in Patient with Sickle Cell Disease. European Journal of Vascular and Endovascular Surgery. 2007. https://www.sciencedirect.com/science/article/pii/S1533316707000192

122 Elsharawy & Moghazy. Peripheral Arterial Lesions in Patient with Sickle Cell Disease. European Journal of Vascular and Endovascular Surgery. 2007. https://www.sciencedirect.com/science/article/pii/S1533316707000192

123 Dinc *et al.* Effects of intravitreal injection of bevacizumab on nitric oxide levels. Eye. 2014. https://www.nature.com/articles/eye2014297

124 Totzeck *et al.* Cardiovascular Adverse Events in Patients With Cancer Treated With Bevacizumab: A Meta-Analysis of More Than 20 000 Patients. Journal of the American Heart Association. 2017. https://www.ahajournals.org/doi/10.1161/JAHA.117.006278

125 Yale University. Stress May Cause Excess Abdominal Fat In Otherwise Slender Women, Study Conducted At Yale Shows. Science Daily. November 23rd, 2000. https://www.sciencedaily.com/releases/2000/11/001120072314.htm

126 National Institute of Diabetes and Digestive and Kidney Diseases. Health Information. Cushing's Syndrome. https://www.niddk.nih.gov/health-information/endocrine-diseases/cushings-syndrome

127 Kelly *et al.* Cortisol and hypertension. Clin Exp Pharmacol Physiol Suppl. 1998. https://www.ncbi.nlm.nih.gov/pubmed/9809193

128 Alice Melao. Arterial Blood Clots May Be First Sign of Cushing's Syndrome, Case Report Shows. Cushing's Disease News. March 12th 2019. https://cushingsdiseasenews.com/2019/03/12/arterial-blood-clots-first-sign-cushings-syndrome-case-report/

129 Jane E. Brody. Steroids' Miracle Comes With a Caveat. NY Times. Nov. 9, 2009. https://www.nytimes.com/2009/11/10/health/10brod.html

130 Etxabe & Vazquez. Morbidity and mortality in Cushing's disease: an epidemiological approach. Clin Endocrinol (Oxf). 1994. https://www.ncbi.nlm.nih.gov/pubmed/8187313

131 Fardet. Risk of cardiovascular events in people prescribed glucocorticoids with iatrogenic Cushing's syndrome: cohort study. BMJ. 2012. https://www.bmj.com/content/345/bmj.e4928

132 Keller *et al.* HPA Axis in Major Depression: Cortisol, Clinical Symptomatology, and Genetic Variation Predict Cognition. Mol Psychiatry. 2017. https://www.ncbi.nlm.nih.gov/pmc/articles/PMC5313380/

133 Joseph & Golden. Cortisol dysregulation: the bidirectional link between stress, depression, and type 2 diabetes mellitus. Ann N Y Acad Sci. 2017. https://www.ncbi.nlm.nih.gov/pmc/articles/PMC5334212/

134 Brown. Atypical Antipsychotics and Insulin Resistance in Acute Mental Illness: A Case Series. Prim Care Companion CNS Disord. 2011. https://www.ncbi.nlm.nih.gov/pmc/articles/PMC3121200/

135 Ana Sandoiu. Heart disease and depression: Scientists find missing link. Medical News Today. March 19 2019. https://www.medicalnewstoday.com/articles/324748

136 Borges *et al.* A systematic review of the activity of the hypothalamic–pituitary–adrenal axis in first episode psychosis. Psychoneuroendocrinology. Volume 38, Issue 5, May 2013. https://www.sciencedirect.com/science/article/pii/S0306453013000048

137 Hennekens *et al.* Schizophrenia and increased risks of cardiovascular disease. Am Heart J. 2005. https://www.ncbi.nlm.nih.gov/pubmed/16338246

138 Newcomer. Metabolic Syndrome and Mental Illness. AJMC. 2007. https://www.ajmc.com/journals/supplement/2007/2007-11-vol13-n7suppl/nov07-2657ps170-s177

139 Calkin *et al.* The relationship between bipolar disorder and type 2 diabetes: more than just co-morbid disorders. Ann Med. 2013. https://www.ncbi.nlm.nih.gov/pubmed/22621171

140 Ana Starcevic. Structural Brain Changes in PTSD. Open Access Peer-reviewed chapter. November 2nd 2016. https://www.intechopen.com/books/a-multidimensional-approach-to-post-traumatic-stress-disorder-from-theory-to-practice/structural-brain-changes-in-ptsd

141 Klaassens. Bouncing back – trauma and the HPA-axis in healthy adults. Eur J Psychotraumatol. 2010. https://www.ncbi.nlm.nih.gov/pmc/articles/PMC3402002/

142 Lauren Biscaldi. Insulin Resistance, Biological Markers of PTSD Increased in Military Veterans. Psychiatry Advisor. July 13, 2017. https://www.psychiatryadvisor.com/home/topics/anxiety/ptsd-trauma-and-stressor-related/insulin-resistance-biological-markers-of-ptsd-increased-in-military-veterans/

143 Paul L. Huang. A comprehensive definition for metabolic syndrome. Dis Model Mech. 2009. https://www.ncbi.nlm.nih.gov/pmc/articles/PMC2675814/

144 Why does PTSD increase the risk of cardiovascular disease? American Physiological Society (APS). July 15, 2015. https://www.sciencedaily.com/releases/2015/07/150715091252.htm

145 UK NHS Information page. Causes – Bipolar disorder. https://www.nhs.uk/conditions/bipolar-disorder/causes/

146 Kathleen Davis. What is Takotsubo cardiomyopathy? Medical News Today. June 28, 2018. https://www.medicalnewstoday.com/articles/309547

147 Dalia *et al.* A Rare Case of Sudden Death in a Patient with Takotsubo Cardiomyopathy Secondary to Cardiac Rupture. Case reports in cardiology. Volume 2019. https://www.hindawi.com/journals/cric/2019/5404365/

148 Mayo Clinic information page. Fibromyalgia. Overview. https://www.mayoclinic.org/diseases-conditions/fibromyalgia/symptoms-causes/syc-20354780

149 Tsai *et al.* Fibromyalgia is associated with coronary heart disease: a population-based cohort study. Reg Anesth Pain Med. Jan-Feb 2015. https://pubmed.ncbi.nlm.nih.gov/25436616/

150 Crises in the Post-Soviet Space From the dissolution of the Soviet Union to the conflict in Ukraine. Edited by Felix Jaitner, Tina Olteanu, Tobias Spöri. ISBN 9780815377245. June 2018.

151 Kristenson *et al.* The LiVcordia Study : Possible causes for the differences in coronary heart disease mortality between Lithuania and Sweden. Dissertation. 1998. https://www.dissertations.se/dissertation/b4d35c6583/

152 Per Bjorntorp. Visceral Obesity: A "Civilization Syndrome." Obesity Research. May 1993. https://onlinelibrary.wiley.com/doi/pdf/10.1002/j.1550-8528.1993.tb00614.x

153 Björntorp & Rosmond. Neuroendocrine abnormalities in visceral obesity. International Journal of Obesity. July 2000. https://www.nature.com/articles/0801285

154 James Ciment. Life expectancy of Russian men falls to 58. BMJ. 1999. https://www.ncbi.nlm.nih.gov/pmc/articles/PMC1116380/

155 Ben Aris. Remembering Russia's 1998 Financial Crisis (Op-ed). The Moscow Times. Aug. 2018. https://www.themoscowtimes.com/2018/08/22/remembering-russias-1998-financial-crash-op-ed-a62595

156 Ana Sandoiu. Financial worries may raise heart attack risk by 13-fold. Medical News Today. November 2017. https://www.medicalnewstoday.com/articles/320037.php

157 Marmot & Elliott. Coronary heart disease epidemiology. From aetiology to public health. Second edition. Oxford University Press. 2005. ISBN 0198525737.

158 Brainerd & Cutler. Autopsy on an Empire: Understanding Mortality in Russia and the Former Soviet Union. Institute for the Study of Labor. January 2005. http://ftp.iza.org/dp1472.pdf

159 World health rankings. https://www.worldlifeexpectancy.com/cause-of-death/coronary-heart-disease/by-country/male

160 NITV. Indigenous life expectancy 'worst in world.' United Nations report. February 1, 2017. http://www.sbs.com.au/nitv/article/2010/01/15/indigenous-life-expectancy-worst-world

161 James Cook University Australia. Media Release. Stress hormones underlie Indigenous health gap in Australia. 2 Feb 2017. https://www.jcu.edu.au/news/releases/2017/february/stress-hormones-underlie-indigenous-health-gap-in-australia

162 MyDr. Diabetes and Indigenous Australians. Tonic Media Network. June 28 2018. https://www.mydr.com.au/diabetes/diabetes-in-indigenous-australians

163 Wang & Hoy. Is the Framingham coronary heart disease absolute risk function applicable to Aboriginal people? Med J Aust. 2005. https://pubmed.ncbi.nlm.nih.gov/15651963/?dopt=Abstract

164 Australian Government. Australian Institute of Health and Welfare. Cardiovascular disease, diabetes and chronic kidney disease – Australian acts: Aboriginal and Torres Strait Islander people. Media Release. 25 Nov 2015. https://www.aihw.gov.au/reports/heart-stroke-vascular-disease/cardiovascular-diabetes-chronic-kidney-indigenous/summary

165 Dr Rock Positano, Health Columnist for the New York Daily News. The Mystery of the Rosetan People. HuffPost Contributor platform. 28 March 2008. https://www.huffingtonpost.com/dr-rock-positano/the-mystery-of-the-roseta_b_73260.html

166 Jin et al. A Chinese Immigrant Paradox? Low Coronary Heart Disease Incidence but Higher Short-Term Mortality in Western-Dwelling Chinese Immigrants: A Systematic Review and Meta-Analysis. J Am Heart Assoc. 2015. https://www.ncbi.nlm.nih.gov/pmc/articles/PMC4845291

167 Nair & Prabhakaran. Why Do South Asians Have High Risk for CAD? Global Heart. Volume 7, Issue 4, December 2012. https://www.sciencedirect.com/science/article/pii/S2211816012001573

168 Enas et al. Coronary heart disease and its risk factors in first-generation immigrant Asian Indians to the United States of America. Indian Heart J. Jul-Aug 1996. https://pubmed.ncbi.nlm.nih.gov/8908818/

169 Williams et al. Subgroup differences in psychosocial factors relating to coronary heart disease in the UK South Asian population. J Psychosom Res. 2010. https://www.ncbi.nlm.nih.gov/pmc/articles/PMC2946562/

170 Heart disease death rates 2017-2019 adults ages 35+ by county. US Centers for Disease Control and prevention. Content source: National Center for Chronic Disease Prevention and Health Promotion, Division for Heart Disease and Stroke Prevention. Last reviewed May 3rd, 2021.
https://www.cdc.gov/dhdsp/maps/national_maps/hd_all.htm

171 British Heart Foundation (BHF) (2021) UK Factsheet. The original reference is BHF/ University of Birmingham calculated rates in partnership with UK statistical agencies:
ONS/NRS/NISRA (2016-18 data). Reproduced with kind permission from, and a donation to, the BHF.

172 Malcolm Gladwell. Outliers. The New York Times. November 28, 2008. https://www.nytimes.com/2008/11/30/books/chapters/chapter-outliers.html

173 Iba *et al*. Coagulopathy in COVID-19. Journal of Thrombosis and Haemostasis. 18 June 2020. https://onlinelibrary.wiley.com/doi/abs/10.1111/jth.14975

174 Rachael Rettner. Mysterious inflammatory syndrome tied to COVID-19 is showing up in adults in their early 20s. Live Science. May 2020. https://www.livescience.com/covid-19-inflammatory-syndrome-mis-c-young-adults.html

175 Cheng *et al*. Cardiovascular Risks in Patients with COVID-19: Potential Mechanisms and Areas of Uncertainty. Curr Cardiol Rep. 2020. https://www.ncbi.nlm.nih.gov/pmc/articles/PMC7189178/

176 Kwong *et al*. Acute Myocardial Infarction after Laboratory-Confirmed Influenza Infection. N Engl J Med 2018. https://www.nejm.org/doi/full/10.1056/NEJMoa1702090

177 Grandel & Grimminger. Endothelial responses to bacterial toxins in sepsis. Crit Rev Immunol. 2003. https://pubmed.ncbi.nlm.nih.gov/14700271/

178 Fisher *et al*. Periodontal disease as a risk marker in coronary heart disease and chronic kidney disease. Curr Opin Nephrol Hypertens. 2010. https://www.ncbi.nlm.nih.gov/pmc/articles/PMC3084591/

179 Lertpimonchai *et al*. Periodontitis as the risk factor of chronic kidney disease: Mediation analysis. J Clin Periodontol. 2019. https://www.ncbi.nlm.nih.gov/pmc/articles/PMC6593715/

180 Varki *et al*. Heart disease is common in humans and chimpanzees, but is caused by different pathological processes. Evol Appl. 2009. https://www.ncbi.nlm.nih.gov/pmc/articles/PMC3352420/

181 Arbustini *et al*. Plaque composition in plexogenic and thromboembolic pulmonary hypertension: the critical role of thrombotic material in pultaceous core formation. Heart. 2002. https://www.ncbi.nlm.nih.gov/pmc/articles/PMC1767204/

182 O'Neal & Thomas. The Role of Pulmonary Hypertension and Thromboembolism in the Production of Pulmonary Arteriosclerosis. Circulation, Volume XII, September, 1955. https://www.ahajournals.org/doi/pdf/10.1161/01.CIR.12.3.370

183 Kristensen *et al*. The effect of statins on average survival in randomised trials, an analysis of end point postponement. BMJ Open. May 2015. https://bmjopen.bmj.com/content/5/9/e007118

184 American College of Cardiology. ASCVD Risk Estimator Plus. http://tools.acc.org/ASCVD-Risk-Estimator-Plus/#!/calculate/estimate/

185 QRISK 3-208 risk calculator. https://qrisk.org/three/index.php

186 NIHR. Leicester Biomedical Research Centre. Ten minutes of walking per day may increase life by three years. July 30 2019. https://www.leicesterbrc.nihr.ac.uk/ten-minutes-of-walking-per-day-may-increase-life-by-three-years/

187 Centers for Disease Control and Prevention. Data and Statistics. Fast Facts and Fact Sheets. Tobacco-Related Mortality. https://www.cdc.gov/tobacco/data_statistics/fact_sheets/health_effects/tobacco_related_mortality/index.htm

188 Orpana *et al*. BMI and mortality: results from a national longitudinal study of Canadian adults. Obesity (Silver Spring). 2010. https://pubmed.ncbi.nlm.nih.gov/19543208/

189 Diabetes.co.uk editor. Diabetes Life Expectancy. 15th January 2019. https://www.diabetes.co.uk/diabetes-life-expectancy.html

190 American Heart Association. Short bursts of high-intensity exercise does more for type 2 diabetes. Science Daily. November 10, 2015. https://www.sciencedaily.com/releases/2015/11/151110093914.htm

191 Diabetes.co.uk editor. Pensioner sends type 2 diabetes into remission with 12-minute workouts. 26th March 2014. https://www.diabetes.co.uk/news/2014/mar/pensioner-sends-type-2-diabetes-into-remission-with-12-minute-workouts-91295470.html

192 Berne. Insulin resistance in hypertension--a relationship with consequences? J Intern Med Suppl. 1991. https://pubmed.ncbi.nlm.nih.gov/2043224/

193 Ozeki et al. Relationship of High-intensity Training and Body Mass Index in Japanese Students. Clinical Journal of Nutrition and Dietetics. Volume 1, Issue 1, 2018. https://asclepiusopen.com/clinical-journal-of-nutrition-and-dietetics/volume-1-issue-1/3.php

194 Akinci et al. Lipodystrophy Syndromes: Presentation and Treatment. Book. April 24, 2018. https://www.ncbi.nlm.nih.gov/books/NBK513130/

195 Jehl et al. Acquired Generalized Lipodystrophy: A New Cause of Anti-PD-1 Immune-Related Diabetes. Diabetes Care. 2019. https://care.diabetesjournals.org/content/42/10/2008

196 McGinnis et al. Biofeedback-Assisted Relaxation in Type 2 Diabetes. Diabetes Care. 2005. https://care.diabetesjournals.org/content/28/9/2145

197 Shelley Wood. Yoga Works for BP Lowering in Cardiac Rehab. Just Don't Call It "Yoga". Report from EuroPRevent conference Prague. Medscape. May 12, 2010. https://www.medscape.com/viewarticle/721720

198 Bornemann et al. Voluntary upregulation of heart rate variability through biofeedback is improved by mental contemplative training. Scientific Reports volume 9, Article number: 7860 (2019). https://www.nature.com/articles/s41598-019-44201-7

199 Eichstaedt et al. Psychological Language on Twitter Predicts County-Level Heart Disease Mortality. Psychol Sci. 2015. https://www.ncbi.nlm.nih.gov/pmc/articles/PMC4433545/

Reproduced with kind permission from, and license paid to, SAGE publications.

200 Burnett et al. Global estimates of mortality associated with long-term exposure to outdoor fine particulate matter. PNAS September 18, 2018. https://www.pnas.org/content/115/38/9592

201 Comini et al. Therapeutic modulation of the nitric oxide: all ace inhibitors are not equivalent. Pharmacol Res. 2007. https://pubmed.ncbi.nlm.nih.gov/17475504/

202 Dimmeler et al. Angiotensin II Induces Apoptosis of Human Endothelial Cells. Protective Effect of Nitric Oxide. Circulation Research. 1997. https://www.ahajournals.org/doi/full/10.1161/01.RES.81.6.970

203 Adler et al. Reduced dietary salt for the prevention of cardiovascular disease. Cochrane Database of Systematic Reviews. 18 December 2014. https://www.cochranelibrary.com/cdsr/doi/10.1002/14651858.CD009217.pub3/full?cookiesEnabled

204 Kotliar *et al.* Lack of RAAS inhibition by high-salt intake is associated with arterial stiffness in hypertensive patients. Journal of the Renin-Angiotensin-Aldosterone System. 2014. https://journals.sagepub.com/doi/full/10.1177/1470320313503692

205 Fels *et al.* Ménage à trois: Aldosterone, sodium and nitric oxide in vascular endothelium. Biochimica et Biophysica Acta (BBA) – Molecular Basis of Disease. Volume 1802, Issue 12, December 2010. https://www.sciencedirect.com/science/article/pii/S0925443910000657

206 Tikellis *et al.* Activation of the Renin-Angiotensin System Mediates the Effects of Dietary Salt Intake on Atherogenesis in the Apolipoprotein E Knockout Mouse. Hypertension. 2012. https://www.ahajournals.org/doi/full/10.1161/hypertensionaha.112.191767

207 Cohen *et al.* Sodium intake and mortality in the NHANES II follow-up study. Am J Med. 2006. https://pubmed.ncbi.nlm.nih.gov/16490476/

208 Harvard Health Publishing. Potassium and sodium out of balance. April 03, 2019. https://www.health.harvard.edu/staying-healthy/potassium_and_sodium_out_of_balance

209 Harvard Health Publishing. Potassium lowers blood pressure. January 23, 2017. https://www.health.harvard.edu/heart-health/potassium-lowers-blood-pressure

210 Tunstall-Pedoe *et al.* Comparison of the prediction by 27 different factors of coronary heart disease and death in men and women of the Scottish heart health study: cohort study. BMJ. 1997. https://www.bmj.com/content/315/7110/722

211 McCallum *et al.* Serum Chloride Is an Independent Predictor of Mortality in Hypertensive Patients. Hypertension. 2013. https://www.ahajournals.org/doi/pdf/10.1161/HYPERTENSIONAHA.113.01793

212 Sukhovershin & Cooke. How may proton pump inhibitors impair cardiovascular health? Am J Cardiovasc Drugs. 2016. https://www.ncbi.nlm.nih.gov/pmc/articles/PMC4864131/

213 Shah *et al.* Proton Pump Inhibitor Usage and the Risk of Myocardial Infarction in the General Population. PLoS ONE. 2015. https://pubmed.ncbi.nlm.nih.gov/26061035/

214 Platt *et al.* Type II diabetes mellitus and hyperhomocysteinemia: a complex interaction. Diabetol Metab Syndr. 2017. https://www.ncbi.nlm.nih.gov/pmc/articles/PMC5359933/

215 Jeanie Lerche Davis. Elderly Dementia Linked to Homocysteine Vitamin Deficiency, Too Little Exercise Raise Alzheimer's Risk. WebMD. February 28 2003. https://www.webmd.com/alzheimers/news/20030228/elderly-dementia-linked-to-homocysteine

216 Hemati *et al.* High plasma homocysteine and insulin resistance in patients with polycystic ovarian syndrome. Iran J Reprod Med. 2011. https://www.ncbi.nlm.nih.gov/pmc/articles/PMC4575758/

217 Nguyen *et al.* Type 3 Diabetes and Its Role Implications in Alzheimer's Disease. Int J Mol Sci. 2020. https://www.ncbi.nlm.nih.gov/pmc/articles/PMC7246646/

218 Jeanie Lerche Davis. Elderly Dementia Linked to Homocysteine Vitamin Deficiency, Too Little Exercise Raise Alzheimer's Risk. WebMD. February 28 2003. https://www.webmd.com/alzheimers/news/20030228/elderly-dementia-linked-to-homocysteine

219 The Heart Outcomes Prevention Evaluation (HOPE) 2 Investigators. Homocysteine Lowering with Folic Acid and B Vitamins in Vascular Disease. NEMJ. 2006. https://www.nejm.org/doi/full/10.1056/nejmoa060900

220 Douaud *et al.* Preventing Alzheimer's disease-related gray matter atrophy by B-vitamin treatment. Proc Natl Acad Sci U S A. 2013. https://www.ncbi.nlm.nih.gov/pmc/articles/PMC3677457/

221 Douaud *et al.* Preventing Alzheimer's disease-related gray matter atrophy by B-vitamin treatment. Proc Natl Acad Sci U S A. 2013. https://www.ncbi.nlm.nih.gov/pmc/articles/PMC3677457/

222 Clarke et al. Effects of homocysteine lowering with B vitamins on cognitive aging: meta-analysis of 11 trials with cognitive data on 22,000 individuals. AJCN. 2014. https://academic.oup.com/ajcn/article/100/2/657/4576556

223 Alzheimer's Research UK. In the news: B vitamins and Alzheimer's disease. Blog. 13 October 2014. https://www.alzheimersresearchuk.org/blog/b-vitamins-andalzheimers-disease/

224 University of Oxford. Taking B vitamins won't prevent Alzheimer's disease. 15 July 2014 https://www.ox.ac.uk/news/2014-07-15-taking-b-vitamins-won't-prevent-alzheimer's-disease

225 University of Oxford. Many mental illnesses reduce life expectancy more than heavy smoking. 25 May 2014. https://www.ox.ac.uk/news/2014-05-23-manymental-illnesses-reduce-life-expectancy-more-heavy-smoking

226 Science Norway. June 7 2019. https://sciencenorway.no/disease-forskningno-mentalhealth/why-do-schizophrenia-patients-die-earlier-than-other-people/1554587

227 Aldecoa *et al.* Role of albumin in the preservation of endothelial glycocalyx integrity and the microcirculation: a review. Ann Intensive Care. 2020. https://www.ncbi.nlm.nih.gov/pmc/articles/PMC7310051/

228 Aldecoa *et al.* Role of albumin in the preservation of endothelial glycocalyx integrity and the microcirculation: a review. Ann Intensive Care. 2020. https://www.ncbi.nlm.nih.gov/pmc/articles/PMC7310051/

229 Ronit *et al.* Plasma Albumin and Incident Cardiovascular Disease. Arteriosclerosis, Thrombosis, and Vascular Biology. 2020. https://www.ahajournals.org/doi/10.1161/ATVBAHA.119.313681

230 Ma *et al.* Association of habitual glucosamine use with risk of cardiovascular disease: prospective study in UK Biobank. BMJ 2019. https://www.bmj.com/content/365/bmj.l1628

231 Melgar-Lesmes *et al.* Treatment with chondroitin sulfate to modulate inflammation and atherogenesis in obesity. Atherosclerosis. 2016. https://www.ncbi.nlm.nih.gov/pmc/articles/PMC4738029/

232 Fonseca & Mourão. Fucosylated chondroitin sulfate as a new oral antithrombotic agent. Thromb Haemost. 2006. https://pubmed.ncbi.nlm.nih.gov/17139379/

233 Teas *et al.* Walking Outside Improves Mood for Healthy Postmenopausal Women. Clinical Medicine: Oncology. 2007. https://journals.sagepub.com/doi/10.4137/CMO.S343

234 Kent *et al.* Effect of sunlight exposure on cognitive function among depressed and non-depressed participants: a REGARDS cross-sectional study. Environ Health. 2009. https://www.ncbi.nlm.nih.gov/pmc/articles/PMC2728098/

235 Budhathoki *et al.* Plasma 25-hydroxyvitamin D concentration and subsequent risk of total and site specific cancers in Japanese population: large case-cohort study within Japan Public Health Center-based Prospective Study cohort. BMJ. 2018. https://www.bmj.com/content/360/bmj.k671

236 Judd & Tangpricha. Vitamin D Deficiency and Risk for Cardiovascular Disease. Am J Med Sci. 2009. https://www.ncbi.nlm.nih.gov/pmc/articles/PMC2851242/

237 Halliday & Byrne. An Unexpected Role: UVA-Induced Release of Nitric Oxide from Skin May Have Unexpected Health Benefits. Journal of Investigative Dermatology. 2014. https://www.sciencedirect.com/science/article/pii/S0022202X15368974

238 Wang *et al.* Nitric Oxide Directly Promotes Vascular Endothelial Insulin Transport. Diabetes. 2013. https://diabetes.diabetesjournals.org/content/62/12/4030

239 Lindqvist *et al.* Avoidance of sun exposure as a risk factor for major causes of death: a competing risk analysis of the Melanoma in Southern Sweden cohort. J Intern Med. 2016. https://pubmed.ncbi.nlm.nih.gov/26992108/

240 Levell *et al.* Melanoma epidemic: a midsummer night's dream? Br J Dermatol. 2009. https://pubmed.ncbi.nlm.nih.gov/19519827/

241 Chandler *et al.* Effect of Vitamin D3 Supplements on Development of Advanced Cancer A Secondary Analysis of the VITAL Randomized Clinical Trial. JAMA. 2020. https://jamanetwork.com/journals/jamanetworkopen/fullarticle/2773074

242 Dunn & Grider. Physiology, Adenosine Triphosphate. StatPearls [Internet]. February 27, 2021. https://www.ncbi.nlm.nih.gov/books/NBK553175/

243 Marcoff & Thompson. The Role of Coenzyme Q10 in Statin-Associated Myopathy: A Systematic Review. Journal of the American College of Cardiology. 2007. https://www.sciencedirect.com/science/article/pii/S0735109707010546

244 Rasmusen *et al.* Arginine and statins: relationship between the nitric oxide pathway and the atherosclerosis development.Ann Biol Clin (Paris). Sep-Oct 2005. https://pubmed.ncbi.nlm.nih.gov/16230278/

245 Anderson *et al.* Phosphodiesterase type-5 inhibitor use in type 2 diabetes is associated with a reduction in all-cause mortality. BMJ Heart. 2016. https://heart.bmj.com/content/102/21/1750.full

246 Making evidence appraisal easy for clinicians. HPS – Statins in secondary prevention & patients with diabetes. 2016. https://nerdcat.org/studysummaries/hps

247 Lundberg. Nitric oxide and the paranasal sinuses. Anat Rec (Hoboken). 2008. https://pubmed.ncbi.nlm.nih.gov/18951492/

248 Medical City Healthcare. How to Have a Healthier Heart Just by Breathing. Blog. January 19, 2021. https://medicalcityhealthcare.com/blog/entry/healthier-heart-breathing

249 Kannel *et al.* Update on fibrinogen as a cardiovascular risk factor. Ann Epidemiol. 1992. https://pubmed.ncbi.nlm.nih.gov/1342296/

250 Seaman *et al.* Does deficiency of von Willebrand factor protect against cardiovascular disease? Analysis of a national discharge register. J Thromb Haemost. 2015. https://pubmed.ncbi.nlm.nih.gov/26368360/

251 Morange *et al.* Endothelial Cell Markers and the Risk of Coronary Heart Disease The Prospective Epidemiological Study of Myocardial Infarction (PRIME) Study. Circulation. 2004. https://www.ahajournals.org/doi/full/10.1161/01.CIR.0000120705.55512.EC

252 Wachira *et al.* n-3 Fatty acids affect haemostasis but do not increase the risk of bleeding: clinical observations and mechanistic insights. Br J Nutr. 2014. https://pubmed.ncbi.nlm.nih.gov/24472372/

253 Kopytina & Cherkesov. Clinical and functional features of the development of myocardial infarction in miners engaged in deep coal mines. Ter Arkh. 1989. https://pubmed.ncbi.nlm.nih.gov/2718115/

254 Harvard Health Publishing. Protect your heart when shoveling snow. January 15, 2011. https://www.health.harvard.edu/blog/protect-your-heart-when-shoveling-snow-201101151153

255 Känel. Acute mental stress and hemostatis: When physiology becomes vascular harm. Thromb Res. 2015. https://www.ncbi.nlm.nih.gov/pmc/articles/PMC4386736/

256 Science quotes by John Hunter. (1728-1793). Today in Science History. https://todayinsci.com/H/Hunter_John/HunterJohn-Quotations.htm

257 Fanelli *et al.* Cardiovascular and cerebrovascular risk with nonsteroidal anti-inflammatory drugs and cyclooxygenase 2 inhibitors: latest evidence and clinical implications. Ther Adv Drug Saf. 2017. https://www.ncbi.nlm.nih.gov/pmc/articles/PMC5455842/

258 Union of concerned scientists. Merck Manipulated the Science about the Drug Vioxx. Case study. Oct 12, 2017. https://www.ucsusa.org/resources/merck-manipulated-science-about-drug-vioxx

259 Enas *et al.* Lipoprotein(a): An independent, genetic, and causal factor for cardiovascular disease and acute myocardial infarction. Indian Heart Journal. March–April 2019. https://www.sciencedirect.com/science/article/pii/S0019483218312781

260 Scholl. Does a ketogenic diet lower a very high Lp(a)? A striking experiment in a male physician. BMJ Nutrition, Prevention & Health. 2020. https://nutrition.bmj.com/content/bmjnph/early/2020/11/19/bmjnph-2020-000189.full.pdf

261 Wood *et al.* Effects of a carbohydrate-restricted diet on emerging plasma markers for cardiovascular disease. Nutrition & Metabolism. 2006. https://nutritionandmetabolism.biomedcentral.com/articles/10.1186/1743-7075-3-19

262 Boffa & Koschinsky. A Role for Pharmacogenetics? Circulation: Genomic and Precision Medicine. 2018. https://www.ahajournals.org/doi/10.1161/CIRCGEN.118.002052

263 Saeed & Virani. Lipoprotein(a) and cardiovascular disease: current state and future directions for an enigmatic lipoprotein. Frontiers In Bioscience, Landmark, 23, 1099-1112, January 2018. https://www.bioscience.org/2018/v23/af/4635/2.htm

264 Khan. Antiphospholipid syndrome is an important modifiable risk factor of stroke in the young. Ann Indian Acad Neurol. 2015. https://www.ncbi.nlm.nih.gov/pmc/articles/PMC4564481/

265 Rodziewicz *et al.* The epidemiology of antiphospholipid syndrome in the UK, 1990-2016. Rheumatology. 2019. https://academic.oup.com/rheumatology/article/58/Supplement_3/kez105.029/5444495

266 NHS Diagnosis. Antiphospholipid syndrome (APS). August 2018. https://www.nhs.uk/conditions/antiphospholipid-syndrome/diagnosis/

267 Shlezinger *et al.* Association between exposure to desalinated sea water and ischemic heart disease, diabetes mellitus and colorectal cancer; A population-based

study in Israel. Environmental Research. 2018. http://www.mgwater.com/files/Shlezinger%20Environmenntal%20Research%20July%202018.pdf

268 Judy Siegel-Itzkovich. 4,000 Israelis die annually due to lack of magnesium. The Jerusalem Post. January 21, 2017. https://www.jpost.com/business-and-innovation/health-and-science/4000-israelis-die-annually-due-to-lack-of-magnesium-479184

269 Khan *et al.* Low serum magnesium and the development of atrial fibrillation in the community: the Framingham Heart Study. Circulation. 2013. https://pubmed.ncbi.nlm.nih.gov/23172839/

270 DiNicolantonio *et al.* Subclinical magnesium deficiency: a principal driver of cardiovascular disease and a public health crisis. Open Heart. 2018. https://www.ncbi.nlm.nih.gov/pmc/articles/PMC5786912/

271 DiNicolantonio *et al.* Magnesium for the prevention and treatment of cardiovascular disease. Open Heart. 2018. https://openheart.bmj.com/content/openhrt/5/2/e000775.full.pdf

272 Carr & Maggini. Vitamin C and Immune Function. Nutrients. 2017. https://www.ncbi.nlm.nih.gov/pmc/articles/PMC5707683/

273 DiNicolantonio *et al.* Thiamine supplementation for the treatment of heart failure: a review of the literature. Congest Heart Fail. Jul-Aug 2013. https://pubmed.ncbi.nlm.nih.gov/23910704/

274 Mayo Clinic. Lead Poisoning. Diagnosis. https://www.mayoclinic.org/diseases-conditions/lead-poisoning/diagnosis-treatment/drc-20354723

275 Peguero *et al.* Chelation therapy and cardiovascular disease: Connecting scientific silos to benefit cardiac patients. Trends in Cardiovascular Medicine. 2014. https://www.sciencedirect.com/science/article/pii/S1050173814000486

276 Atwood *et al.* Why the NIH Trial to Assess Chelation Therapy (TACT) Should Be Abandoned. Medscape J Med. 2008. https://www.medscape.com/viewarticle/570625

277 Larry Husten. NIH Trial Gives Surprising Boost To Chelation Therapy. Forbes. Nov 4, 2012. https://www.forbes.com/sites/larryhusten/2012/11/04/nih-trial-gives-surprising-boost-to-chelation-therapy/?sh=3d771e384c91

278 Kumbhani. The Trial to Assess Chelation Therapy – TACT. American College of Cardiology. July 30, 2014. https://www.acc.org/latest-in-cardiology/clinical-trials/2014/07/30/10/56/tact

279 Sharma *et al.* The Role of Enhanced External Counter Pulsation Therapy in Clinical Practice. Clin Med Res. 2013. https://www.ncbi.nlm.nih.gov/pmc/articles/PMC3917995/

280 Weng *et al.* Can machine-learning improve cardiovascular risk prediction using routine clinical data? PLoS ONE. 2017. https://journals.plos.org/plosone/article?id=10.1371/journal.pone.0174944

INDEX

323

About the author

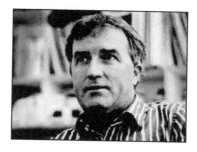

Dr Malcolm Kendrick graduated from medical school in Aberdeen and trained as a General Practitioner in Scotland. After ten years he split his time between General Practice and education. On the doctor side, Malcolm currently lives and works in Cheshire in General Practice, Intermediate Care and Out of Hours. On the education side, Malcolm set up the on-line educational system for the European Society of Cardiology, working with the European Commission and also set up the first website for the National Institute for Clinical Excellence (NICE) in the UK.

Malcolm is an early member of the Centre for Evidence Based Medicine (CEBM) in Oxford and of The International Network of Cholesterol Sceptics (THINCS). The latter comprises a group of scientists, doctors and researchers who share the belief that cholesterol does not cause cardiovascular disease.

This is the field of medicine for which Malcolm is best known. His long-term interest in the epidemiology of cardiovascular disease has resulted in many publications in journals such as the BMJ, Medical Hypotheses, Pulse and PharmacoEconomics. His breadth and depth of expertise in this area led to his election to Who's Who in 2009.

The Great Cholesterol Con was the book that firmly placed Malcolm on the world stage of the 'diet-cholesterol-heart' hypothesis and his army of followers are eagerly awaiting his next bout of wit and wisdom. Malcolm blogs at drmalcolmkendrick.org and lectures by invitation.

Married with two children and two cats, Malcolm would like more people to challenge the status quo, and never just accept the party line. He likes to ski, golf, sail, play squash, walk in the hills and drink... not necessarily in that order.